The WAHLS PROTOCOL
Cooking for Life

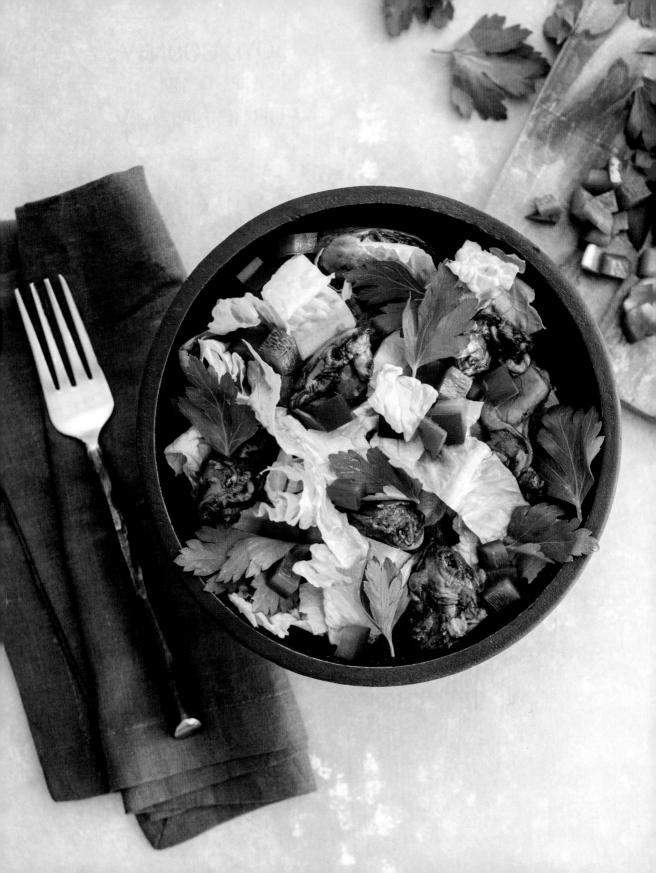

The WAHLS PROTOCOL
Cooking for Life

The Revolutionary Modern Paleo Plan
to Treat All Chronic Autoimmune Conditions

Terry Wahls, M.D.

with Eve Adamson

AVERY
an imprint of Penguin Random House
New York

Ⓐ
AVERY

an imprint of Penguin Random House LLC
375 Hudson Street
New York, New York 10014

Most Avery books are available at special quantity discounts for bulk purchase
for sales promotions, premiums, fund-raising, and educational needs.
Special books or book excerpts also can be created to fit specific needs.
For details, write SpecialMarkets@penguinrandomhouse.com.

Library of Congress Cataloging-in-Publication Data

Names: Wahls, Terry L., author. | Adamson, Eve, author.
Title: The Wahls protocol cooking for life : the revolutionary modern Paleo plan
to treat all chronic autoimmune conditions. / Terry Wahls with Eve Adamson.
Description: New York : Avery, an imprint of Penguin Random House, 2017.
Identifiers: LCCN 2016054066 (print) | LCCN 2017004112 (ebook) |
ISBN 9780399184772 (paperback) | ISBN 9780399184789 (ebook)
Subjects: LCSH: Wahls, Terry L.–Health. | High-protein diet–Recipes. |
Reducing diets–Recipes. | Prehistoric peoples–Nutrition. | Cooking
(Natural foods) | Autoimmune diseases–Diet therapy. | BISAC: COOKING / Health &
Healing / General. | HEALTH & FITNESS / Diseases / Musculoskeletal. | HEALTH &
FITNESS / Diseases / Nervous System (incl. Brain). | LCGFT: Cookbooks.
Classification: LCC RM237.65 .W34 2017 (print) |
LCC RM237.65 (ebook) | DDC 641.5/637–dc23
LC record available at https://lccn.loc.gov/2016054066
p.   cm.

Printed in the United States of America
1   3   5   7   9   10   8   6   4   2

Book design by Ashley Tucker

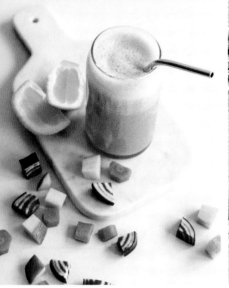
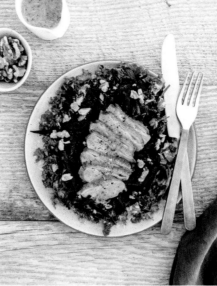
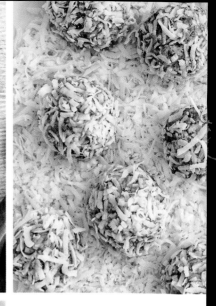
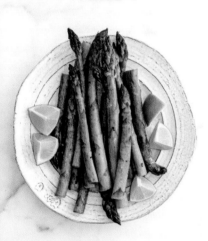
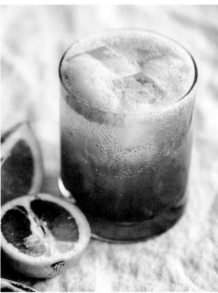
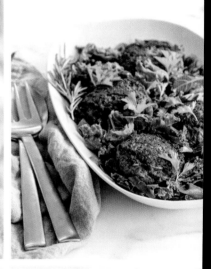
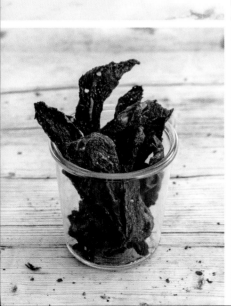
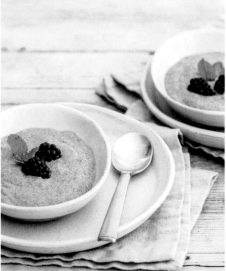
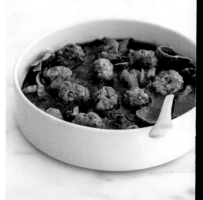

CONTENTS

INTRODUCTION 1

1 | WAHLS PROTOCOL REVIEW 11

2 | YOUR WAHLS KITCHEN AND BASIC RECIPES 23

3 | SENSATIONAL SMOOTHIES 59

4 | BEYOND WATER: GREEN JUICES, TEAS, AND OTHER BEVERAGES 87

5 | GRAIN-FREE GRANOLA AND PORRIDGE 127

6 | MAIN COURSE SALADS, SIDE SALADS, AND WRAPS 153

7 | SUCCULENT SOUPS 195

8 | SAVORY SKILLETS 225

9 | DELECTABLE DESSERTS 253

10 | SNACKS IN A SNAP 281

11 | WAHLS HOLIDAYS 295

12 | HOUSEHOLD AND PERSONAL CARE RECIPES 329

FINAL WORDS 337 · RECIPE LIST 339 · RESOURCES 345
ACKNOWLEDGMENTS 349 · INDEX 351

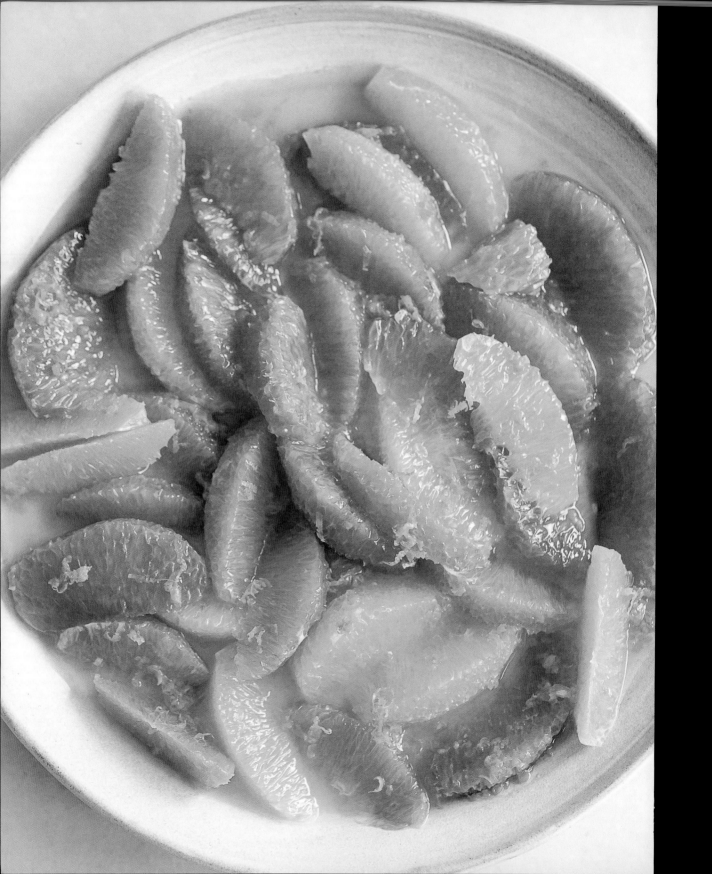

INTRODUCTION

I WAS A YOUNG DOCTOR AND PASSIONATE ATHLETE when I was diagnosed with multiple sclerosis in 2000. I declined rapidly, and within four years, my back and stomach muscles were so weak and my mobility had become so impaired that I needed a tilt/recline wheelchair. This was how I did my rounds at the hospital, tilt-reclined and barely able to move, with clouded thinking and intermittent severe face pain that felt like a cattle prod on my cheekbone. I lost the joy of interacting with my family and friends. I spent much of my time on the sidelines of the active life I had once embraced, fighting to join in and be my old self but failing miserably. I saw a life of increasing disability, becoming bedridden, dying young. I became increasingly isolated, depressed, and lost.

But being a stubborn and curious (mostly stubborn) person with medical knowledge, I finally decided that this could not be the end for me. I would not go down this way. I fought my disease by learning everything I could about the most cutting-edge nutritional studies that could in any way impact the brain, nerves, and muscles. I experimented on myself with supplements, then with nutritionally dense whole foods, then with electrical stimulation. I gave myself a crash course in functional medicine. I read, tested, experimented, and ate obsessively. I was determined to fight.

And I began to get better. Slowly, then more quickly, I began to regain mobility and function. First I sat upright. Then I got out of the wheelchair. Then I began to walk with a cane, then without a cane. Then I began to ride my bicycle. I took back my freedom from the crippling effects of multiple sclerosis, and it changed everything about the way I practice medicine. I was a transformed woman and a transformed doctor. Because I knew so many others with similar disabling conditions (including a lot of my own patients), I knew I couldn't keep this information to myself.

The first thing I did was begin to organize and conduct clinical trials to prove that the protocol I had developed for myself would work for others who had multiple sclerosis or similar issues, from other autoimmune diseases to traumatic brain injuries. I also wrote *The Wahls Protocol* so those who didn't want to wait for the results of the clinical trials could get started changing their bodies, brains, and lives right away.

That's the short version. You can read more about my story in *The Wahls Protocol*. That is also where I laid out a complete and detailed three-tier program for anyone who wants to heal their brain and their body, who struggles with autoimmunity, or who is living with a chronic disease or injury, especially of a neurological or psychological nature. In that book, I presented not only my own story and the protocol that changed my body, brain, and life but hundreds of studies that underlie the rationale behind my program, including much cutting-edge research, the conclusions from which have not yet made their way into the doctor's office or into the standard of care for hospitals.

That was then, and much has happened since I finished writing *The Wahls Protocol*. We have now completed the first clinical trial in which I had participants with progressive multiple sclerosis use the same lifestyle interventions that I used for my recovery. We taught them how to follow the Wahls Diet (the first level of the Wahls Protocol) and how to use self-massage and meditation to lower their stress. We designed exercise and electrical stimulation programs that were specific to their levels of function. What we observed is that people could adopt and sustain the diet, stress reduction, exercise, and electrical therapy for the twelve-month duration of the study. (This alone is significant because, as many researchers well know, getting test subjects to comply with difficult or unpleasant therapies is a challenge—our subjects actually enjoyed their therapies, so compliance was high.) We also observed that people who were overweight lost weight without being hungry, and that their levels of fatigue (a significant problem for MS patients) steadily declined. In fact, we observed the largest reduction in fatigue in the most severely disabled group of MS-fatigued patients studied to date, and the biggest improvement in energy that has ever been reported with any therapeutic intervention for MS-related fatigue.

I've also integrated many aspects of the Wahls Protocol into my work at the VA hospital where I see patients and am the medical director for the therapeutic lifestyle clinic. In that clinic, we teach veterans about the link between lifestyle/environment and genetics. I explain to them how our environment speaks to our genes, and can turn genes "on" and "off," shifting what should have been a healthy, robust, disease-resistant body into an inflamed, sickly, disease-prone body, or doing the reverse: transforming an inflamed, disease-prone body into a healthier, more robust body. I explain how each of us gets to choose, based on our lifestyle, which way we want to progress. I also explain how, as a society, we have radically changed our environment, including the types of foods we eat, making healthful, natural living more difficult, but not impossible. I explain that the way we engineer our own individual environments—the foods we eat, the physical activity we do, the social and family networks we maintain, the home and work environments we live in, the chemicals we are exposed to, the personal care products we use, and the life purpose we have—speaks to our genes, and shifts which of those genes will become active and which will remain silent. What we do and how we live sends a direct message to our bodies about how to respond: with vitality, or with decline.

Next, I show them that lifestyle also impacts things that are more obvious to us than genetic switches. Lifestyle impacts how our cells function and, in turn, how responsive our organs will be. If we practice lifestyles that deprive the body of nutrients, introduce inflammatory substances, and induce stress, things can begin to malfunction. For example, when the body produces too many inflammatory molecules, the immune system can overreact. Blood pressure and blood sugar can rise, weight can increase, the body can become insulin-resistant, memory can decline, and we can become irritable, anxious, depressed, and/or have joint pain, breathing problems, skin rashes, and more. Life becomes increasingly uncomfortable and unpleasant. When there is enough damage for a physician to make an actual diagnosis, we may then be prescribed medication, with its own set of side effects, to control symptoms. But sadly, many—if not most—of those medical professionals so ready to prescribe drug therapies will never even mention the powerful and potent intersection of diet and lifestyle with health or disease.

Then we get more specific. The next thing I teach the people in my clinic is how dietary tweaks like eating more vegetables (especially those that are sulfur rich, leafy green, and deeply colored), along with the elimination of common inflammatory foods like gluten and dairy, can help reduce the inflammation that is often at the heart of pain, mood problems, weight issues, and autoimmune conditions. And time and time again, as people adopt the Wahls Protocol, they experience reduced pain, increased energy, mood stabilization, and a normalization of both blood pressure and blood sugar. Often, their need for medication steadily declines as well.

In our classes, we also have a demonstration kitchen, in which we teach our veterans how to prepare foods that are healing and health promoting, and can be made in minutes. We talk about ingredient quality and easy, quick cooking methods. We talk about how to easily integrate more vegetables, which fruits are best, and how to take advantage of the superior protein and other nutrients animal foods offer us. We talk about fermenting cabbage and making homemade yogurts and kefir from coconut milk or nut milks (easier than most people think), and we even teach them about gardening, composting, and foraging for wild food. Our classes are steadily growing in size, and I am currently beginning to train other practitioners at our VA hospital so they can also help teach our therapeutic lifestyle clinic.

I've seen profound changes in many of the veterans in our clinic. They are eating differently and moving differently, and the results are visible. Many have planted container gardens, raised-bed gardens, or traditional gardens. Others have backyards that are heavily shaded, and instead are planting berry bushes and mushroom gardens in those shady spots. Some go out on country roads and public hunting areas to forage for wild foods like mushrooms and hunt for venison. And they are beginning to cook again, and share what they've learned, telling one another how to make smoothies, soups, and skillet meals.

They are a thrifty bunch, too. Many of my veterans as well as my followers (whom we call Wahls Warriors) are on disability. Even if they are ready to make radical changes in their diets and lifestyles to follow the Wahls Protocol, they encounter many barriers, including money, energy, and strength. They may not be able to afford a lot of unusual or hard-to-find ingredients, not to mention pay extra for organic produce (or even be able to find it). They can't use complex recipes that require a lot of standing or chopping and other handwork. They are already exhausted. Or they may live in what we call a food desert, where there is no local grocery store that carries good-quality fresh vegetables and fruit. But together we find ways to make this program work for them.

As they continue to transform, I see the spark reigniting in them. They begin not just to help themselves, but to reach out to help others. The people who are old-timers in our lifestyle clinics tell the newbies how they have been able to stop taking the narcotics they had relied on for years because of severe pain, or that their brain fog and fatigue are gone, and that they are happy for the first time in years. They are spreading the word for me.

As for me, I have continued to speak around the country and around the globe about the critical role of diet and lifestyle in creating health. In each place I go, I find that people are hungry for information and strategies that will help them implement the Wahls Protocol. They want to know how to stock their pantries, how to shop, and how to prepare a meal in minutes without using packaged, processed food. Many people ask me how I did it. How did I, as a busy working person with health issues, manage to begin cooking, not to mention get my family on board with the meals I make for myself? Most of us have many demands upon our time and simply cannot spend hours preparing meals. Or we are tired due to our health challenges. So how did I do it? How can they do it? How can you do it, too?

I've heard from thousands of you, and I already know you want more—more recipes, more ideas, more lifestyle tips, more advice. You want to know more about others who are living the Wahls Protocol, and you want to keep going and keep feeling better and better as the years pass. In this book, I will remind you of the basics of the three levels of the Wahls Protocol, but then I will help you integrate your goals into your life with recipes, tools, tips, and strategies to help you reimagine your relationship with food. You'll learn easy ways to sharpen your shopping, cooking, gardening, and even foraging skills. From new skillet and smoothie ideas to what to eat on holidays, from homemade personal care product recipes to cleaning solutions made with ingredients from your own kitchen (and no toxic chemicals), you'll find it all between the covers of this book.

I created the Wahls Protocol because I could not wait for modern medicine to solve my health problems. I had to take action myself, and when my strategies worked, I felt compelled to let others with chronic pain and chronic disabling medical, neurological, and psychological conditions know that there is hope for them, too. I was compelled to share what I learned with others who also were not willing or able to wait for a medical future where food and lifestyle are part of the prescription to address chronic disease. I wanted people to know that they could begin eating for health right away.

Now I find that it is time to take the next step. Whether you have already begun the Wahls Protocol or you are new to this community, ask yourself: How would you like to live your life? Do you hunger for a diet and lifestyle that is both fulfilling and therapeutic? Do you crave renewed strength, mobility, and vitality? And if you have already begun to gain those things through the Wahls Protocol, how do you keep going, not just for a few weeks or months, but for life? This cookbook will help you take your Wahls Protocol to the next level with more ideas, more guidance, more options, and more delicious food than I've ever offered before.

In this book, I share many of those tips, tricks, and techniques, not just from my own experience but based on what I teach in our lifestyle classes at the VA hospital. You will learn about some of my family's favorite meals and treats, how I typically cook, how I hardly ever waste any part of a vegetable, and how easy and quick it is to make the meals in this book. Most of them come together in thirty minutes. That's faster than going out to eat, and also tastier and much less costly, not to mention vastly superior in terms of health benefits.

You will also find that these meals are tasty enough that teenagers and children enjoy them. Speaking of children, I encourage you to get the kids in your life involved in meal preparation in some way, as soon as they are old enough to hold a wooden spoon. Children can mix, stir, help set the table, and, as they get older, chop, slice, and use the stove and oven. When children grow up learning to cook—especially cooking and eating vegetables—they will be more likely to continue those healthful habits throughout their lives and will give themselves a better shot at good health as they get older. The mealtime was a daily family ritual when I was growing up, and it is still a family ritual in my household today. We all take turns doing the preparation and the cleanup. Both of my children, Zach and Zebby, are excellent cooks. They like to text photos to me of the wonderful meals they prepare for each other when Jackie and I are traveling. Those photos always make me smile. Of course, you don't have to have children to have a family meal—it is also an excellent time to touch base with your partner, parents, siblings, or friends.

We have an epidemic of disease, but what we need is an "epidemic" of health. Reclaiming health isn't about early diagnosis or drug therapy or screening or imaging or testing. It is about providing an environment for cells to function in the most optimal way possible, so that our bodies can function optimally. We need to learn how to shop for high-quality ingredients, how to get back in the kitchen and cook food that nourishes us and tastes great, and how to adapt favorite recipes so they are more nutrient dense and less inflammatory.

The Wahls Protocol is not a diet. It is a lifestyle, and this is the book to help you live it. You have the power to minimize your symptoms or stop the progression of your disease. And then you can focus on the end goal: building a satisfying and meaningful life. As you begin to feel better, your other passions, motivations, and important pursuits will emerge. Teaching my medical colleagues and the public that we can take powerful steps to control our own health is what gives my life meaning. It's why I write books, do research, spread the word on social media, and speak around the globe.

Some of our Wahls Warriors have gone on to study nutrition or the culinary arts so they could teach others how to use food to heal. Your path might be much different, but I urge you to seek it. I invite you to take the next step on the journey to a meaningful life as you continue on your healing journey. Your journey will be different from mine, but no less meaningful, no less impactful, no less courageous.

My dream is to witness and be a part of creating this epidemic of health. I imagine a future where grandparents, parents, and children all understand that health depends on preserving the quality of our whole foods—a future in which policy makers understand that health care costs will not be contained unless we become well, and that becoming well requires that we cook at home and eat real, whole food.

But the government can't accomplish this. The health insurance companies can't do this, and neither can our employers. It's up to us—you and me, right down here at the grassroots level. Person to person, talking to our families, friends, and coworkers, sharing food and ideas with them—that

WAHLS WARRIORS SPEAK

Last year I was desperate, and then I found you. Thank you for your book and your passion. You give me hope.

—Wahls Warrior CLAUDIA

is how we make change. We can use social media to spread our stories of cooking and healing. We can cook delicious meals, and teach our children how easy and enjoyable cooking at home can be, so the next generation will do better than we have. To achieve this vision, this epidemic of health, I am recruiting an army of Wahls Warriors to tell the world about their health recovery stories. Will you enlist in this noble cause, to reclaim the health of your family, your community, your country, and your world? Let this cookbook be your guide to changing the current paradigm, one meal at a time.

I welcome you, fellow Wahls Warrior, to a meaningful life in which you help to create a worldwide epidemic of health. We are on the noblest of journeys together. Let us begin.

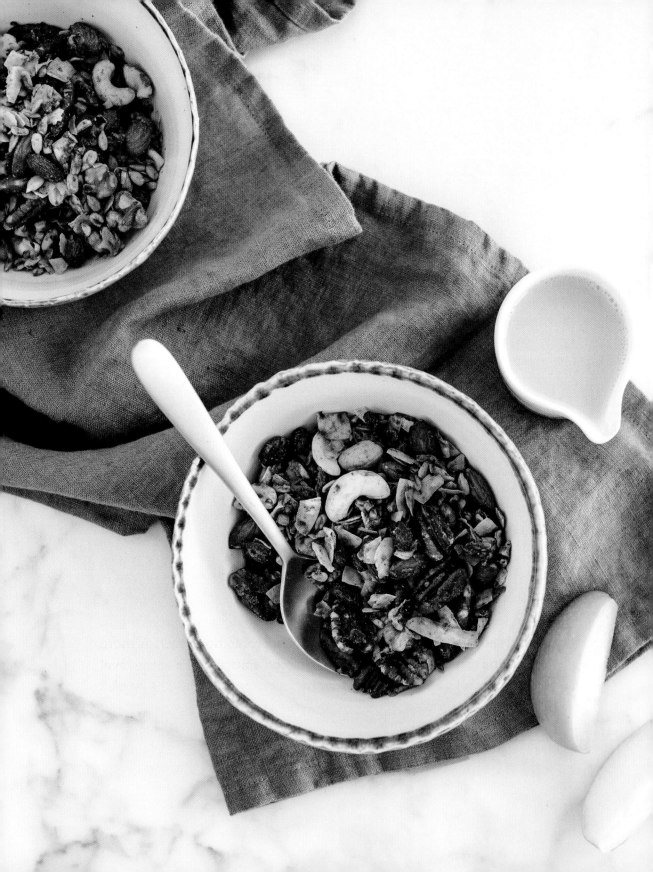

WAHLS PROTOCOL REVIEW

IF YOU HAVE BEEN ON THE WAHLS PROTOCOL FOR YEARS and you know it inside and out, you probably don't need this chapter, but if you are just learning about it or think you could benefit from a review of the guidelines for each of the three levels, look over this chapter and refer back to it whenever you need a reminder or help staying on track.

There are three levels to the Wahls Protocol:

The first level, the Wahls Diet, is the most accessible and will be the only level some people ever need. Many people do quite well living on the Wahls Diet, with its high volume of vegetables and fruits and its elimination of gluten-containing grains and dairy foods. However, for others, it is a stepping-stone to Wahls Paleo.

The second level, Wahls Paleo, has additional elements, such as organ meats and sea vegetables, as well as additional prohibitions, such as more limited grains, fruits, and other high-carb food sources. This is the level that I recommend as a goal for most of my autoimmune patients, as well as those suffering from other chronic diseases, including obesity.

Finally, for those whose autoimmune diseases are still causing them difficulty at the Wahls Paleo level, and especially for those people grappling with neurological problems (such as dementia, epilepsy, brain injury,

THE KETOGENIC DIET

A ketogenic diet is a diet that gets you into ketosis and keeps you there. Ketosis is simply a fancy way of saying that your cells are burning fat instead of sugar in the mitochondria. Also, ketones make excellent brain fuel, especially for those suffering from neurological issues like MS, epilepsy, and dementia. Consuming more fat, especially fat from coconuts, which is rich in medium-chain triglycerides, makes it easier to get into and stay in ketosis.

Using fat instead of sugar as an energy source seems to have healing properties. Physicians originally used ketogenic diets to treat refractory seizures back in the 1920s. Scientists are now researching the use of ketosis-producing (ketogenic) diets to treat progressive brain disorders like Parkinson's, Alzheimer's, Huntington's, Lou Gehrig's (ALS), and MS; psychiatric disorders like depression, bipolar, schizophrenia; and metabolic and hormonal issues like diabetes, obesity, and polycystic ovarian syndrome.

I use my version of a ketogenic diet with my patients, and I stay in ketosis myself seasonally, about ten months out of the year, because I have found it has a profound effect on disease symptoms, including my own MS symptoms. This is the goal at the Wahls Paleo Plus level of my diet—the most advanced level, and the level I recommend for the most severe levels of chronic disease. Decreasing the amount of protein and carbohydrates in the diet and ramping up the amount of fat, while getting sufficient vitamins, minerals, phytonutrients, and fiber to maintain optimal nutrition, is the ideal way to practice a ketogenic diet. You can track whether your body is in ketosis with simple test strips from your local pharmacy, which test the ketones in your urine. For more details on the benefits of ketosis and how to achieve ketosis while maintaining optimal nutrition, see *The Wahls Protocol.*

WAHLS WARRIORS SPEAK

Something recently began to click for me, and I have been adopting more of the components of the Wahls Protocol over the last couple of months. Perhaps my gut flora are changing. I also know it's Dr. Terry Wahls's steady, no-nonsense information about the benefits of following the protocol. Thank you!

—Wahls Warrior RAYE

---

and Parkinson's), I recommend working up to the third level, Wahls Paleo Plus. This level is a ketogenic diet, characterized by very high fat levels and very low carbohydrate levels. This can be difficult for some to follow, but has dramatic results for many of those who stick to it.

FUEL FOR YOUR CELLS, YOUR ORGANS, YOUR LIFE

The Wahls Protocol begins with the mitochondria. These tiny organelles inside the cells are like engines delivering energy to the cells and, by extension, the organs and the body itself. Mitochondria are fueled by the food you eat, so healthy, well-nourished mitochondria can only develop if you eat healthy food. They are the key to creating strong, resilient cells.

Each level of the Wahls Protocol is specifically formulated to infuse cells with intense nutrition while also eliminating food ingredients that are most likely to cause reactivity, especially in people with autoimmune conditions and/or who may have a compromised gut lining (i.e., leaky gut syndrome). This two-pronged approach calms down inflammation and autoimmune overreaction while also providing the building blocks for cells to heal, rebuild tissues, and reestablish healthy organ function. In a nutshell, the Wahls Protocol creates the ultimate environment for self-healing, which your body is always trying to do, but which is so often impeded by lifestyle choices.

WAHLS WARRIORS SPEAK

I was on the Wahls Diet for five months, and I wasn't looking to lose weight, but I lost 30 pounds. Also, my brain fog disappeared and my energy returned. Then I went off the diet during Christmas. Bad mistake! I feel like crap. I'm back on the diet today and can't wait to feel better again.

—Wahls Warrior TONYA

PICK YOUR LEVEL

In general, I recommend that most people begin with the Wahls Diet, especially if they currently have a very poor diet. The Wahls Diet introduces the body to a better way to live and is closer to how most people currently eat than either Wahls Paleo or Wahls Paleo Plus. However, if you are currently in a serious disease state, I recommend starting with Wahls Paleo. Eventually, you can work up to Wahls Paleo Plus, if it feels necessary or if your health could still use some improvement.

Look at the guidelines for each level of the diet and decide how doable they will be in your life. This book will include lifestyle tips throughout, but changing your diet always comes with some challenges. And the challenges are a little tougher to navigate if you are following the second- or third-level plan. Some things to think about:

- What will your family eat? Adherence to any diet is much easier if everyone in the family follows the plan, and the Wahls Diet in particular is healthful and nourishing for anyone, but what if your family isn't willing to do this with you?

- What will you do at restaurants, or when you are socializing?

- What will you eat when you travel? How will you maintain your healthful practices on the road?

- How will you handle craving and exposure to foods that are non-compliant with your health plan?

There are solutions to all of these issues and I will discuss them throughout this book, but if you foresee issues and you don't feel quite ready to tackle them yet, start with the Wahls Diet—it is the least likely to feel difficult and has the most flexibility for situations like restaurants, socializing, and travel.

But if you are gung-ho to jump in and see fast results and don't plan to let anything stop you, start with Wahls Paleo. This is a truly transformative diet that will give you results faster than you will see on the Wahls Diet.

Now let's look at the guidelines for each level of the Wahls Protocol.

WAHLS DIET (LEVEL 1)

Whenever possible, choose organic produce, grass-fed meat, free-range poultry, and wild-caught seafood.

ADD

- 9 cups of fruits and vegetables every day, broken down as follows:
  - 3 cups tightly packed (or 6 cups loosely packed) raw or cooked leafy greens, such as kale, collards, chard, Asian greens, and lettuces (the darker green, the better)
  - 3 cups deeply colored vegetables and fruits, such as berries, tomatoes, peppers, beets, carrots, and winter squash
  - 3 cups sulfur-rich vegetables, such as broccoli, cabbage, mushrooms, asparagus, Brussels sprouts, turnips, radishes, onions, and garlic

  Note: Eat "white fruits" (apples, pears, bananas) only *after* you have eaten your 9 cups.

- 16 ounces omega-3-rich fish (such as salmon, herring, and sardines) per week

- 6 to 12 ounces meat, fish, poultry, and/or game per day

- Up to 2 tablespoons flaxseed oil, hemp oil, or walnut oil per day. Eat coconut oil, animal fat (including clarified butter, which has had its dairy solids removed), extra-virgin olive oil, and other cold-pressed fats freely. *Do not cook with any plant oils other than coconut oil.* Plant oils should be eaten cold, in the form of salad dressings and dips.

WAHLS KITCHEN TIPS

For those of you on the metric system who are not familiar with cups, or for those of you who just don't like to measure, use this system to measure 3 cups: Cover a dinner plate completely with your vegetables, cooked or raw, so you can't see the surface of the plate. That is approximately 3 cups of vegetables!

- All gluten-containing grain products. That includes anything made with wheat or wheat flour (wheat bread, wheat pasta, rolls, bagels, etc., and also most baked goods, unless specifically gluten-free). This also includes anything made with barley, rye, spelt, or any other wheat-related grains.

- All dairy products. That means milk and anything made with cow's, goat's, or sheep's milk (such as cheese, ice cream, yogurt, and many processed foods). Use plant milks instead, such as almond and coconut milk. (If you use soy milk, be sure it is organic.)

- All eggs and egg-containing products.

- All artificial sweeteners.

- Limit non-gluten flour and grain products (such as rice, gluten-free pasta, gluten-free bread, etc.) to one serving per day. (One serving equals ½ cup cooked grain or pasta, or one small piece of bread.)

- Limit all types of added sweeteners (honey, maple syrup, sugar, sorghum, etc.) to no more than 1 teaspoon per day.

WAHLS PALEO (LEVEL 2)

At this level, follow all the guidelines for the Wahls Diet (Level 1), as well as these additional guidelines:

ADD

- 12 ounces organ meats and whole seafood (which includes the organs) per week, including mussels, sardines, oysters, liver, gizzards, heart, and kidneys.

- Seaweed or algae food products (such as kelp, spirulina, nori, and kombu) once or twice a week as part of a meal (such as in sushi rolls, seaweed salads, and added to soups and stews).

- One serving per day of nondairy, non-grain fermented foods (like lacto-fermented sauerkraut, pickles, kimchi, kvass, and kombucha tea).

- Raw foods whenever you can, including raw vegetables but also raw soaked and sprouted seeds and nuts, and raw animal protein (such as sushi, ceviche, and even steak tartare).

- Up to (but no more than) 4 ounces raw nuts and seeds per day, especially almonds, sunflower seeds, and sesame seeds. When possible, soak them overnight, rinse, and dry on paper towels (or in a dehydrator) before eating. Soaking nuts and seeds for 6 to 24 hours initiates the germination process and reduces the content of lectins and phytates. Phytates can interfere with the body's absorption of minerals, and lectins can increase inflammation in genetically susceptible people.

- Meat, fish, poultry, and game, increasing servings to 6 to 20 ounces per day.

WAHLS WARRIORS SPEAK

My mother and I started the Wahls Paleo Plus a year ago after I was hospitalized for debilitating pain during my period (endometriosis and fibroids). I decided to give it a shot even though I don't have MS. My mother, who has crippling rheumatoid arthritis and has tried everything under the sun over the past forty years, decided to join me. Within a month my pain was gone. More astounding were my mother's results. Within a month she started noticing improvements in her vision, some arthritic nodules she had on her elbows went away, her pain was way, way down, and she cut her methotrexate dosage in half. She also no longer gets recurring urinary tract infections. She can walk on the beach barefoot now. The swelling in her hands is down so much that her rings are suddenly too large. Even her shoe size is down. Her energy is up and so is her mood. This has been nothing short of a miracle for my seventy-year-old mother.

—Wahls Warrior CARMEN (and her mother)

- All soy products, including tofu, edamame, tempeh, and processed products like veggie burgers and veggie "dogs" that contain soy.

- Reduce all non-gluten grains, legumes (like beans, lentils, peas, and peanuts), and potatoes—in other words, all starchy foods—to just two servings per week total.

WAHLS KITCHEN TIP: LACTO-FERMENTATION

Many foods are fermented—some with yeast, such as wine and beer, and some with vinegar, such as the pickled vegetables commonly available in conventional grocery stores. Lacto-fermentation, however, uses natural bacteria (the kind that are good for you to eat) to ferment foods without yeast or vinegar. You can use a starter that you purchase in a health food store, but I often use a probiotic capsule. I just mix it with salt water and soak the food (such as cabbage or beets) in the salt water for a few days at room temperature, and you will have a healthful fermented food product. (This is how I will advise you to make your own lacto-ferments in the recipes in this book.)

Lacto-fermented foods are traditional in most cultures around the world, and they are an excellent way to nurture and replenish your own gut bacteria. Later in this book, you will learn more about how to lacto-ferment your own food as part of the Wahls Protocol, and I will provide you with some recipes. I do this frequently with vegetables from my own garden. It's easy and interesting.

WAHLS PALEO PLUS (LEVEL 3)

At this level, you will continue to follow all the guidelines for the two previous levels, with these exceptions and additions—with the goal of getting you into and keeping you in ketosis:

ADD

- Coconut oil and full-fat coconut milk every day. Aim for 4½ tablespoons coconut oil (or medium-chain triglyceride oil—labeled MCT oil—which you can find in health food stores) per day, or up to

1½ (14-ounce) cans full-fat coconut milk per day. Wahls Paleo Plus should consist of a large proportion of coconut fat because it is the type of fat most effective at keeping the body in ketosis. Level 3 is a high-fat diet … and it's good for you!

- Increase nondairy, non-grain lacto-fermented foods (such as sauerkraut, kimchi, kombucha, and kvass) to two servings per day.

ELIMINATE

- All grains, legumes, and potatoes (including white, yellow, red, blue, and sweet potatoes as well as yams). Anything that is high in starch is not appropriate at this level.

- All legumes, including beans, peas, soy products, lentils, or peanuts. These are too starchy, and at this level of the diet, you also want to stay away from lectins and phytates as much as possible.

- All added sweeteners, including natural sweeteners.

- Reduce vegetable consumption to 6 cups per day, divided evenly among leafy greens, deeply colored vegetables, and sulfur-rich vegetables. This is reduced from the 9 cups required at the Wahls Diet level because the goal of Wahls Paleo Plus is for you to remain in ketosis, which requires lower carbohydrate consumption.

- Reduce cooked starchy vegetables (winter squashes like butternut squash, acorn squash, and pumpkins, as well as root vegetables like carrots and beets) to two servings per week maximum, and only eat them with fat, such as butter or coconut oil. Even better, eat them raw—I prefer this because it makes the starch even less available, but feeds your gut bacteria. I have found that a nice way to eat starchy vegetables raw is to use a spiralizer to make them into noodles.

- Reduce fruit to one serving per day, berries only. Sweet fruits like grapes and pineapples and white-fleshed fruits like apples, pears, and bananas are too high in sugars for Level 3. (I might occasionally eat half a red grapefruit or a small peach and be able to stay in ketosis, but see what works for you. Some people can do this, and others really can't.)

- Reduce meat, fish, poultry, and game consumption to 6 to 12 ounces per day (this is back to the Wahls Diet level).

- Eat just twice per day, and fast 12 to 16 hours each night. This gives your body lots of healing time, without the added burden of digestion. Personally, I tend to eat breakfast and dinner, then wait 12 to 16 hours between dinner and breakfast.

LET'S GET STARTED

Once you have decided on your starting level and are familiar with the rules, you can eat anything you want—as long as it fits into the guidelines. The recipes in this book will make this much easier to do. Every recipe will include modifications for each level or will note if it is not appropriate for a particular level. (This is most often the case for Wahls Paleo Plus, as some recipes contain too many carbohydrates for most people to maintain ketosis.)

Now let's get into the kitchen!

A NOTE ABOUT A NEW EATING DISORDER

Orthorexia is the medical term for an obsession with eating only the food that one considers healthful, or that complies with a particular dietary regimen (such as Paleo, vegan, etc.). This obsession becomes so extreme that the person's physical and/or mental health suffers—they constantly fear the presence of unknown bits of "forbidden" food, or rearrange their entire lives to fit a diet's particular schedule or rules. Some fear every bite of food, and will severely limit their social exposure and activities in case the food available might not comply with their diet plan. There is evidence that some people become so controlling of their own diets that they get severely stressed, or so restrictive that they become starved for nutrients and their health declines.

Unfortunately, any diet plan can trigger this condition in susceptible people, and I have encountered this now in a few people following the Wahls Protocol. Sometimes, the line is blurry—if you have a serious health condition, following a therapeutic diet and not "cheating" is important for your healing. However, when this crosses the line into anxiety or becomes obsessive, that's a problem.

In this book, I calculate vegetable servings for you in those recipes containing vegetables, but I worry a little sometimes about how some people might react to this. Although the Wahls Diet is known for its "9 cups" and I strongly believe it is good to include a lot of different vegetables in the human diet every day, I don't want you to get so rigid about this that you become overly stressed or obsessed if, for example, you only get in 6 cups or you eat an apple before you eat your 9 cups or your percentage of leafy greens was smaller than your percentage of colored vegetables, or you do something else you perceive as "wrong." I do not want you to make your meals into accounting systems or subjects of obsession. This exacerbates stress, and stress is dangerous for your health. I want you to think about the big picture, not get caught up in the minutiae. The goal of 9 cups of vegetables per day (or 6 cups for Wahls Paleo Plus and petite people), split approximately equally among greens, color, and sulfur-containing vegetables, is a guideline, not a law. Because of our unique health history and genetics, these recommendations may need to be personalized, and I never expect anybody to precisely hit these exact targets every single day for the rest of their lives. Putting that kind of pressure on yourself will drive you crazy and go against what we are trying to do for your health, so go easy. Eat your vegetables, yes, but don't make yourself ill.

Where I *do* want you to be more rigid is when it comes to being gluten-free, dairy-free, and (for most, especially with autoimmunity) egg-free. These foods really can undo all your progress and cause damage if you suffer from an autoimmune disease or neurological disorder, even if you "just have a little." This is important, but you can also be strict with yourself without becoming obsessive. Just focus on vegetables and high-quality protein, and breathe. Remember, stress management is another important arm of the Wahls Protocol, so again, your meals should *not cause you stress.*

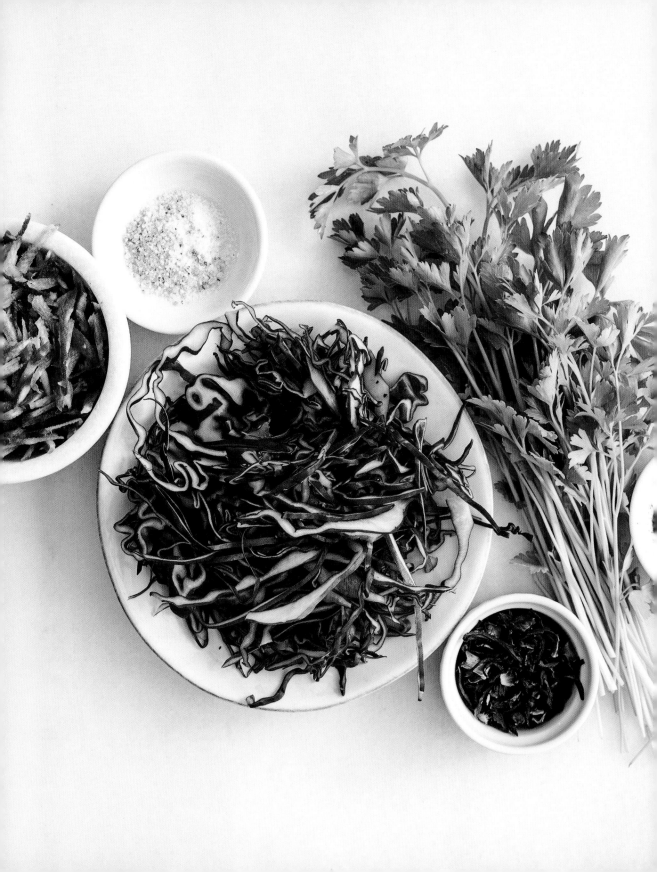

YOUR WAHLS KITCHEN AND BASIC RECIPES

I THINK THE REASON WHY SO MANY PEOPLE, especially those struggling with chronic health conditions, are resistant to cooking is that they don't have the right tools and ingredients to make it easier. In this chapter, I'll help you set up your Wahls kitchen so that you have the tools and basic pantry staples you need to make every recipe in this book. Beyond that, all you will need to buy is fresh food—meats, veggies, and fruits—which you can of course also freeze if you buy in bulk or get a good deal at the farmers' market or from a local meat producer. (I'll talk more about how to store food throughout this book.)

This chapter also provides some basic recipes for staples that you will use often throughout this book, such as bone broth, nut milk, and cheese substitutes.

KITCHEN TOOLS AND EQUIPMENT

These are the tools and equipment I have in my own kitchen that I use most frequently. I find it is useful to have them all in cabinets that are easy to reach. I keep the equipment I use almost daily out on my counter. Where you store your equipment can make all the difference when it comes to whipping up a meal with ease.

- **Aprons, oven mitts, hot pads**
- **Custard cups or ramekins**
- **Cutting board**
- **Food processor** with blades for chopping, grating, matchstick cuts, and slicing
- **Ice cube trays,** for freezing treats
- **Knives:** Four basic knives should cover all knife work: a good chef's knife or Santoku knife, small paring knife, butcher's knife for cutting meat, and a serrated knife for cutting things you don't want to crush, like tomatoes. All should be kept sharp.
- **Ladle,** for soup
- **Large glass or ceramic mixing bowls,** for fermentation as well as general mixing
- **Measuring cups** (dry and liquid) and spoons
- **Metal colander**
- **Quart and gallon wide-mouth glass jars with lids,** for fermentation
- **Salad spinner**
- **Spoons:** wooden for stirring and slotted for fishing food out of water
- **Springform pan,** for making cheezcakes (pages 266, 270, and 271) and other Paleo-style desserts
- **Stainless-steel or ceramic cookware with lids:** small skillet, large skillet, small saucepan, large saucepan, stockpot, and some sort of lidded casserole dish. Look for types without plastic parts so you can also put skillets in the oven. *Avoid all nonstick surfaces and hardened or anodized aluminum.*
- **Tea kettle,** for boiling water
- **Tea strainer or tea ball**
- **Vitamix** or other high-speed blender (Blendtec is another good option, but use what you have) with dry mix attachment (or a separate grinder for seeds, spices, and coffee if you drink it).
- **Wide-mouth funnel,** for filling jars
- **Wide-mouth lidded glass jars in various sizes** (½ pint, pint, quart) for storing food

WAHLS KITCHEN TIP: MATCHA

Matcha is a powdered form of green tea. Unlike regular tea leaves, which are discarded after being steeped, matcha is actually ingested, so you get more caffeine, but you also get more potent nutrition, especially antioxidants called polyphenols, which help regulate blood sugar and blood pressure, and may protect against cancer and heart disease. Matcha is the type of tea used in Japanese tea ceremonies. Look for pure matcha powder, not mixes that contain sugar.

- **Activated charcoal water filter or reverse-osmosis system** to treat your water. This isn't necessary if you have good-quality water, but good water is increasingly rare. You could also purchase water, but buying a filtration system is more cost-effective over time.

- **Dehydrator,** for easy drying of vegetable chips, raw crackers, and meat. You can also use your oven, but a dehydrator, while it does take up a lot of counter or cabinet space, will do this without requiring the same kind of supervision you would need with the oven.

- **Juicer,** if you like juicing (although as you will see in chapter 3, I generally recommend "juicing" in a Vitamix rather than through a juicer)

- **Nut milk bag,** if you want to filter your nut milk (I don't bother, but some people prefer a smoother texture, and a nut milk bag will give you a product more like the nut milk you would buy in the store)

- **Occupational therapy tools,** if needed because of weak hands. This site has many useful tools: www.lifesolutionsplus .com. Click on "Kitchen Aids."

- **Stool with back** for sitting and working at the counter/table/stove, if you get tired from standing

- **Tamper, wooden:** Useful for fermentation, to push vegetables beneath the liquid, but not strictly necessary.

PANTRY FOODS

These are the items I keep regularly stocked in my pantry. Sometimes I need to buy additional things for special recipes, but these are the things I use frequently. Having them on hand at all times is very useful for cooking quickly and easily.

BAKING ITEMS

- **Almond flour**
- **Cocoa powder or raw cacao powder,** unsweetened and organic only
- **Coconut flour**
- **Tapioca flour or minute tapioca**

BEVERAGES

- **Coffee, organic,** if you drink coffee
- **Teas,** especially green tea and herbal teas

- **Matcha green tea powder**

DRIED FOODS

Note: Do not consume dried fruit if you are following Wahls Paleo Plus. Dried coconut is just fine for all levels of the Wahls Protocol.

- **Dried plums (prunes)**
- **Raisins**
- **Dried cranberries** (try to find unsweetened or at least naturally sweetened)
- **Dried unsweetened coconut flakes**

FATS AND OILS

- **Coconut oil**
- **Ghee**
- **Extra-virgin olive oil, flaxseed oil, hemp oil**
- **MCT oil (page 26)**

FERMENTED FOODS

- **Fermented garlic and ginger** (if available, or use the recipe on page 34 to make your own)
- **Fermented horseradish**

PANTRY FOODS CONTINUES

- **Fermented vegetables** (such as sauerkraut, pickles, and kimchi)

FLAVORING AND NUTRITIONAL BOOSTS

- **Coconut aminos** (or gluten-free soy-based aminos, preferably organic, such as Bragg Liquid Aminos–this is one of the few instances where a soy product is okay)
- **Nutritional yeast**
- **Sea salt**
- **Seaweed flakes or powder** (I like flakes the best), especially kelp, dulse, and mixed seaweed blends (Maine Seaweed Company tests for heavy metals–find them at www.seaveg.com/shop)
- **Unflavored gelatin or collagen, or agar-agar** (a sea vegetable product), if you are vegetarian or vegan
- **Vinegars,** especially apple cider and balsamic

- **Mustard**
- **Canned coconut milk**
- **Canned coconut cream**
- **Fresh citrus juice**
- **Minced garlic**

NATURAL SWEETENERS, if you are using sweeteners

- **Brown rice syrup**
- **Honey**
- **Maple syrup, pure**
- **Molasses**

NUTS AND SEEDS

- **Almond butter**
- **Almonds**
- **Brazil nuts**
- **Cashew butter**
- **Chia seeds** (purchase whole seeds)
- **Flaxseeds** (purchase whole seeds and grind them yourself in a spice grinder immediately before use, to prevent oxidation)
- **Pumpkin seeds**

- **Sesame butter** (or tahini)
- **Sunflower butter**
- **Sunflower seeds**
- **Walnuts**

DRIED HERBS AND SPICES

- **Basil**
- **Black pepper,** freshly ground
- **Cardamom**
- **Celery seed**
- **Cloves**
- **Cinnamon**
- **Cumin**
- **Coriander**
- **Fresh ginger** (I keep it in the refrigerator)
- **Herbes de Provence** (a mix of herbs)
- **Nutmeg**
- **Oregano**
- **Red pepper flakes**
- **Rosemary**
- **Savory**
- **Thyme**

WAHLS KITCHEN TIP: MCT OIL

MCT stands for medium-chain triglycerides. It is a type of fat that I recommend for people following Wahls Paleo Plus because it is converted to ketones in the liver, making it easier to get to and stay in ketosis. Coconut oil contains a large quantity of MCT fatty acids, but you can also buy MCT oil in health food stores. I suggest that people on Wahls Paleo Plus use 1 to 2 tablespoons of MCT oil or warmed coconut oil in their smoothies. A few people will have GI upset or loose stools as they get accustomed to MCT oil, so start with 1 teaspoon and gradually increase to 1 tablespoon. Make sure you are able to tolerate it before trying to add 2 tablespoons to any smoothie recipe.

- **Turmeric**
- **Vanilla**
- **And others according to your preference**

- **Canned salmon, sardines, oysters, mussels**
- **Dried powdered beets**
- **Dried powdered green algae such as chlorella/ spirulina.** I no longer recommend wheatgrass, barley grass, and other cereal grasses because I have found that some very gluten-sensitive people react to these, even though they are technically gluten-free. There must be some other structures in the cereal grasses that are also stimulating the immune system in an adverse way. I also no longer recommend wild blue-green algae, as there have been reports of wild algae blooms associated with neurotoxicity. Stick with chlorella and spirulina for best results and nutritional density.
- **Paleo meat bars or sticks** (preferably without added sugar)
- **Powdered coconut milk**

YOUR WAHLS-REQUIRED VEGETABLE SERVINGS MADE EASY

Everyone on the Wahls Protocol knows the importance of getting those requisite cups of greens, sulfur-containing vegetables, and deeply colored vegetables. To make your life a little easier, every recipe in this book that contains vegetables (frankly, that includes most of them) has a note at the top to tell you how many cups of vegetables you get in one serving of that recipe. I also note if the cup amounts are different for different levels of the diet (for example, many Wahls Paleo Plus recipes contain fewer vegetables, and fewer are required at that level in order to stay in ketosis). This will help you keep track of your daily allowance and you won't even have to do any math!

However, also note that these measurements may not always be totally precise. There are many different sizes when it comes to vegetables. Consider, for example, a cucumber or a sweet potato or a tomato. Some are very small and some are very large. In general, the following list summarizes how we translated some common vegetables into cups for you. If you know the vegetables you are using are especially large or small, you can choose to adapt this or measure them yourself. Otherwise, this is a good average, and you can use it whenever you are making your own recipes out of the templates.

1 avocado = 1 cup	6 stalks celery = 3 cups	1 pound mushrooms = 5 cups
1 beet = 1 cup	1 large cucumber = 3 cups	1 onion = 1 cup
1 pound Brussels sprouts = 5 cups	2 cloves garlic = 1 cup (see page 57; note that you get extra veggie credit for those little garlic cloves!)	1 rutabaga = 1½ cups
1 cabbage = 6 cups		1 medium tomato = ¾ cup
1 small to medium carrot = ½ cup; 1 large carrot = 1 cup		1 large yam or sweet potato = 3 cups
1 large head cauliflower = 4 cups	4 lettuce leaves = 1 cup (1 to 2 large green leaves for wraps = ½ cup)	

STAPLE RECIPES

These recipes are used as ingredients often throughout this book. I make them frequently so I always have them around. Each recipe also tells you the best storage strategy so you can make staples in bulk.

You will use this recipe frequently throughout the book. I like to make a big batch every few weeks, divide it into portions for soup or other recipes I plan to make, and freeze them. This is also just a nourishing and rejuvenating snack. Heat up a cup and sip. The gelatin/collagen in the broth adds the rich flavor and is part of what gives the broth its healing and antiaging properties. Collagen is the building block of connective tissue in the body and we lose collagen as we age, causing our tissue to sag and skin to wrinkle. Keeping connective tissue optimally functioning and healthy decreases injury and can make us "youthen."

When choosing bones for the bone broth, the more cartilage, the better, as this is what dissolves most readily into the broth and nourishes you. The amount of bone doesn't really matter—a chicken or turkey carcass, a few big beef bones like knuckle bones or marrow bones, or save bones from your T-bone steaks and pork chops in the freezer until you have several. Use whatever will fit in your soup pot or stockpot. Ask your butcher for pig's feet and chicken feet. These items are often discarded and can be quite inexpensive. You may also be able to find them in ethnic grocery stores.

Also note that bone broth is an excellent place to use greens you might otherwise discard. You can leach the nutrients out of radish tops, beet tops, carrot tops, or any other clean edible trimmings from the vegetables you eat. I store my trimmings in an airtight container in the refrigerator until I am ready to make my weekly batch of stock. It's economical and waste minimizing, and it adds even more nutrition to your stock.

BASIC BONE BROTH

MAKES ABOUT 8 CUPS
Note: The yield will vary based on the volume of water used and the length of time the broth simmers.

3 to 5 pounds bones, or 1 poultry carcass

1 pig's foot, or 4 to 8 chicken feet

1 to 3 tablespoons powdered beef gelatin (optional, to add even more richness; ideally, use organic gelatin from grass-fed cows)

¼ cup apple cider vinegar, to help dissolve the cartilage and release the minerals from the bone

1 onion, quartered

1 celery stalk, quartered

1 carrot, quartered

1 to 4 garlic cloves

1 teaspoon dulse flakes, or ¼ teaspoon kelp powder

Herbs of your choice (I particularly like bay leaf, celery seed, savory, thyme, and 1 whole clove, or try bay leaf, oregano, chives, basil, or herbes de Provence or any herbs from your culinary tradition)

RECIPE CONTINUES

TO MAKE: Put the bones in a soup pot or stockpot. Add water to cover the bones. Add the remaining ingredients. Heat over medium heat until steaming but not quite simmering. Cook for 6 to 12 hours–whatever is convenient with your schedule. Do not boil. Skim off any foam that develops. (Alternatively, make the broth in a slow cooker–you can cook it on high for six hours or put it on low and leave it for up to 24 hours.)

Strain the broth, discarding the solids, and serve or use immediately, or divide into portions and freeze.

Chicken Broth Variation: **Use a chicken carcass as your only source of bones.**

Fish or Shellfish Broth Variation: **For a fish stock, use a fish carcass from a white fish (this works better than a carcass from an oily fish like salmon and tuna), preferably with the cartilage-rich head on. For a shellfish stock, add shrimp, crab, lobster, and/or mussel shells. Saffron is a good spice to add to seafood-based stocks.**

Thicker Broth Variation: **Strain the broth but reserve the vegetables. Puree them and stir them back into the broth for a rich and nutritious stock.**

WAYS TO ENJOY BONE BROTH

Here are some of the things I like to add to my bowl of Bone Broth for more nutrition, texture, and taste:

1. Chopped scallions and fresh cilantro
2. Fermented cabbage
3. Kimchi
4. Chopped onions (for onion soup—you can sauté them first in some coconut oil)
5. Coconut milk, a little grated fresh ginger, and a pinch of turmeric
6. Fermented cabbage mixed with fermented beets
7. Coconut milk and chopped fresh raw beet stalks

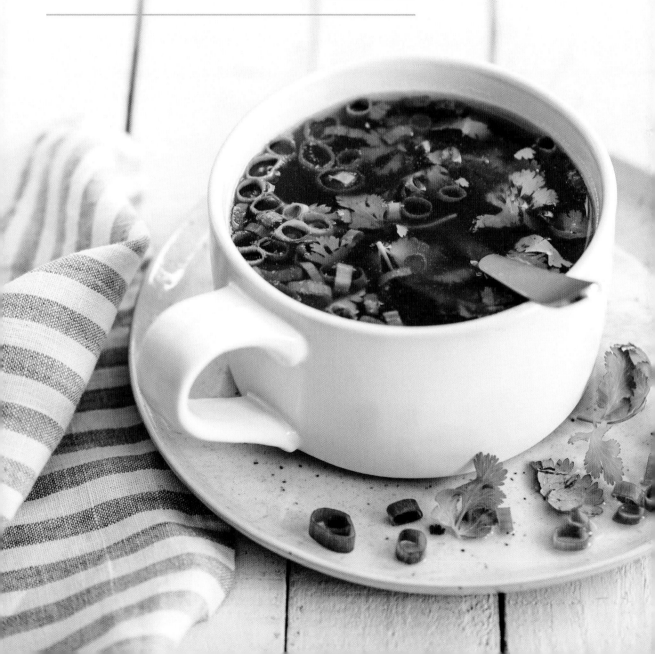

Fermentation is a fun project, and I hope you will try it! Serving and eating a vegetable you fermented yourself is rewarding and impressive, not to mention excellent for your digestion and healthy gut bacteria load. I always keep a homemade ferment in the refrigerator to garnish soups or skillets, and sometimes I just eat them for a snack. They are quick and easy to grab, and delicious, especially once you get used to the taste. As I often discuss (see *The Wahls Protocol*), the beneficial bacteria in fermented vegetables is an incredible boon to health, edging out the gut microbes you don't want and populating your gut with the bacteria that boost immunity, aid digestion, and contribute to many other internal functions. Although you can buy excellent fermented vegetables (Bubbies is a popular brand I enjoy), they are so easy to make that you might as well give it a try. All you have to do is mix some simple ingredients together and let them sit for a while. This recipe is for fermented cabbage, but you could use any vegetable.

The best way to start a ferment is to use a fermented vegetable of the same type, because it already has the starter culture in it. For example, if you are fermenting cabbage, you could use some cabbage from a jar of Bubbies sauerkraut. If you don't have any fermented vegetables to use, you can use some starter ferment (look for this in health food stores) or a probiotic capsule.

I do not recommend fermenting greens like kale or collard greens. They do not ferment well. Most other firm vegetables will work, however. I've tried carrots and beets. Experiment to find the types you like best. If you use cabbage, you might also try combining it with some other vegetables or fruit, like thinly sliced onions or carrots, chopped apples, or chopped pears. Just be sure the mixture is at least 80 percent cabbage. In this recipe, I use carrots, herbs, and aronia berries or cranberries—colorful and nutritious! The green herbs are optional.

Also note that if you make this recipe with green cabbage and use the hibiscus or aronia berries, your fermented cabbage will be pinkish or purple. My daughter enjoys when we make it this way and especially likes the purple color.

FERMENTED RED CABBAGE

MAKES 4 SERVINGS
1 serving = 1 Wahls veg/fruit cup

1 cup fermented cabbage (I like Bubbies brand), or 1 probiotic capsule (such as VSL#3)

1 head red cabbage, 2 or 3 large outer leaves reserved, remainder shredded

½ cup aronia berries, or 1 cup cranberries (optional, but very nice to include)

1 tablespoon dried hibiscus leaves (optional, if not using aronia, to give the ferment a more vibrant purple color)

1 or 2 large heirloom purple carrots or orange carrots, grated

1 bunch parsley or dill, minced (include the stems as well, to prevent waste)

2 tablespoons sea salt

1 teaspoon dulse flakes (optional, but adds a nice flavor)

TO MAKE: In a very large non-metal bowl, combine all the ingredients. Use a wooden spoon to stir until thoroughly combined. (Don't use any metal on the mixture—it can ruin the ferment. You can also mix it up with your clean hands.) Let sit for 15 minutes to 1 hour. Wash a wide-mouth 2-quart glass jar and lid (or two 1-quart jars and lids) carefully in hot soapy water and rinse well. Pack the cabbage mixture into the jar(s). (You could use a crock that has an air lock or allows you to put a plate over the top to keep the cabbage submerged under the liquid—whatever works for you.) Push everything down with a clean hand or a wooden spoon so there are no air pockets. Cover the top with the reserved whole cabbage leaves and put a glass filled with water (tap water is fine) or some other clean heavy object that will fit in the mouth of the jar on top to keep the cabbage submerged.

If there is not enough cabbage juice to cover the cabbage after you let the cabbage sit in the salt, you could gently add salt water (made by mixing 1 teaspoon salt per 1 cup water) to just cover the cabbage.

Cover the jar(s) with a clean tea towel and set aside in a corner of the kitchen. Check it in 3 to 5 days. Take a small spoonful out and taste it to see if you like the flavor. If you do, screw the lid on the jar and put it in the refrigerator. If it doesn't taste sufficiently tangy enough for you, allow it to ferment for 2 to 3 days more and taste again.

FERMENTATION AND SALT

Salt is used in fermented vegetables because it inhibits the growth of all bacteria other than the beneficial types in the Lactobacillus family. When you use salt to ferment your vegetables, you can be sure you are getting the good bacteria and none of the bad, even when you leave your ferment on your counter for a week or more.

If some mold develops on the wall of the jar, wipe it away. The ferment should still taste good. In the rare case that it tastes bad or develops an odor that seems rancid to you, throw it on the compost heap and start over. However, most of the time it will be fine—don't let a little mold scare you away! I rarely see any mold if I ferment the cabbage for no more than 5 days. Keeping all the cabbage completely submerged in liquid will drastically reduce the likelihood of mold, but do wipe away anything you see forming along the rim above the water line and you should have a delicious final product.

The cabbage will shrink down as it ferments, so you won't have as much as you started with. This will keep in the refrigerator for many months.

Kimchi Variation: Do not use the hibiscus flowers or the berries. Instead, add 1 tablespoon minced fresh ginger, 6 minced garlic cloves, and 1 teaspoon hot pepper flakes (use more hot pepper flakes if you like it extra spicy) to the cabbage mixture, to transform it into kimchi. You could also add one grated Granny Smith apple to the mixture to make the kimchi a bit mellower.

FERMENTED GARLIC-GINGER SAUCE

Every 2 cloves of garlic = 1 Wahls vegetable serving

One of my favorite condiments for meat or skillets is my homemade Fermented Garlic-Ginger Sauce. Fill a quart jar with peeled garlic cloves and slices of peeled fresh ginger, 1 tablespoon salt, and about ¼ cup of starter ferment from a previous batch or enough probiotic capsules to equal at least 50 billion CFUs (the amount per capsule should be on the bottle). I sometimes also add 1 teaspoon seaweed flakes. Barely cover the mixture with filtered, chlorine-free water, seal the jar, and leave it on the counter for 1 to 2 weeks. Open the jar, pour everything into a food processor, and pulse to mince. Return to the jar, add 1 tablespoon whole black peppercorns, and refrigerate. (Do not wash or rinse the jar, as chlorine in tap water will kill some of the Lactobacillus bacteria you have been growing in the ferment.) You can mix this chutney-like sauce with a little extra-virgin olive oil to make a drizzle for meat or vegetables, or spoon it on top of anything and everything.

WAHLS KITCHEN TIP: PROBIOTIC CAPSULES FOR FOOD PREP

In some recipes I call for using a probiotic capsule. I like to do this because it adds beneficial bacteria to whatever you are making, whether it is homemade yogurt or garlic-ginger chutney or chia pudding or homemade fermented beets. The probiotic capsule I prefer is called VSL#3, so I will often refer to VSL#3 in this book. You can buy this at Walgreens in the refrigerated section, or online. If you can't find or don't want to use VSL#3, you could use any probiotic capsule with at least 50 billion CFUs (colony-forming units), or enough capsules to equal this amount. When making fermented vegetables, I prefer using ½ cup of the same fermented vegetables from a previous recipe (or a good-quality purchased fermented vegetable—such as fermented cabbage in a cabbage recipe, beets for a beets recipe, etc.). However, if you don't have any fermented vegetable, or if you are making yogurt, kefir, or fermented chia pudding (pages 38, 277), the VSL#3 is the best choice.

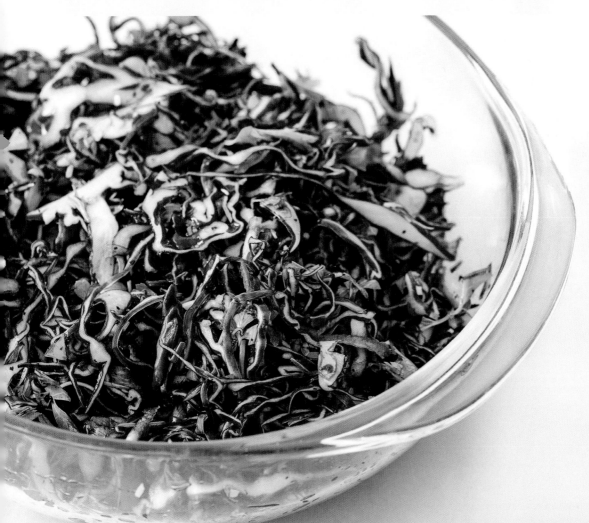

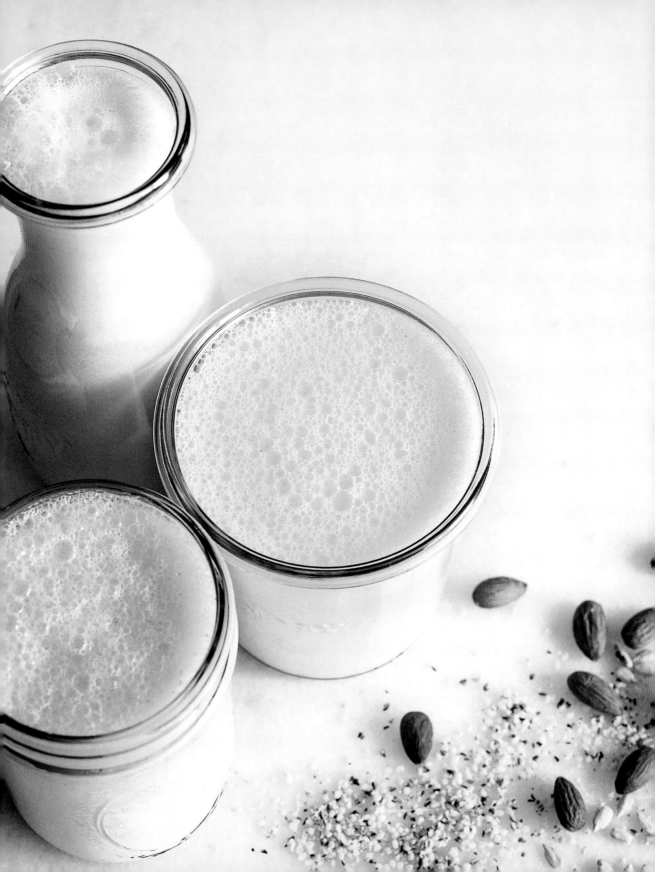

Many recipes in this book, especially those for smoothies and some for soups, use nut milk. You can of course buy nut milk easily in the grocery store, but it is cheaper and purer (i.e., without added sweeteners, preservatives, and thickeners) if you make it yourself. Fortunately, this is easy to do. I often make nut milk out of nut or seed butter (page 39), so I don't even have to blend the nuts. Homemade nut milk will be a little gritty unless you filter it through a nut milk bag (widely available at health food stores and online) or two or three layers of cheesecloth. I don't bother filtering my nut milk—I'd rather keep the grit and the associated nutrients, and in a smoothie, I don't even notice the grit.

Sometimes I eliminate an additional step and just add soaked nuts or seeds directly to my smoothie recipe with some water, so I only blend once—I am always looking for ways to save time and effort in the kitchen.

NUT MILK

MAKES ABOUT 2 CUPS

¼ cup nuts, soaked in water overnight and drained,
or 2½ to 3 tablespoons nut or seed butter

TO MAKE: Combine the nuts or nut butter and 2 cups water in a Vitamix or other high-speed blender and blend until smooth. Add more nuts/seeds/butter if you want richer milk, or more water if it seems too thick. Experiment to find your ideal ratios.

Strain the nut milk through a nut milk bag or 2 or 3 layers of cheesecloth in a colander, if desired. Transfer the nut milk to a glass jar and store in the refrigerator for up to 1 week. Shake before drinking.

YOGURT MILK

| MAKES 4 CUPS

1 tablespoon powdered gelatin or agar-agar

3 cups nut milk or coconut milk

1 probiotic capsule (such as VSL#3)

TO MAKE: Heat 1 cup water in a small saucepan just until warm. Stir in the gelatin or agar-agar until dissolved. Add the nut milk or coconut milk. Let cool to body temperature. Empty the probiotic capsule into the mixture and stir until incorporated. Place in a quart jar, cover with a clean tea towel, and leave on the counter for 12 to 24 hours. After fermentation, screw the lid on tight and refrigerate. Store in the refrigerator for up to 2 weeks.

Note: The yogurt milk may separate in the refrigerator, so you may need to stir it prior to eating. The gelatin makes the yogurt thick. If you want a thicker or thinner texture, simply adjust the amount of gelatin. I like to flavor this with 1 to 2 tablespoons fresh lemon or lime juice. You could also flavor this by adding fresh or frozen berries, or other fruit like peaches or oranges, chopped or pureed. You could also stir in some savory spices like ground turmeric, ground cumin, and ground coriander for a nice Indian-spiced yogurt to use on vegetables or meats.

Kefir Milk Variation: Eliminate the gelatin or agar-agar for a tangy, probiotic-rich beverage. You can also add fruit to this. When I do, I combine the water, nut milk or coconut milk, and fruit in a Vitamix and blend to combine before adding the probiotic capsule. Let ferment as directed in the yogurt recipe, then cover and refrigerate. Shake the jar or stir the kefir milk before consuming.

FERMENTED NUT OR COCONUT MILK

Fermenting your nut or coconut milks adds bacteria to boost your gut health, and gives them a nice tangy taste. This recipe and the kefir version use a probiotic capsule. These recipes are a great way to get your Wahls-required fermented food into your diet, especially if you aren't a big fan of fermented vegetables.

If you thought you liked almond butter before, just wait until you try it fresh from your own food processor. I use nut or seed butter to make my own nut or seed milk, but I also use it for dips, dressings, or as a spread on vegetables. If you are on the Wahls Diet, you could also put this on gluten-free crackers or mix it into gluten-free oatmeal.

NUT OR SEED BUTTER

MAKES ABOUT ¾ CUP NUT OR SEED BUTTER
Note: You can double or triple this recipe—in general, every 1 cup of nuts or seeds makes about ¾ cup nut or seed butter.

TO MAKE: Process 1 cup nuts or seeds in a food processor. They will eventually break down into a rich, delicious butter. If it is too thick, drizzle in a little bit of raw, cold-pressed nut oil, just 1 teaspoon at a time. Store in an airtight container in the refrigerator for up to 2 weeks, or at room temperature for up to 1 week.

Whenever I cook liver and onions for a skillet meal (page 247), I always cook twice what I plan to eat and use half to make pâté. Here's how I do it. Note that the nut butter isn't required, but it does add a very nice subtle flavor and texture to this pâté.

WAHLS PÂTÉ

MAKES ABOUT 8 SERVINGS

½ pound any cooked liver (chicken liver will be the mildest flavored)

1 large onion, cut into rings and cooked in coconut oil until soft

1 to 3 tablespoons extra-virgin olive oil, depending on how silky you like the texture (if you are on Wahls Paleo Plus, use coconut oil instead)

2 tablespoons nut or seed butter of your choice (optional)

Sea salt, to taste

TO MAKE: Process all the ingredients in a food processor until smooth. Pack into an airtight container and store in the refrigerator. This keeps for 3 to 4 days in the refrigerator. Enjoy it with sliced vegetables, in a lettuce wrap, or just by the spoonful.

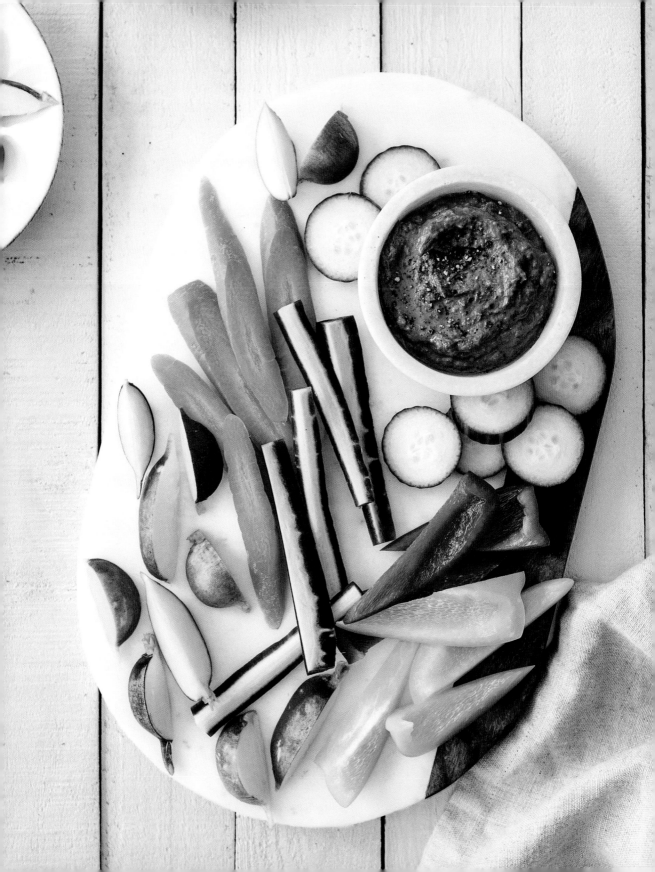

This recipe was in *The Wahls Protocol,* but I include it here because it is such a versatile and popular recipe. You can sprinkle Rawmesan anywhere you would sprinkle Parmesan cheese. The nutritional yeast provides the cheese-like flavor. It is also a very rich source of B vitamins and RNA (ribonucleic acid), both of which provide excellent nutrition for your brain cells.

RAWMESAN

| MAKES ABOUT 1 CUP

½ cup nutritional yeast   ½ teaspoon sea salt
½ cup ground walnuts

TO MAKE: Combine all the ingredients in a food processor and pulse briefly until the mixture resembles grated Parmesan cheese.

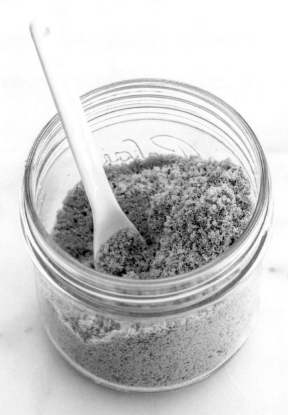

This creamy combination of coconut milk and gelatin has a cream cheese- or goat cheese-like consistency, and you can use it anywhere you would use those cheeses, depending on how you flavor it. I like to mix it with minced garlic, chopped chives, and various fresh or dried herbs for a goat-cheesy experience, or with vanilla extract and cinnamon for use as a dessert cream. I have used it as a topping for soup, on vegetables, or just in a bowl with a few berries.

SOFT CHEEZ

MAKES ABOUT 1½ CUPS

1 (14-ounce) can full-fat coconut milk

1 to 2 tablespoons powdered gelatin
(more will make a thicker cheez)

1 probiotic capsule (such as VSL#3)

Optional add-ins

Sea salt and freshly ground black pepper

Minced garlic

Minced fresh herbs

Spices

Extracts

TO MAKE: Combine all the ingredients except the probiotic capsule in a Vitamix or other high-speed blender and blend on high until fully combined. Open the probiotic capsule and sprinkle the contents into the blender. Blend on low until combined. Pour into a ceramic or glass bowl and cover with a towel. Let it sit on the counter overnight. In the morning, stir in salt, pepper, garlic, herbs, spices, or extracts to taste. Store in an airtight container in the refrigerator for up to 1 week.

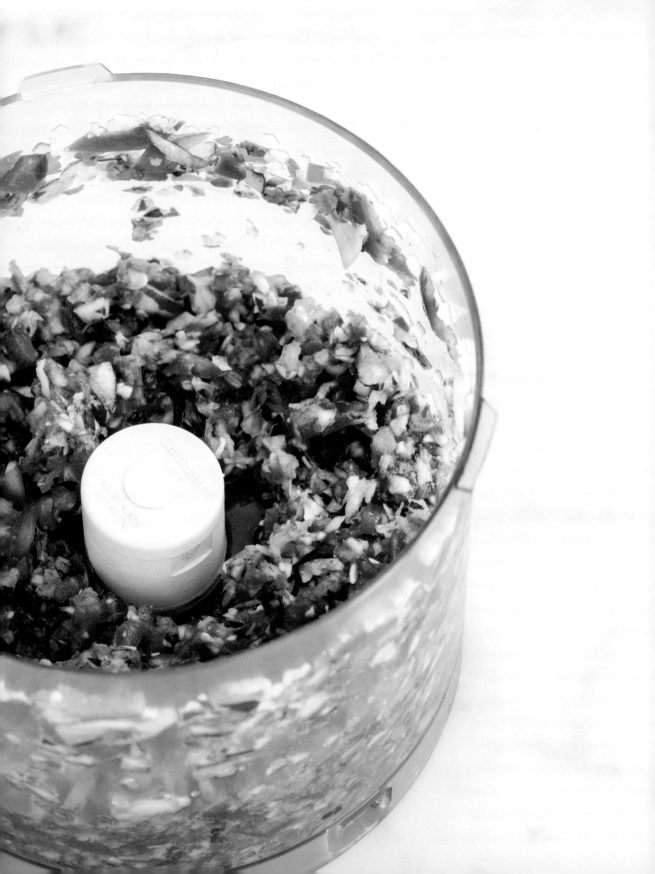

I try to grow tomatoes, parsley, and peppers in my garden so that during the summer, I can pick vegetables and herbs to make a delicious, fresh salsa. Like nut milk, the homemade version of salsa is far superior to anything you can buy in the store, and it's easy to make. You can chop the ingredients with a knife, but this recipe is much easier to make with a food processor or large food chopper. Use this recipe for any recipe in this book that calls for salsa.

FRESH SALSA

MAKES 6 SERVINGS
1 serving = 1 Wahls veg/fruit cup

4 garlic cloves, or 1 tablespoon minced (or fermented) garlic

3 medium tomatoes, cored and quartered

1 onion, quartered

1 jalapeño or banana pepper, quartered and seeded

1 cup fresh cilantro or flat-leaf parsley leaves (it's okay if a few stems remain)

Juice of 1 lime, or 1 tablespoon fresh lime juice

Sea salt

TO MAKE: Put the garlic in a food processor and process until finely chopped. Add the tomatoes, onion, pepper, and cilantro and pulse until mixed thoroughly. Pour into a bowl or storage container and stir in the lime juice and sea salt to taste. Eat immediately or store in an airtight container in the refrigerator for up to 2 days.

WAHLS TACO SEASONING

You can create many of your own custom herb and spice mixtures, but one I find myself using again and again is this basic taco seasoning.

Combine 1 tablespoon chili powder, 1 teaspoon ground cumin, 1 teaspoon paprika, and ¼ teaspoon dried oregano. If you want a saltier mix, add ½ teaspoon sea salt. Store in an airtight container in a cool, dark place (it will keep indefinitely) and use to flavor taco meat.

NIGHTSHADE SUBSTITUTION GUIDE

Some of my patients and many of my readers report that they don't do well eating nightshade vegetables. Nightshades are a family of plants that includes all types of tomatoes and tomatillos, eggplants, all types of peppers (sweet and hot), and potatoes (except sweet potatoes and yams, which are a different branch of this family and don't seem to be problematic). The people most likely to have trouble with nightshades are those with autoimmune conditions affecting their joints, such as rheumatoid arthritis or systemic lupus. (For more details on this, see *The Wahls Protocol.*) While most people can eat these nutritious vegetables—and I recommend them all, other than starchy white potatoes—those who find that nightshades increase their pain should avoid them. However, you can still enjoy delicious approximations of these foods. Here are some ideas.

TOMATO REPLACEMENT

Carrots, squash, or pumpkin with an added beet or 1 tablespoon aronia berries for color will work in almost any recipe that calls for tomato sauce or chopped tomatoes.

EGGPLANT REPLACEMENT

Sliced zucchini works in almost any recipe that calls for sliced eggplant. The cooking time would be about half of what would be required for eggplant.

HOT PEPPER REPLACEMENT

Coarsely ground black pepper, ground ginger, or minced fresh ginger will add heat to any recipe that calls for hot peppers. Horseradish root would also add heat to any recipe that calls for hot peppers.

POTATO REPLACEMENT

Starchy root vegetables like turnips, rutabaga, winter squash, and yams work in almost any recipe that calls for white or yellow potatoes.

CILANTRO SALSA

This is a delicious green salsa for those who love the taste of cilantro. I recommend adding the optional jicama or zucchini for more interest (and more vegetables).

> **MAKES 2 SERVINGS, OR 4 WITH ADDED JICAMA OR ZUCCHINI**
> 1 serving = 1 Wahls veg/fruit cup

1 onion, chopped

2 garlic cloves, minced

1 tablespoon chopped fresh chives

1 tablespoon chopped fresh parsley

½ cup chopped fresh cilantro

1 cup chopped jicama or zucchini (optional)

Coarsely ground black pepper

TO MAKE: Stir together the onion, garlic, chives, parsley, and cilantro. If desired, stir in the jicama or zucchini. If you prefer a finer texture, transfer the salsa to a food processor and pulse until you reach the desired texture. Add spice with black pepper.

WATERMELON GAZPACHO

Watermelon has more lycopene than tomatoes and is more readily absorbed by the body. It tastes sweet, but it doesn't raise your blood sugar the way some fruits do. If you have a Vitamix, then you don't need to remove the seeds—the Vitamix will completely break them down.

MAKES 6 SERVINGS
1 serving = 1 Wahls and Wahls Paleo veg/fruit cup
Note: This recipe is not appropriate for Wahls Paleo Plus.

6 cups cubed watermelon

2 tablespoons high-quality extra-virgin olive oil

1 tablespoon fresh lime juice

Sea salt and freshly ground black pepper

Diced cucumber, zucchini, and jicama, for serving

Minced fresh cilantro or parsley, for garnish

TO MAKE: Combine the watermelon, olive oil, and lime juice in a blender or food processor and blend until liquefied. Season with sea salt and pepper. Refrigerate until very cold and serve in bowls topped with cucumber, zucchini, and jicama. Garnish with cilantro.

TOMATO-FREE RED SAUCE

If you can't eat tomatoes, try this delicious and nutrient-dense sauce instead. It's great on Cauliflower Cranberry Rice (page 313) or gluten-free pasta.

MAKES 12 SERVINGS
1 serving = 1 Wahls veg/fruit cup

2 large carrots

2 medium onions, chopped

1 cup sliced mushrooms

1 small beet, peeled and chopped, or 1 tablespoon aronia berries if you don't like beets

1 tablespoon chopped fresh basil

1 tablespoon chopped fresh oregano

4 garlic cloves

Sea salt and freshly ground black pepper

TO MAKE: In a large sauté pan or soup pot, combine the carrots, onions, mushrooms, beet, basil, oregano, and 1½ cups water. Bring to a simmer and cook, adding more water just to keep the vegetables covered and stirring occasionally to prevent sticking, until the vegetables are all soft, about 15 minutes. Put the garlic in a food processor and pulse to mince. Add the cooked vegetable mixture and process until smooth or just slightly chunky, depending on your preference. (You can add more water if it's too thick.) Taste and season with sea salt and pepper.

I'm a big fan of guacamole, not just because of the delicious taste but because of the healthy fats and fiber in avocados. Use this in any recipe that calls for guacamole.

WAHLS GUACAMOLE

MAKES 5 SERVINGS
1 serving = 1 Wahls veg/fruit cup

2 avocados, pitted, peeled, and mashed

1 teaspoon fresh lemon or lime juice

1 garlic clove, minced, or
½ teaspoon fermented garlic

1 small jalapeño, minced
(optional, if you like it spicy)

1 small tomato, minced

TO MAKE: Combine all the ingredients and serve immediately.

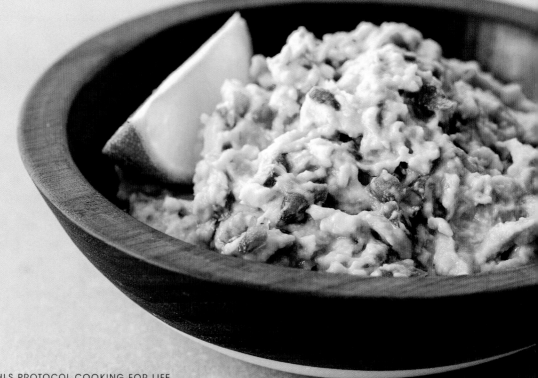

I use these as a side vegetable with my meal. I top them with herbed extra-virgin olive oil, ghee, or coconut oil. Another way of using these vegetables is to blend them with bone broth using a Vitamix or other high-speed blender to make a lovely and tasty pureed soup.

SLOW-COOKER ROASTED ROOT VEGETABLES

MAKES 4 SERVINGS
1 serving = 1 Wahls veg/fruit cup

4 cups bite-size pieces mixed root and other vegetables (rutabaga, turnips, yams, winter squash, whole garlic, quartered onions, Brussels sprouts, beets, and/or carrots)

1 tablespoon herbes de Provence *or*
1 teaspoon each dried oregano, basil, and thyme

1 garlic clove, minced, or ½ teaspoon fermented garlic

1 teaspoon sea salt

½ teaspoon freshly ground black pepper or culinary herbs of your tradition

2 tablespoons warmed ghee or coconut oil

TO MAKE: Put the vegetables in a large bowl. Sprinkle with the garlic, salt, pepper, and herbs and drizzle with the ghee. Stir to coat the vegetables. Put them in a slow cooker, without adding any liquid, and cook on low for 8 to 12 hours. Alternatively, spread them over a baking sheet and bake in a preheated 350°F oven for 45 minutes to 1 hour, or until tender and golden brown.

For grain-free eaters who miss pasta, one solution is spaghetti squash, a delicious and curiously pasta-like vegetable that you can top with all kinds of delicious sauces. Making it is simple if you use your slow cooker. The advantage to this is that you don't have to wrestle with trying to cut the squash in half. Just plop the whole thing in the slow cooker and set a timer. However, oven-roasting is also easy, once you get the squash halved. You can roast or use your slow cooker to prepare all winter squash, such as butternut, acorn, and delicata.

SLOW-COOKER SPAGHETTI SQUASH

MAKES 4 SERVINGS
1 serving = 1 Wahls veg/fruit cup

1 medium spaghetti squash

1 tablespoon ghee, melted

¼ cup nutritional yeast

Sea salt and freshly ground black pepper

TO MAKE: Put the spaghetti squash in the slow cooker, cover, and cook on low for 8 to 10 hours, or until the squash feels soft. Remove the squash and let it cool until you can handle it. Cut it in half lengthwise, scoop out the seeds, and scrape out the pasta-like strands with a fork.

Alternatively, preheat the oven to 375°F. Cut the squash in half lengthwise, scoop out the seeds, put the halves cut-side down in a large roasting pan or on a rimmed baking sheet, and roast for about 40 minutes, or until you can easily pierce the squash with a fork. Use a fork to scrape out the pasta-like strands.

Put the spaghetti squash "noodles" in a large bowl and drizzle with the ghee, then sprinkle with the nutritional yeast, and sea salt and pepper to taste. You can also try topping this with your favorite Bolognese sauce (marinara sauce with ground meat).

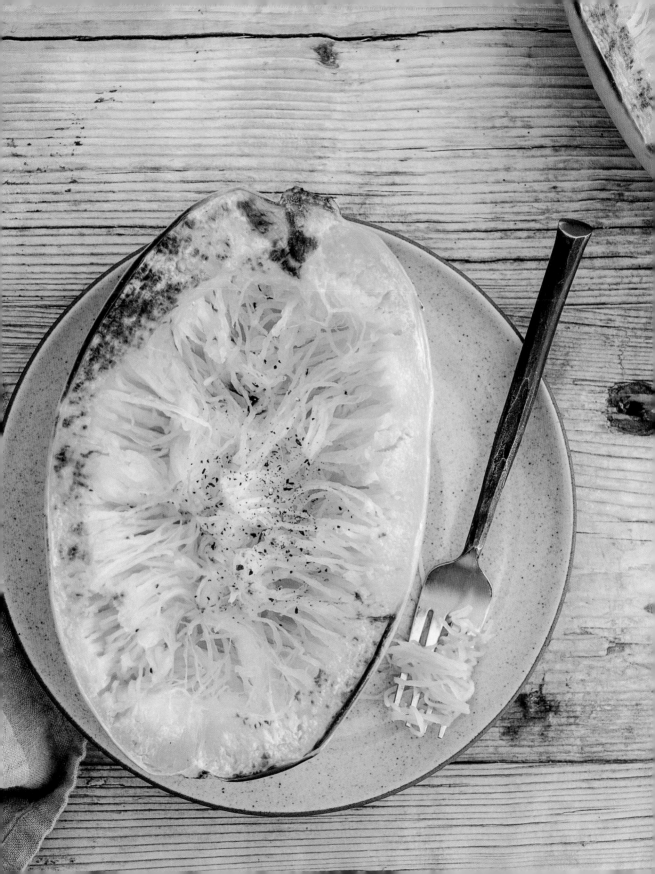

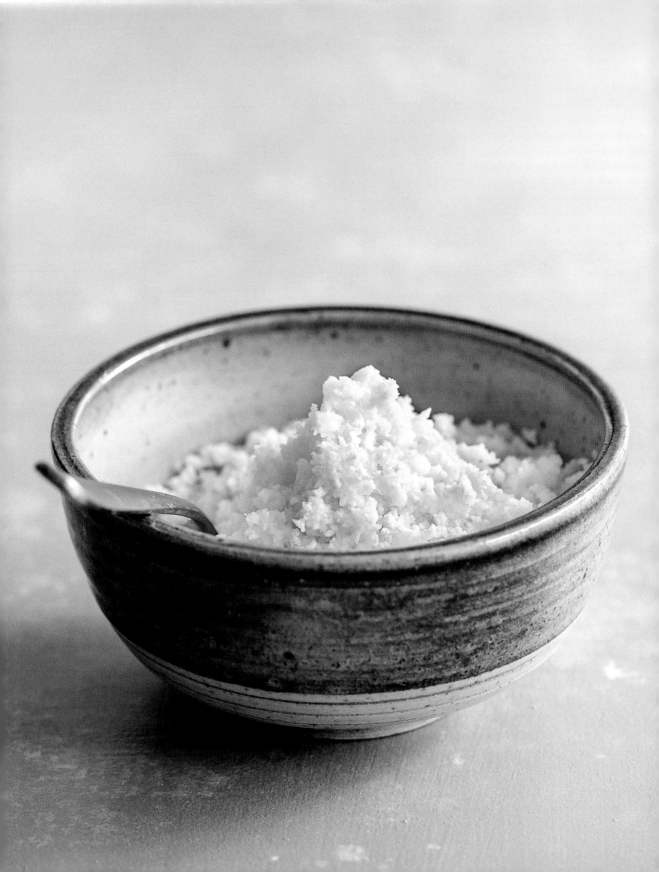

If you've given up or drastically reduced your rice consumption, you may miss having a starchy grain as a base for your meat and vegetables. Instead, try cauliflower or broccoli rice! It couldn't be simpler.

CAULIFLOWER/BROCCOLI RICE

MAKES 4 SERVINGS
1 serving = 1 Wahls veg/fruit cup

TO MAKE: Trim and break up one raw head of cauliflower or broccoli and process it in batches in a food processor until it is about the size of rice or couscous grains. (I include the leaves and core—an excellent way to reduce food waste!) Serve it raw or sauté it briefly in a large sauté pan with about a tablespoon of ghee and a teaspoon of sea salt, for more flavor and warmth. Use this as you would regular rice or couscous, and enjoy the extra nutrition and the lower carbohydrate load. This is excellent to add to a soup to which you would normally add rice. If you do this, stir it in at the end, just prior to consuming, so it maintains the correct texture. If cooked for more than a minute or two, it will get too soft and in a soup, it will dissolve.

HERBED OLIVE OIL

Make your own custom gourmet herbed olive oil by putting any good-quality extra-virgin olive oil into a clean glass bottle or jar and adding fresh sprigs of herbs. Herbs with woody stems work best. Try rosemary, oregano, tarragon, or lavender. You can also put freshly peeled garlic cloves and/or ginger slices into the bottle. Use this oil to drizzle over your skillet meals, soups, or salads. I also like to make an olive oil sauce by blending extra-virgin olive oil with different fresh herbs, with or without garlic and/or spring onions. This is wonderful over vegetables or meat.

WAHLS KITCHEN TIPS: EXTRA-VIRGIN OLIVE OIL

You may have heard in the news recently that up to 70 percent of olive oils available on supermarket shelves are fake, meaning that they are either diluted with non-olive oil or don't even contain any olive oil at all! Cheap vegetable oils are inflammatory, so be very careful about which extra-virgin olive oil you purchase. Real, high-quality extra-virgin olive oil contains a high phenol content, which is not only valuable for preserving the vitamin E content in olive oil but also serves as a potent anti-inflammatory and free-radical scavenger. But how do you know if your olive oil is authentic and high quality?

When tested, the olive oils most likely to be authentic were those from small companies, especially single-family or small co-op companies. Large olive oil companies (like the kinds that produce most of your supermarket brands), including many in Italy where you might think olive oil would be authentic, often sell their oil to distributors who may do the diluting and adulteration.

If you are lucky enough to live near a local olive oil producer, that's your best bet. If not, there are many excellent oils from small family producers available in specialty olive oil or gourmet food stores, and also online. There is an ultra premium olive oil store right here in Iowa City, Iowa, where I live, and where I can purchase 200 ml of olive oil for $12 or 375 ml for $17. If I can do this in Iowa, you might just have a reliable source in your city or town, but if not, do go online. I like a very good olive oil from Greece called Koroneiki. I have ordered three 750-ml bottles for $49 from this producer. Paying a higher price for a good container of extra-virgin olive oil is worth the investment—it should last you a long time since you will only use it for salad dressings and drizzling (remember never to cook with olive oil, as you lose some of the antioxidants contained in olive oil when it is heated for cooking. Also, when you fry with olive oil, it develops toxic properties due to the high heat, so stick with coconut oil or ghee for cooking).

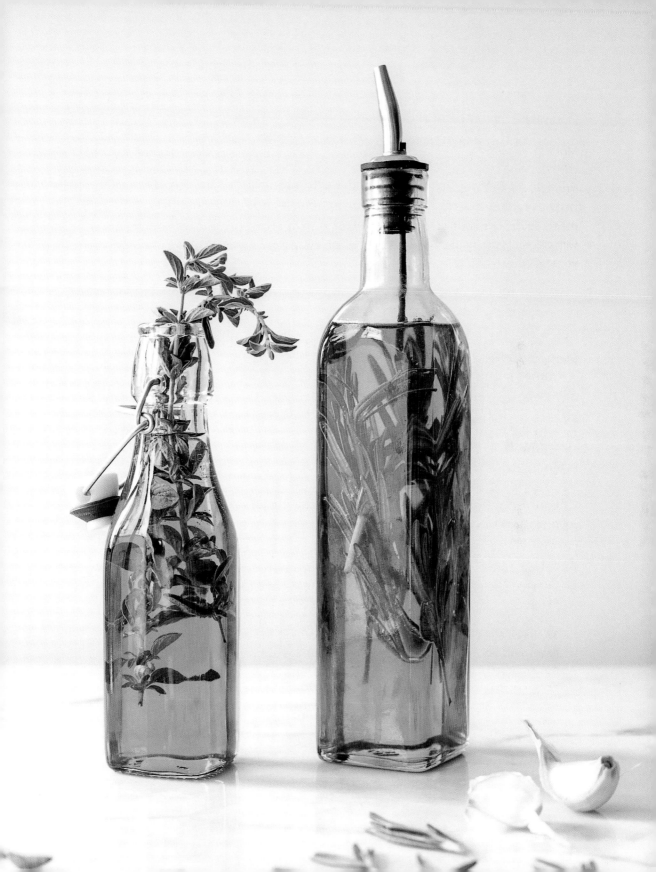

ABOUT THE RECIPES

For most of the rest of the recipes in this book, I will be using a format that is different from most cookbooks you have probably seen. First, I include a basic template for every food category (such as smoothies, soups, or skillets) that allows you to create your own recipe using the ratios I list. Each template has an ingredient chart with three columns, one for each level of the Wahls Protocol (Wahls Diet, Wahls Paleo, and Wahls Paleo Plus), so you can easily see how much of each type of ingredient to use for the level of the diet you are currently using. For example, if you are on Wahls Paleo and you want to make soup, the Wahls Paleo column of the soup template will tell you exactly how much liquid, meat, greens, other vegetables, and seasonings you can use to comply with your diet, and which types of liquids, meat, greens, vegetables, and seasonings are appropriate for you. And then you can get creative!

In addition to the general template recipes, I'll give you specific recipes in each section, for those of you who prefer to take the guesswork out of cooking. I'll also break out the ingredients you should use according to the level of the plan you are following. Each recipe includes a chart that has a column for each level of the Wahls Protocol, with ingredients customized for your level of the diet. It's a simple way for you to adapt every recipe in this book to your own nutritional needs. (Recipes that are appropriate for all levels of the Wahls Protocol will appear in a more standard format.) When a recipe is not appropriate for a certain level of the diet—for example, some of the recipes in this cookbook are not appropriate for Wahls Paleo Plus—I eliminate that column and make a note of it above the chart. If you are following Wahls Paleo Plus, just ignore those few recipes that are not for you.

A few extremely simple recipes in this book will not use a template but instead will be in boxes. For these recipes, I will note if they are not acceptable for Wahls Paleo Plus, but in most cases, all the recipes in this book are adaptable to all levels of the Wahls Protocol.

Although this format may seem unusual to you, I believe you will find it simple and useful, especially if you are practicing one level of the diet and working on transitioning to the next. The ingredient charts will give you all the information you need to successfully prepare delicious, nourishing food that is appropriate for each level of the Wahls Protocol.

DOING YOUR WAHLS VEG/FRUIT CUP MATH

Also, please note a few more important bits of information about the recipes in this book:

- At the beginning of most recipes, you will see the number of servings and the number of Wahls vegetable or fruit cups that count toward your daily 9 cups (6 for Paleo Plus), per serving. This will help you track your progress toward your vegetable/fruit goal. For example: 1 serving = 1 Wahls veg/fruit cup.

- In figuring these Wahls veg/fruit cups, note that when the recipe includes optional additions, I did not include these in the count. If you add more vegetables or fruits, you may be able to increase the cups you get from that recipe.

- In these recipes, 1 serving does not always equal 1 cup, and 1 cup doesn't always equal 1 Wahls veg/fruit cup, depending on density and preparation. Also, 2 garlic cloves equals 1 Wahls veg/fruit cup, so you get more credit toward your goal when a recipe contains garlic. A lot of non-veg or fruit items (like nuts, seeds, fats, and gluten-free grains) in a recipe will also affect how many Wahls veg/fruit cups you get per serving. When a recipe doesn't contain any vegetables or deeply colored fruits (such as some of the granola recipes or certain Paleo Plus versions of recipes), I did not include any information on Wahls veg/fruit cups, since those recipes don't contain any. They are good for your health for other reasons (like healthy fats).

- Note that in some cases, when the total count came out slightly more than 1 cup, I rounded down. If a recipe contains a very small amount of something, such as ¼ avocado or 1 tablespoon dried fruit, I did not count it toward the total cups.

- Finally, remember: Don't obsess. These counts are estimates, and your personal count can also be an estimate. I don't want anyone to become stressed out about or obsessed with the exact number of cups they get. Shoot for 9, or 6, or whatever your goal is. If you approximately get there, that is totally fine.

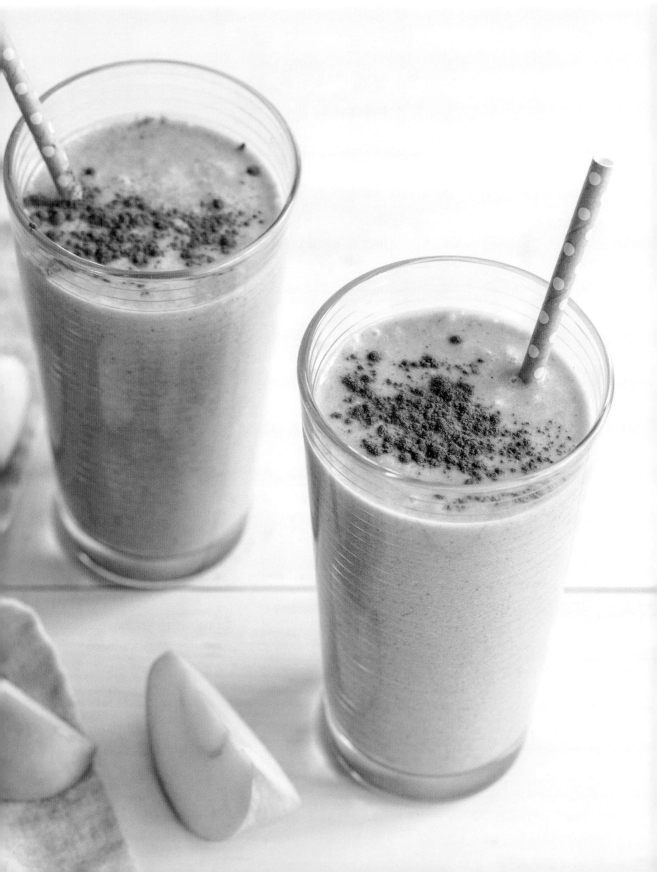

3 SENSATIONAL SMOOTHIES

I ALMOST ALWAYS START MY DAY WITH A SMOOTHIE. Smoothies are such an easy way to take care of breakfast. Just throw some things in a blender, and in minutes you have a nutrient-dense, satisfying breakfast. If you aren't a smoothie person and you are used to a breakfast you can really chew, or if you like to skip breakfast, I urge you to give the smoothie lifestyle a try. Smoothies are easier to consume than "chewed food" first thing in the morning, and you can pack a lot more nutrients into your breakfast than you could into a regular meal (imagine consuming 2 cups of greens every morning in the form of a pleasant drink—a great way to start your day nutritionally). If you are used to skipping breakfast, you will enjoy a new boost of energy and a feeling of well-being before you start your day.

As with the rest of the chapters in this book, I will begin this chapter with a template. This template is your guide for how to make any smoothie. Use whatever ingredients fit the template to create your own recipes without worrying that you are going off-plan. As long as you are adhering to the choices appropriate for your plan level (see *The Wahls Protocol*, or chapter 1 of this book for a review), you will be fine.

But I won't leave you at the mercy of your own creativity, because I know that many of us are fatigued and have brain fog, especially in the

COUNTING UP YOUR SMOOTHIE VEGGIES

Note that when you are making replacements in these smoothie recipes (such as when greens might make the smoothie an unpleasant color or are too bitter for you as you get used to them), 1 cup greens = ½ cup chopped solid vegetables (like chopped carrots or beets) or stems (like parsley, cilantro, or kale stems).

early stages of healing. So I will also provide you with recipes. For each recipe, I will show you how to adapt it to your plan level. But I do strongly encourage you to experiment with whatever fruits and greens are seasonal and fresh in your area when you feel comfortable.

Note that while most of the recipes in this chapter (and most smoothies I recommend) do include greens and I hope you will soon learn to love the taste, you will find a few recipes with the greens either omitted or listed as optional. If you aren't getting greens in your morning smoothie, be sure you are getting plenty of greens later in the day.

Here are some tips to guide you:

- **Gradually increase your greens.** Not everybody likes leafy greens, but when you stash them in a smoothie, you won't even taste them … as long as you get the ratio right. When you first start getting used to green smoothies, you can easily hide greens in fruit smoothies when you have approximately two to three times more sweet fruit—such as oranges, melons, peaches, or grapes—than greens. As you get used to the taste of greens, slowly begin to increase your greens-to-fruit ratio. Eventually, for those following the Wahls Diet or Wahls Paleo, the goal is to get to a greens-to-fruit ratio of 3:1. Take your time working up to this, but do aim to get there.

- **Add citrus juice.** The bitterness of greens is a reflection of their alkalinity. You can minimize this taste by adding more acid to your smoothie in the form of fresh lemon or lime juice. Just a tablespoon of citrus juice can markedly decrease the bitterness in your green smoothie by lowering its pH.

For flavor without sugar or carbs, try food-grade essential oils and pure extracts in your smoothies. This is a great option for Wahls Paleo Plus smoothies that can't contain fruit. Choose essential oils and extracts that are high in quality, food grade, and don't contain additives your body doesn't need or that could be harmful.

Essential Oils: These should be cold-pressed or steam-distilled and have the natural aroma of the plant. They should be obtained from organic or wild plants and they should be diluted with almond oil, flaxseed oil, coconut oil, or MCT oil to avoid irritation that could result from inferior industrial-grade oils. Two companies, called Young Living and doTerra, produce high-quality food-grade essential oils. Both companies also provide guidance about which oils are safe to consume, as well as featuring their oils. If you are looking at other brands, please know that the term *therapeutic grade* does not have a legal definition, and I can't say for sure that *food-grade essential oil* does, either. If you are going to consume any essential oil, be sure that the label clearly states that particular oil is suitable for internal consumption.

Extracts: Extracts such as vanilla, peppermint, and orange are widely available and can be a good way to flavor a smoothie without adding carbs. Most extracts contain an extremely small amount of alcohol and either propylene glycol or glycerine. Both are sugar alcohols that have a sweet taste but a lower glycemic index than sugar. Many dietitians advocate the use of sugar alcohols as a good alternative to sugar, and these products are considered safe by the government. While propylene glycol is an ingredient in antifreeze, you would likely have to ingest a very large amount for it to have any toxic effect. Glycerine is likely harmless. Even so, I still would like to see an extract without any sugar alcohols, which can produce gastric discomfort in some people. One brand that does not contain propylene glycol but may include glycerine in some flavors is Olive Nation, which makes a variety of fruit-flavored extracts, like watermelon, pineapple, blackberry, raspberry, strawberry, mango, and peach. Silver Cloud Estates also makes propylene glycol–free extracts.

Go ahead and try them if you don't mind a few drops of sugar alcohol and perhaps a little glycerine in your smoothie. I use them on occasion, but in general, I use either real fruit or essential oils instead.

- **Avoid mixing berries with greens.** When you are using lower-sugar fruits such as berries, the greens can overpower the fruit. When I use berries, I don't include greens (I know I will get them in some other form later). Instead, I use other vegetables, usually carrots or beets, which have a milder flavor (and give the smoothie a nicer color).

- **Add fat.** Fats add nutrition and a great texture to smoothies. Fat also mellows out the bitterness of greens. Try adding a little extra-virgin olive oil, MCT oil, food-grade essential oils, full-fat coconut milk, flaxseeds, avocado oil, or nut butter. Note that nut butter can give many smoothies an unattractive color. I only use it in my "orange" smoothies (those made with mangos, peaches, or oranges).

Smoothies on Wahls Paleo Plus: If you are following Wahls Paleo Plus, you have a stricter goal. I would like you to be drinking smoothies with no fruit at all, to keep your carb intake lower. Make your smoothies with greens and a can of full-fat coconut milk along with 1 cup water and any herbs or spices you would like (no fruit other than a maximum of 1 tablespoon fresh lemon or lime juice, and of course no added sweetener). Additional fat such as 1 tablespoon nut butter or avocado will help reduce the bitterness even more. Experiment to determine how much fat and citrus juice you like best (you can also add citrus essential oils or fruit extracts to add a fruit flavor), but I find that greens and coconut milk are a lovely combination

DON'T FORGET THE FAT

I recommend adding some type of fat to every smoothie. This slows down the release of fruit and vegetable sugars. I often use full-fat coconut milk for this purpose, but there are many options, like nut butter, avocado, extra-virgin olive oil, flaxseed oil, hemp oil, MCT oil, or Brazil nuts. I like all my patients to have one or two Brazil nuts per day to get the daily 100 to 200 mcg of selenium recommended for healthy thyroid function. (Don't have more than four Brazil nuts in one day, or you will get too much selenium. The upper limit for daily intake is 400 mcg per day, and four Brazil nuts is right at this maximum.)

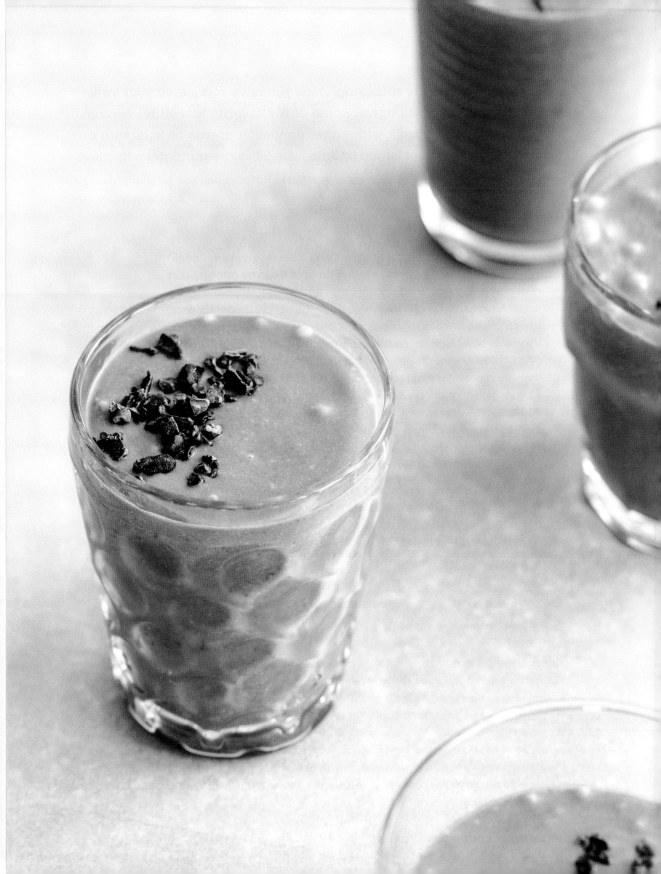

TROPICAL SMOOTHIE

MAKES 2 SERVINGS

1 serving = 2 Wahls veg/fruit cups

1 serving = 1½ Wahls Paleo veg/fruit cups

1 serving = 1 Wahls Paleo Plus veg/fruit cup

TO MAKE: Put all the ingredients in a Vitamix or other high-speed blender and blend until smooth. Add water as needed if you prefer a thinner smoothie.

	WAHLS DIET	WAHLS PALEO	WAHLS PALEO PLUS
FRUIT	2 cups frozen unsweetened tropical fruit blend, or 2 tangerines	1 cup frozen unsweetened tropical fruit blend, or 1 tangerine	None
	½ cup papaya	½ cup papaya or mango	
	½ cup mango		
GREENS/ VEGETABLES	1 cup chopped fresh parsley, or ½ cup parsley stems	2 cups chopped parsley, or 1 cup parsley stems	2 cups chopped parsley, or 1 cup parsley stems
FAT	1 tablespoon nut butter, or 1 Brazil nut	2 tablespoons nut butter, or 2 Brazil nuts	1 to 2 tablespoons MCT oil or coconut oil, warmed, or 4 Brazil nuts
LIQUID	2 cups water	2 cups water	1 (14-ounce) can full-fat coconut milk, plus enough water to make 2 cups
FLAVORINGS	None	None	1 to 2 tablespoons fresh lemon juice
			1 to 3 drops any tropical fruit food-grade essential oil, or 1 teaspoon extract

CITRUS SMOOTHIE

MAKES 2 SERVINGS

1 serving = 2 Wahls and Wahls Paleo veg/fruit cups

1 serving = ½ Wahls Paleo Plus veg/fruit cup

TO MAKE: Put all the ingredients in a Vitamix or other high-speed blender and blend until smooth. Add water as needed if you prefer a thinner smoothie.

	WAHLS DIET	WAHLS PALEO	WAHLS PALEO PLUS
FRUIT	2 cups frozen mangos	1 cup frozen mangos	None
GREENS/ VEGETABLES	1 cup coarsely chopped parsley or spring mix blend, or ½ cup parsley stems	2 cups coarsely chopped parsley with stems or spring mix blend, or 1 cup parsley stems	1 cup coarsely chopped parsley with stems or spring mix blend, or ½ cup parsley stems
FAT	1 tablespoon almond butter, or 1 Brazil nut	2 tablespoons almond butter, or 2 to 3 Brazil nuts	2 tablespoons MCT oil or coconut oil, warmed, or 4 Brazil nuts
LIQUID	1 cup pink grapefruit juice, no sugar added 1 cup nut milk, or ½ cup full-fat unsweetened coconut milk, plus ½ cup water	1 cup pink grapefruit juice, no sugar added 1 cup full-fat unsweetened coconut milk, or ½ (14-ounce) can full-fat coconut milk, plus enough water to make 1 cup	1 (14-ounce) can full-fat coconut milk, plus enough water to make 2 cups
FLAVORINGS	None	None	1 tablespoon orange or grapefruit zest, 1 to 4 drops of citrus food-grade essential oil, or 1 teaspoon any citrus extract

STRAWBERRY OR RASPBERRY CARROT SMOOTHIE

MAKES 2 SERVINGS

1 serving = 1 Wahls and Wahls Paleo veg/fruit cup

1 serving = ½ Wahls Paleo Plus veg/fruit cup

TO MAKE: Put all the ingredients in a Vitamix or other high-speed blender and blend until smooth. Add water as needed if you prefer a thinner smoothie.

	WAHLS DIET	WAHLS PALEO	WAHLS PALEO PLUS
FRUIT	2 cups frozen unsweetened strawberries or raspberries	1 cup frozen unsweetened strawberries or raspberries	None
GREENS/VEGETABLES	1 medium carrot, chopped	2 medium carrots, chopped	2 medium carrots, chopped
FAT	1 tablespoon extra-virgin olive oil	2 tablespoons extra-virgin olive oil	1 to 2 tablespoons MCT oil or coconut oil
	1 Brazil nut	2 Brazil nuts	2 Brazil nuts
		2 tablespoons almond butter, or ½ cup soaked almonds	
LIQUID	2 cups water	2 cups water	1 (14-ounce) can full-fat coconut milk, plus enough water to make 2 cups
FLAVORINGS	None	None	1 to 3 drops berry food-grade essential oil, or 1 teaspoon extract

I am a thirty-three-year-old mother of three with Hashimoto's and MS. I actually started the Wahls Protocol (modified) before my MS diagnosis. In October 2011, I suddenly lost most of my vision in my right eye. I kept going to work and figured that it would go away. My mother convinced me to go to the ER and get checked out. After a series of vision checks, I was admitted under the care of the neurology department and put on a steroid IV drip for three days. They told me that their primary concern was MS and did a full MS work-up. My MRI and spinal tap were clean. There was nothing to indicate MS. I was sent home with an oral taper of steroids and told to follow up with the neurologist. The neurologist cleared me and told me to come back if I had any MS-like symptoms in the future.

Shortly after my episode of optic neuritis, I became pregnant with my daughter. It was the hardest pregnancy I have had. I had terrible fatigue, brain fog, and moodiness. Toward the end of the pregnancy my labs showed that my thyroid was slightly underactive. I was put on a "baby dose" of Synthroid. I felt a little better and just pushed through it. The year after I had my daughter was the hardest of my life. I tried to treat my hypothyroidism naturally and ended up gaining weight on top of baby weight, getting sick frequently with no sick days left at work, and generally struggling to be a halfway-decent mom. The following spring, I saw my physician's assistant. She advised me to read *Wheat Belly* and try gluten-free. She also put me on Armour Thyroid. I started to feel better and lose weight, but never really felt like my old self again.

In August 2014, I started to feel numbness/tingling in my left hand. I also felt electric shocks down my back when I bent my chin to my chest. I knew that these were signs of MS. Unfortunately, the neurologist that I went to did not. I was diagnosed with carpal tunnel—twice! While I got the runaround from the hospital system, I found *The Wahls Protocol* and read it. I was sold, but it would not be an easy transition for me. I had been a vegetarian since the age of nine. Giving up grains wasn't terrible, since I had already gone gluten-free. I was able to modify my smoothie regimen to get most of my veggies in. Adding meat was harder. I was fine with chicken and turkey (I had never given up fish). Eating bacon again was great. I still have to force myself to eat steak. I tried to make liver and onions one time. I'm not there yet.

It's now been eight months since I started my version of the Wahls Protocol. I was finally diagnosed with MS just over a month ago (after having my PCP order an MRI of my cervical spine and then refer me to a neurologist). I got an infusion of steroids for my hand, and it's mostly better. I have also started treatment with Copaxone. I am hopeful that, between diet and disease-modifying drugs, I can limit relapses and enjoy a mostly normal life. I am also hopeful that I will be able to implement a stricter version of the Wahls Protocol. I am thankful to Dr. Wahls for giving me the power to change my quality of life. Even my version of the diet has made a huge difference. I'm now back to my pre-baby (all three) weight. I have more energy. I'm a better mom. I do miss pizza, though.

—Wahls Warrior ELIZABETH

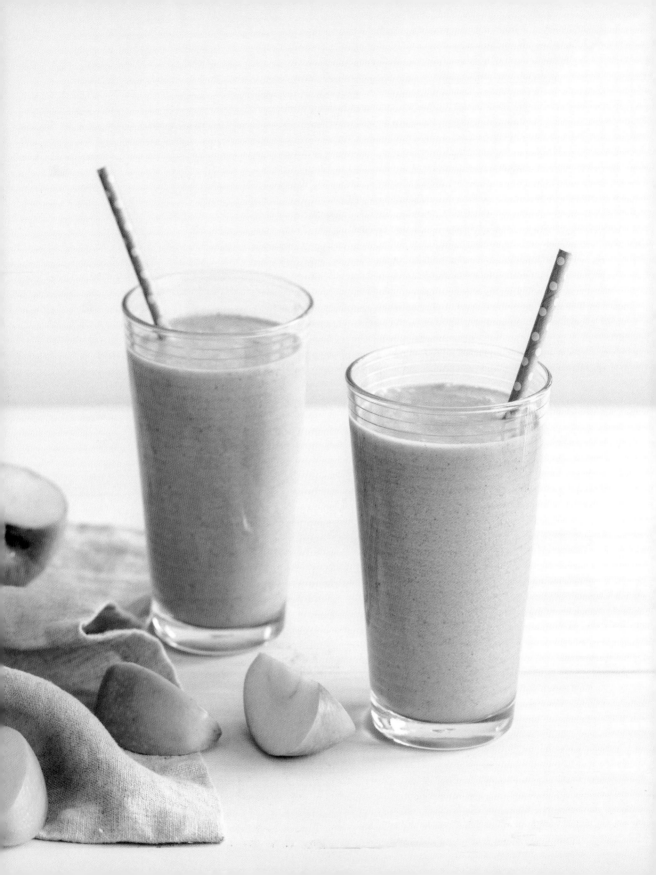

APPLE OR PUMPKIN PIE SMOOTHIE

MAKES 2 SERVINGS

1 serving = 1 Wahls and Wahls Paleo veg/fruit cup

1 serving = ½ Wahls Paleo Plus veg/fruit cup

TO MAKE: Put all the ingredients in a Vitamix or other high-speed blender and blend until smooth. Add water as needed if you prefer a thinner smoothie.

	WAHLS DIET	WAHLS PALEO	WAHLS PALEO PLUS
FRUIT	2 medium Granny Smith apples, cored and chopped, or 1 cup pumpkin puree	1 medium Granny Smith apple, cored and chopped, or ½ cup pumpkin puree	None
GREENS/ VEGETABLES	1 medium carrot, chopped	2 medium carrots, chopped	2 medium carrots, chopped
FAT	1 tablespoon almond butter, or 1 or 2 Brazil nuts	2 tablespoons almond butter	1½ tablespoons almond butter 1½ tablespoons MCT oil or coconut oil, melted
LIQUID	2 cups unsweetened plant milk (such as almond milk), or 1 cup full-fat canned coconut milk plus 1 cup water	2 cups unsweetened plant milk (such as almond milk), or 1 cup full-fat canned coconut milk plus 1 cup water	1 (14-ounce) can full-fat coconut milk, plus enough water to make 2 cups
FLAVORINGS	1 teaspoon ground cinnamon ½ teaspoon ground nutmeg Pinch of ground cloves 1 tablespoon nutritional yeast (optional)	1 teaspoon ground cinnamon (optional) ½ teaspoon ground nutmeg (optional) Pinch of ground cloves (optional) 1 tablespoon nutritional yeast (optional)	2 teaspoons pumpkin pie spice 1 to 2 tablespoons nutritional yeast (optional) ½ teaspoon ground turmeric, for color (optional)

CHOCOLATE SMOOTHIE

MAKES 2 SERVINGS

1 serving = 1½ Wahls veg/fruit cups

1 serving = ½ Wahls Paleo veg/fruit cup

1 serving = ¼ Wahls Paleo Plus veg/fruit cup

TO MAKE: Put all the ingredients in a Vitamix or other high-speed blender and blend until smooth. Add water as needed if you prefer a thinner smoothie.

	WAHLS DIET	WAHLS PALEO	WAHLS PALEO PLUS
FRUIT	2 frozen very ripe bananas, chopped	1 frozen very ripe banana, chopped	None
	1 cup frozen cherries	½ cup frozen cherries	
GREENS/ VEGETABLES	1 cup frozen greens (optional)	1 cup frozen greens (optional)	1 carrot, chopped, or 1 cup chopped greens, or a combination of the two (optional)
FAT	2 teaspoons unsweetened cocoa powder or raw cacao nibs	1 tablespoon unsweetened cocoa powder or raw cacao nibs	1 tablespoon unsweetened cocoa powder or raw cacao nibs
	1 teaspoon coconut oil	1 tablespoon coconut oil	2 tablespoons coconut oil or MCT oil
LIQUID	1 cup full-fat coconut milk	1 cup full-fat canned coconut milk and 1 cup water, or 2 cups boxed coconut milk	1 (14-ounce) can full-fat coconut milk, plus enough water to make 2 cups
	1 cup water		
FLAVORINGS	1 teaspoon ground cinnamon (optional)	1 teaspoon ground cinnamon (optional)	2 teaspoons ground cinnamon (optional)

A few weeks after being diagnosed, I thankfully found Dr. Wahls's book. I jumped right into the deep end and cut out dairy, gluten, and processed food. I continued to exercise the way I always had, started on supplements, and tried to keep stress at bay. After a few months, I had so much energy and the brain fog was gone. My right leg was declining fast, but since the lifestyle changes it has gotten better. I can't thank her enough.

Here's a tip from me. I found I was wasting a lot of greens, so now I buy lots and freeze them. When I'm making my daily smoothies, I always have either fresh or frozen in the house. This summer, I loaded up on fresh local organic blueberries and froze them, too. They are great for snacking on right out of the freezer and of course they go into my smoothies, too.

Other lifestyle changes have helped me, too. I've started dry brushing every morning before my shower to help my largest organ detox. Since I cannot run anymore, I attend a Spin class at least once or twice a week to get the blood flowing. If I miss a week, I notice a decline. I am always stretching either at home or at a yoga class.

Thank you, Dr. Wahls, for all your hard work helping us figure out this crazy path we've been put on!

—Wahls Warrior JESSIE

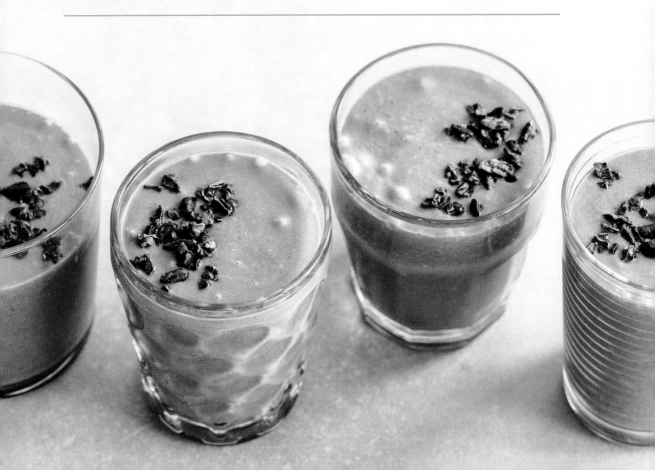

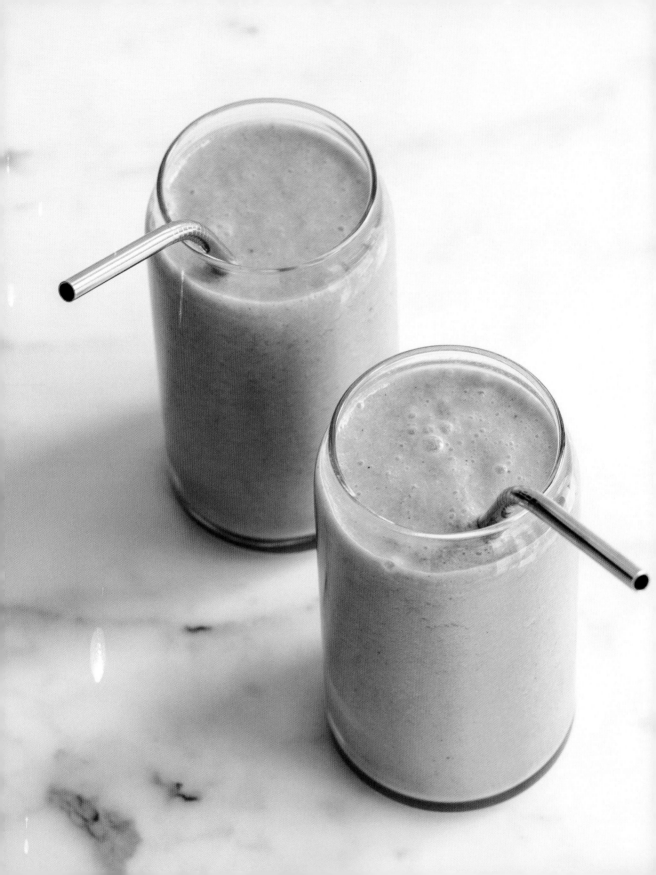

CARROT GINGER SMOOTHIE

MAKES 2 SERVINGS

1 serving = 1 Wahls and Wahls Paleo veg/fruit cup

1 serving = ½ Wahls Paleo Plus veg/fruit cup

TO MAKE: Put all the ingredients in a Vitamix or other high-speed blender and blend until smooth. Add water as needed if you prefer a thinner smoothie.

	WAHLS DIET	WAHLS PALEO	WAHLS PALEO PLUS
FRUIT	2 oranges	1 orange	None
GREENS/ VEGETABLES	1 medium carrot, chopped	2 medium carrots, chopped	2 medium carrots, chopped
FAT	1 tablespoon unsweetened sunflower butter or soaked sunflower seeds	2 tablespoons unsweetened sunflower butter, or ⅓ cup soaked sunflower seeds	2 tablespoons unsweetened sunflower butter or soaked sunflower seeds 2 tablespoons coconut oil
LIQUID	½ cup full-fat coconut milk and 1½ cups water, or 2 cups boxed unsweetened coconut milk	1 cup canned full-fat coconut milk 1 cup water	1 (14-ounce) can full-fat coconut milk, plus enough water to make 2 cups
FLAVORINGS	½ teaspoon grated fresh ginger Twist of black pepper	1 (¼-inch) piece fresh ginger, minced Twist of black pepper	½ teaspoon grated fresh ginger Twist of black pepper

This is one of my favorite recipes, and I often use kale stems to make it. Less waste! The sweetness of the grapes cuts the bitterness of the greens, and in the Wahls Paleo Plus recipe, the richness of the coconut milk serves the same purpose. The black pepper gives this smoothie a surprising spiciness, but feel free to leave it out.

GREEN GODDESS GRAPE SMOOTHIE

MAKES 2 SERVINGS
1 serving = 1½ Wahls and Wahls Paleo veg/fruit cups
1 serving = 1 Wahls Paleo Plus veg/fruit cup

TO MAKE: Put all the ingredients in a Vitamix or other high-speed blender and blend until smooth. Add water as needed if you prefer a thinner smoothie.

	WAHLS DIET	WAHLS PALEO	WAHLS PALEO PLUS
FRUIT	2 cups green grapes	1 cup green grapes	None
GREENS/ VEGETABLES	1 cup kale leaves, or ½ cup coarsely chopped kale stems	2 cups kale leaves, or 1 cup coarsely chopped kale stems	2 cups kale leaves, or 1 cup coarsely chopped kale stems
FAT	¼ avocado	¼ avocado	¼ avocado
LIQUID	2 cups boxed nut milk, or 1 cup full-fat coconut milk, plus enough water to make 2 cups	2 cups boxed nut milk, or 1 (14-ounce) can full-fat coconut milk, plus enough water to make 2 cups	1 (14-ounce) can full-fat coconut milk, plus enough water to make 2 cups
FLAVORINGS	1 tablespoon fresh lime juice	1 tablespoon fresh lime juice	1 tablespoon fresh lime juice
	1 (¼-inch) piece fresh ginger, minced	1 (¼-inch) piece fresh ginger, minced	1 (¼-inch) piece fresh ginger, minced
	Twist of black pepper (optional)	Twist of black pepper (optional)	Twist of black pepper (optional)

Note: On the Wahls Paleo Plus level, this smoothie must contain coconut milk.

Variation for Wahls Diet and Wahls Paleo: Use 2 cups water and ice instead of boxed nut milk or coconut milk.

THE MAGIC OF BLACK PEPPER

Black pepper may seem like a relatively uninteresting and everyday spice to you, but research shows that, even in small amounts, it greatly increases the body's absorption of the healing compounds in spices like turmeric and ginger. Because of this, I often add a twist of black pepper to any smoothie, juice, or food recipe that includes turmeric or ginger. Not only is it useful nutritionally, but it adds an interesting, subtle hint of spice that I think you will enjoy.

PEACH CARROT SMOOTHIE

MAKES 2 SERVINGS

1 serving = 1 Wahls and Wahls Paleo veg/fruit cup

1 serving = ½ Wahls Paleo Plus veg/fruit cup

TO MAKE: Put all the ingredients in a Vitamix or other high-speed blender and blend until smooth. Add water as needed if you prefer a thinner smoothie.

	WAHLS DIET	WAHLS PALEO	WAHLS PALEO PLUS
FRUIT	2 peaches, pitted, or 2 cups frozen peaches	1 peach, pitted, or 1 cup frozen peaches	None
GREENS/ VEGETABLES	1 medium carrot, chopped	2 medium carrots, chopped	2 medium carrots, chopped
FAT	1 tablespoon coconut oil	1 tablespoon coconut oil	1 to 2 tablespoons MCT oil or warmed coconut oil
LIQUID	2 cups water	2 cups water	1 (14-ounce) can full-fat coconut milk, plus enough water to make 2 cups
FLAVORINGS	1 teaspoon ground cinnamon (optional)	1 teaspoon ground cinnamon (optional)	1 teaspoon ground cinnamon (optional)
			1 or 2 drops peach food-grade essential oil, or 1 teaspoon extract

ORANGE SMOOTHIE

MAKES 2 SERVINGS

1 serving = 1½ Wahls veg/fruit cups

1 serving = ¾ Wahls Paleo veg/fruit cup

1 serving = 1 Wahls Paleo Plus veg/fruit cup *only if you use optional parsley*

TO MAKE: Put all the ingredients in a Vitamix or other high-speed blender and blend until smooth. Add water as needed if you prefer a thinner smoothie.

	WAHLS DIET	WAHLS PALEO	WAHLS PALEO PLUS
FRUIT	2 oranges 2 tangerines	1 orange 1 tangerine	None
GREENS/ VEGETABLES	1 cup chopped fresh parsley, including stems (optional)	2 cups chopped fresh parsley, including stems (optional)	2 cups chopped fresh parsley, including stems (optional; omit if you want more noticeable orange flavor)
FAT	1 heaping tablespoon soaked almonds, or 1 Brazil nut	2 heaping tablespoons soaked almonds, or 2 Brazil nuts	2 heaping tablespoons soaked almonds, or 2 Brazil nuts
LIQUID	1 cup canned full-fat coconut milk 1 cup water	1 cup canned full-fat coconut milk 1 cup water	1 (14-ounce) can full-fat coconut milk, plus enough water to make 2 cups
FLAVORINGS	1 (⅛-inch) piece fresh ginger, minced (optional) Twist of black pepper (optional)	1 (⅛-inch) piece fresh ginger, minced (optional) Twist of black pepper (optional)	1 (⅛-inch) piece fresh ginger, minced Twist of black pepper (optional) 1 tablespoon orange zest, 1 to 3 drops orange, lemon, lime, grapefruit, or other citrus food-grade essential oil, or 1 teaspoon extract ½ teaspoon ground turmeric, for color (optional)

BLACKBERRY SMOOTHIE

MAKES 2 SERVINGS

1 serving = 1 Wahls veg/fruit cup

1 serving = 1½ Wahls Paleo veg/fruit cups

1 serving = ½ Wahls Paleo Plus veg/fruit cup

TO MAKE: Put all the ingredients in a Vitamix or other high-speed blender and blend until smooth. Add water as needed if you prefer a thinner smoothie.

	WAHLS DIET	WAHLS PALEO	WAHLS PALEO PLUS
FRUIT	1 frozen ripe banana 1 cup fresh or frozen blackberries	1 cup fresh or frozen blackberries	None
GREENS/ VEGETABLES	1 medium carrot, chopped 1 tablespoon chopped or shredded beets (peeling is optional; use raw or cooked)	2 medium carrots, chopped 2 tablespoons chopped or shredded beets (peeling is optional; use raw or cooked)	2 medium carrots, chopped 2 tablespoons chopped or shredded beets (peeling is optional, but beets must be raw)
FAT	1 to 2 tablespoons MCT oil or warmed coconut oil	1 to 2 tablespoons MCT oil or warmed coconut oil	1 to 2 tablespoons MCT oil or warmed coconut oil
LIQUID	2 cups water	2 cups water	1 (14-ounce) can full-fat coconut milk, plus enough water to make 2 cups
FLAVORINGS	1 teaspoon ground cinnamon	1 teaspoon ground cinnamon	1 teaspoon ground cinnamon 1 to 3 drops any berry essential oil, or 1 to 2 teaspoons any berry extract

Note: On the Wahls Paleo Plus level, this smoothie must contain coconut milk in order for you to stay in ketosis.

I'm twenty-eight years old and I live on the Gold Coast of Australia. I've constantly battled with my weight my entire life. My health issues started at around three years old, with chronic constipation. At around age ten, I started getting severe skin irritation. I had heavy periods starting at age eleven and became very anemic by the age of twelve, so that I had to be put on birth control pills. Next came allergies and face swelling. As an adult, I developed a serious food addiction, and I was always tired, moody, and hungry. When I began to turn my diet around, I realized that I was practically living off dairy foods, morning, noon, and night. I began an exercise program but got injured. Finally, I began to discover information that worked for me.

Now my lifestyle has saved me from myself! I am eating better, exercising without punishing my body, and learning to be gentle with my body and grateful for all that I have. My food addiction, constipation, allergies, menstrual issues, and itchy skin are all gone. I am no longer on any medication, and I feel healthy, vibrant, and energized every day. Now I continue to grow stronger, healthier, and more passionate about life every day because I possess the right tools to start my own family and know that I can give my future children the best possible start to life. I have educated myself and I have learned to listen to my body and fill it with nutrient-dense food filled with quality fat. Knowledge is power, and these days, none of us has any excuse not to educate ourselves. Here is one of my favorite recipes:

POWER PIÑA COLADA

MAKES 2 SERVINGS • 1 SERVING = 4 WAHLS VEG/FRUIT CUPS

1 avocado

2 celery stalks

1 cucumber

2 slices fresh pineapple

1 (14-ounce) can full-fat coconut milk

2 teaspoons maca powder (find this at health food stores)

1 teaspoon powdered gelatin

2 tablespoons sauerkraut juice

2 cups raw baby spinach

2 cups coarsely chopped kale

To make: Blitz it all in a Vitamix, then top with water! I have this nearly every day for lunch.

—Wahls Warrior SHAE

BEET MANGO SMOOTHIE

MAKES 2 SERVINGS

1 serving = 1½ Wahls and Wahls Paleo veg/fruit cups

1 serving = ¼ Wahls Paleo Plus veg/fruit cup

TO MAKE: Put all the ingredients in a Vitamix or other high-speed blender and blend until smooth. Add water as needed if you prefer a thinner smoothie.

	WAHLS DIET	WAHLS PALEO	WAHLS PALEO PLUS
FRUIT	2 cups mango	1 cup mango	None
GREENS/ VEGETABLES	½ cup sliced or chopped beets (peeling is optional; use raw or cooked)	½ cup sliced or chopped beets (peeling is optional; use raw or cooked)	½ cup sliced or chopped raw beets (peeling is optional) (or up to 1 cup for a more intense beet taste)
		1 medium carrot, chopped (or just use 1 cup beets, no carrots)	
FAT	1 tablespoon coconut oil, 1 Brazil nut, or ¼ avocado	2 tablespoons coconut oil, or 2 or 3 Brazil nuts	2 tablespoons MCT oil or warmed coconut oil
LIQUID	1 fresh orange (peeled, or unpeeled if organic), blended with enough water to make 2 cups	1 fresh orange (peeled, or unpeeled if organic), blended with enough water to make 2 cups	1 (14-ounce) can full-fat coconut milk, plus enough water to make 2 cups
FLAVORINGS	1 teaspoon grated fresh ginger	1 teaspoon grated fresh ginger	1 teaspoon grated fresh ginger
	Twist of black pepper	Twist of black pepper	Twist of black pepper
			4 drops orange food-grade essential oil, or 1 teaspoon extract

Variation for Wahls Diet and Wahls Paleo Plus: Instead of blending the orange with water, use 2 cups water or 2 cups nut milk, or a combination equaling 2 cups total liquid.

This excellent smoothie is a bit unusual because the watermelon and ice provide all the liquid. Watermelon contains a lot of water naturally, and the ice makes this smoothie cold and slushy, which is very refreshing. Watermelons have even more of the antioxidant lycopene than tomatoes, although tomatoes get all the glory for being lycopene rich.

WATERMELON SMOOTHIE

MAKES 2 SERVINGS
1 serving = 2½ Wahls veg/fruit cups
1 serving = 2 Wahls Paleo veg/fruit cups
Note: This recipe is not appropriate for Wahls Paleo Plus.

TO MAKE: Put all the ingredients in a Vitamix or other high-speed blender and blend until smooth. Add water as needed if you prefer a thinner smoothie.

	WAHLS DIET	WAHLS PALEO
FRUIT	4 cups cubed watermelon (seedless unless you are using a Vitamix, which will pulverize the harmless seeds)	2 cups cubed watermelon (seedless, unless you are using a Vitamix, which will pulverize the harmless seeds)
GREENS/ VEGETABLES	1 cup fresh mint, including stems	2 cups fresh mint, including stems
FAT	1 heaping tablespoon any soaked nuts or seeds, or 1 Brazil nut	2 heaping tablespoons any soaked nuts or seeds, or 2 Brazil nuts
LIQUID	1 cup water or boxed unsweetened almond or coconut milk	1 cup water or boxed unsweetened almond or coconut milk
FLAVORINGS	None	None

BLACKBERRY GRAPE SMOOTHIE

MAKES 2 SERVINGS

1 serving = 1 Wahls veg/fruit cup

1 serving = ¾ Wahls Paleo veg/fruit cup

Note: This recipe is not appropriate for Wahls Paleo Plus.

TO MAKE: Put all the ingredients in a Vitamix or other high-speed blender and blend until smooth. Add water as needed if you prefer a thinner smoothie.

	WAHLS DIET	WAHLS PALEO
FRUIT	1 cup blackberries	½ cup blackberries
	1 cup black grapes	½ cup black grapes
GREENS/ VEGETABLES	1 medium carrot, chopped	1 medium carrot, chopped
		¼ cup chopped beets (peeling is optional; raw or cooked)
FAT	1 tablespoon coconut oil, 1 Brazil nut, or ¼ avocado	2 tablespoons coconut oil, or 2 or 3 Brazil nuts
LIQUID	1 cup canned full-fat coconut milk	1 cup canned full-fat coconut milk
	1 cup water	1 cup water
FLAVORINGS	½ teaspoon ground cinnamon (optional)	½ teaspoon ground cinnamon (optional)
	¼ teaspoon ground nutmeg (optional)	¼ teaspoon ground nutmeg (optional)

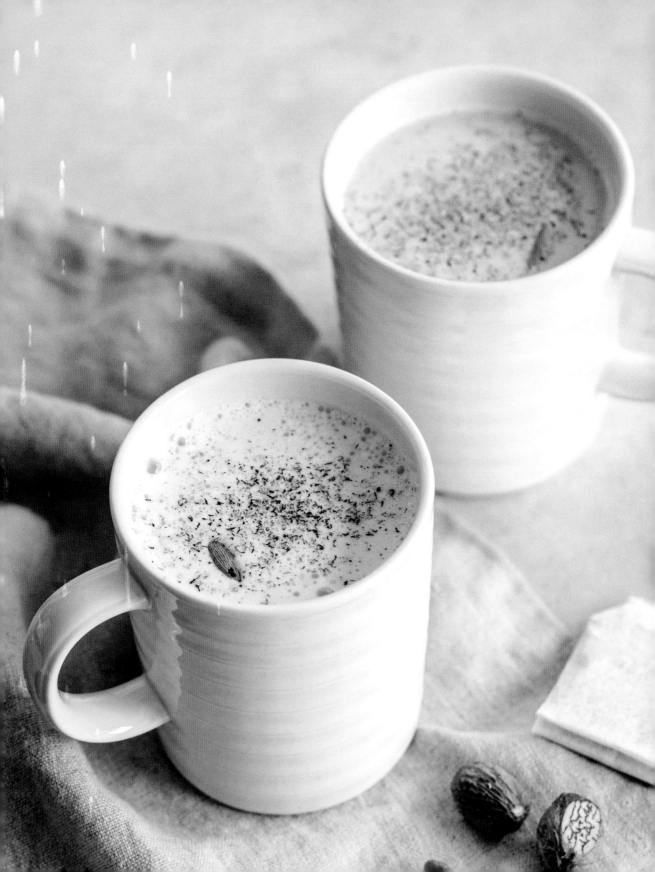

BEYOND WATER: GREEN JUICES, TEAS, AND OTHER BEVERAGES

WATER IS THE MOST VALUABLE BEVERAGE YOU CAN DRINK. Without enough water each day, your organs won't be able to function at peak capacity. Your body's waste management system can break down because your liver, kidneys, and lymphatic system need plenty of water to keep the waste products from digestion and metabolism moving out of your body. For some, not getting enough water can even lead to anxiety.

However, sometimes you may want to mix it up and drink something different from just plain water. In this chapter, I'll give you some ideas to load up your water with even more nutrients as well as flavor. Juicing, spritzers, and tea are all great options for both hydration and healing.

Let's begin by talking about the trendy but often overdone favorite beverage of cleansers, detoxers, and dieters: fresh juice.

JUICE

I never recommend purchased, pasteurized juice in a bottle or carton as a healthful dietary choice. These juices are concentrated sources of sugar and (even in the case of vegetable juices) salt, and the processing has removed many of the beneficial nutrients. However, if you want to make your own juice, there are some things I would like you to consider.

First of all, it's true that fresh juice straight out of a juicer (whether at home or at a juice bar) is a concentrated source of fruit and vegetable nutrients. However, in the case of fruit juice, it is also a concentrated source of sugar. Juicing removes the fiber from the fruit and vegetables, leaving the water and sugars. The natural sugar–delivery system in a piece of fruit or a vegetable has been bypassed, and those fruit sugars will go into your system quickly. Fructose, the sugar in fruit, is not a problem for most people when it is part of the fruit and its associated fiber. But straight fructose without fiber, as you get from juice (or beverages containing high-fructose corn syrup), can lead to fatty liver, central obesity, insulin resistance, and overt diabetes. Vegetables don't necessarily get a pass, either. Even juice from vegetables contains a significant amount of sugar, albeit less than what you get from fruit. When the fiber is stripped away, the sugars become more available and more quickly absorbed, no matter what plant you are running through your juicer.

So the problem is really sugar without fiber, protein, or fat to slow down its delivery into your bloodstream. High sugar intake will also increase the fat that is stored around the belly, and it is this type of fat that is particularly damaging to our health. Belly fat markedly increases your risk of developing a damaged liver, clogging of the arteries, diabetes, and problems with early memory loss. If you have a chronic health issue, keeping blood sugar stable and avoiding belly fat is important, so I advise skipping all forms of pure fruit juice.

For Sugar Addicts

Some of my clients have struggled with substance abuse, and I find that an "addiction" to sugar manifests itself in a similar way. To these people, who insist their smoothies and desserts must be very sweet, I use a metaphor. If I had a patient who was an alcoholic and I was trying to help that patient get off alcohol, I would not give them narcotics to keep them away from the bottle. When I try to help my patients break their addiction to sugar, I find that artificial sweeteners, even stevia, as well as a lot of sweet fruits, will simply feed the brain's need for that sweet taste. Instead, I like to help them avoid sweet tastes altogether, substituting higher fat tastes instead. Fat definitely helps with sweet cravings. If you believe you have a sweet tooth you can't control, I recommend not only avoiding all added sweeteners, but limiting fruit to no more than one serving per day, or even no fruit (other than lime and lemon, which are very low in sugar) at all for two months, which is when the sweet cravings typically subside.

But there are two sides to every story. Freshly prepared vegetable juice (even if it contains a small amount of low-sugar fruit like berries or tart green apple) can be quite a good way to deliver vitamins, minerals, and other phytonutrients, especially if the 9 cups of fruits and vegetables a day on the Wahls Diet is simply too much for you. In our clinical trials, some of our physically smaller subjects chose to juice the balance of vegetables that they couldn't consume. Other clients have trouble with the large amount of fiber in 9 cups of fruits and vegetables, especially at first. In these cases, juicing is useful. It's also easy, if you have a juicer. Many of my patients also quickly adjust to the concept of savory juice—green juice without any fruit at all. If you think of juice as sweet, an all-vegetable juice may not sound very appealing, but it can be quite delicious once you adjust to the taste.

But even juicing vegetables will cause too much of a blood-sugar rise in some people, and if you are on Wahls Paleo Plus, I don't recommend ever drinking any kind of juice from a juicer, even vegetable juice.

However, there is another way to make juice without sacrificing the fiber, and it's my favorite method: using a Vitamix or other high-speed blender. When you add vegetables (and some fruit) to a Vitamix and blend with water until they are completely liquefied, you retain the fiber, which slows the release of sugar into the bloodstream. Fiber also nourishes the health-promoting bacteria in your bowels, your gut microbiome, so that's another benefit. It's a nice compromise between eating all those vegetables and fruits whole and juicing them. A Vitamix helps break down the fiber so that it is, essentially, doing some of the digestion for you. Vitamix "juice" tastes like a cross between juice from a juicer and a smoothie. If it's too thick for your taste, simply add more water to the recipes or halve the amount of fruit. Not incidentally, a Vitamix is also a lot easier and quicker to clean than a juicer. I recommend juicing this way if you want to juice. Now for some more tips on how to make the most of your juice.

Juicer vs. Vitamix Prep

In general, a Vitamix is easier to use and clean than a juicer. However, one advantage to a juicer is that your vegetables, fruits, and other ingredients don't need to be prepped quite as thoroughly as when you use a Vitamix. For example, a juicer can process stems, seeds, and peels.

A word about peels—many of you have been peeling vegetables such as carrots, beets, and ginger before use. But the plant places much of its defense against the world in the peel, and for that reason, it has the highest concentration of beneficial antioxidants (if your produce is not organic, keep peeling).

The benefit to a high-speed blender like a Vitamix is that it can actually pulverize materials like edible peel (including citrus peel) or seeds, and completely liquefy these ingredients, so you will get nutrients you wouldn't otherwise consume. Just be sure to avoid seeds from apples, pears, and citrus fruits, because they contain a very small amount of cyanide (if you accidentally swallow one whole, don't worry—it will pass undigested, but you don't want to pulverize them). Other edible seeds (including watermelon and those from all squash) actually contain more antioxidants than the fruit, so there is definitely a benefit to including the seeds from

one or two fruits a day. Not only do you get a nutrient boost, but you will be wasting less food and getting more fiber. However, also remember that it is much better to have no more than one or two fruits a day. Rely much more on vegetables than on fruits.

Finally, whether you juice or blend, look over the vegetables and fruits you use to be sure that you have cut away anything that shows evidence of spoilage: softening, discoloring, or molding. The foods you use should have their normal texture, color, and scent.

Tips for Delicious, Nourishing Juices

The tips in this section are all suggestions—or troubleshooting. You don't need to use any of them, but they can all make your juices more nutritious and/or tastier:

- **Add oil:** A trick I like to use, especially because I try to stay in ketosis, is to add oil to my juice. This might sound strange, but once I have blended the juice in my Vitamix so it is completely liquefied, I add 1 teaspoon MCT oil or extra-virgin olive oil (you can use food-grade essential oils, too). The oil slows down your body's absorption of the sugars, adds to the satiety the juice provides, and blunts a rise in insulin, preventing a blood-sugar crash. In addition, the oil helps your body absorb the fat-soluble vitamins in the vegetables and fruits. Especially if you are on Wahls Paleo Plus, I recommend adding oil if you want to make juice in your Vitamix.

- **Create a vibrant color:** As with smoothies, I like to consider the color of my juices. Mixing greens with red or orange fruits creates an unappealing color, so I typically mix greens with green fruits (like kiwi and grapes), carrots with orange fruits, and beets or carrots (or a combination) with red or purple fruits.

- **Don't forget the peel:** Citrus peel has many benefits. If you are using organic oranges, you do not need to discard the peel (although you will need a high-speed blender to pulverize it).

Citrus contains many aromatic flavonoids (antioxidants) with tremendous health benefits, and the highest concentration of flavonoids is often in the peel. For example:

- Naringin, an antioxidant particularly high in grapefruit, mandarin orange, and lemon peels, has been shown to be helpful in fighting cancer. However, be aware that it can affect how your body metabolizes certain drugs. (It can reduce the efficiency of how some drugs are processed, causing the drug level in your blood to rise, which could cause adverse side effects—ask your doctor if you are concerned about this.)

- Hesperidin, which is found in the white inner layer of the peel, has been shown to inhibit bone loss and improve cholesterol in animal models of menopause.

- D-limonene, which gives citrus fruit its unique smell, has been shown to be protective against many types of cancer, as well as to lower cholesterol and reduce the risk of gallstones.

Note that even though fruit is in the template, *not all these juice recipes include fruit.* For example, the Cooling Cucumber Mint Juice does not call for any fruits. In fact, I encourage you to drink all-vegetable juices at all levels of the Wahls Protocol, especially when you cannot finish your 9 cups (or 6 cups for Wahls Paleo Plus). Once you get used to the idea that juices don't have to be sweet, I think you will find having vegetable-only juices quite refreshing. They are also tremendously good for your cells.

Special Juicing Guidance for Wahls Paleo Plus

Juicing can be more of a challenge for those on Wahls Paleo Plus because of the importance of keeping sugars low to stay in ketosis. I do not recommend using any fruit other than a little organic lime or lemon juice, which reduces the pH and the bitterness of green juices so they taste better without adding very many carbs. Even vegetable juices should be relatively limited. However, we are all unique. Each of us has an individual tolerance for how many carbohydrates and how much fat and protein we can eat at a meal and remain in ketosis. If you are staying in ketosis using

Wahls Paleo Plus, you will need to pay close attention to how the juices impact your ability to stay in ketosis. Some will find that using a Vitamix or other high-speed blender and keeping all the fiber from the vegetable or fruit will be enough to stay in ketosis. Others will need the addition of MCT oil to stay in ketosis. And some will find that they are not able to stay in ketosis if they use any juices, even Vitamix juices. You will do best if you pay attention to your response to the foods you eat. For more specific guidance on how to monitor if you are staying in ketosis, please see *The Wahls Protocol.*

The bottom line is that "juice," if it retains the fiber, can, in most cases and for most people, be a good way to add nutrients to your meal and get all your daily required vegetables and fruits into your diet. Try making your own creations from the template in this chapter, or try any of the recipes that are suitable for your level of the Wahls Protocol.

Use this template to make up your own juice recipes, according to the level of the Wahls Protocol you are following.

BASIC JUICE TEMPLATE

MAKES 2 SERVINGS

TO MAKE: Put all the ingredients in a Vitamix or other high-speed blender and blend until liquefied. Add water as needed if you prefer a thinner juice. Store the juice in an airtight container in the refrigerator to best preserve nutrients. Sip the juice throughout the day and finish it within 24 hours.

	WAHLS DIET	WAHLS PALEO	WAHLS PALEO PLUS
FRUIT	2 cups	1 cup	None
GREENS/VEGETABLES	1 cup greens, or ½ cup stems or other vegetables	2 cups greens, or 1 cup stems or other vegetables	2 cups greens, or 1 cup stems or other vegetables
HERBS, SPICES, AND FLAVORINGS	As recipe indicates, or as desired	As recipe indicates, or as desired	As recipe indicates, or as desired
WATER	4 cups	4 cups	4 cups

Note for Wahls Paleo Plus: You may add up to ½ cup berries or ½ small Granny Smith apple to this smoothie, but if you do, that is your entire fruit serving for the day.

Variation for Wahls Paleo Plus: Add 1 teaspoon to 2 tablespoons MCT oil as needed to stay in ketosis.

This juice is perfect for spring when strawberries are in season. If you make it in the winter, when oranges are in season, but you can't find good strawberries, you can use thawed frozen strawberries you have saved from the summer garden or farmers' market (or purchased frozen organic strawberries).

STRAWBERRY ORANGE JUICE

MAKES 2 SERVINGS
1 serving = 1 Wahls and Wahls Paleo veg/fruit cup
1 serving = ½ Wahls Paleo Plus veg/fruit cup

TO MAKE: Put all the ingredients in a Vitamix or other high-speed blender and blend until liquefied. Add water as needed if you prefer a thinner juice. Store the juice in an airtight container in the refrigerator to best preserve nutrients. Sip the juice throughout the day and finish it within 24 hours.

	WAHLS DIET	WAHLS PALEO	WAHLS PALEO PLUS
FRUIT	1 cup hulled fresh strawberries	½ cup hulled fresh strawberries	None
	1 orange, seeded and peeled if not organic	1 orange, seeded and peeled if not organic	
GREENS/ VEGETABLES	1 medium carrot, chopped	2 medium carrots, chopped	2 medium carrots, chopped
HERBS, SPICES, AND FLAVORINGS	2 sprigs fresh mint (optional, but adds a nice flavor)	2 sprigs fresh mint (optional, but adds a nice flavor)	1 teaspoon to 1 tablespoon orange zest, 1 to 3 drops of food-grade orange essential oil, or 1 teaspoon orange extract
WATER	4 cups	4 cups	4 cups

Variation for Wahls Paleo Plus: Add 1 teaspoon to 2 tablespoons MCT oil as needed to stay in ketosis.

COOLING CUCUMBER MINT JUICE

MAKES 2 SERVINGS

1 serving = 1½ Wahls veg/fruit cups

1 serving = 3 Wahls Paleo and Wahls Paleo Plus veg/fruit cups

TO MAKE: Put all the ingredients in a Vitamix or other high-speed blender and blend until liquefied. Add water as needed if you prefer a thinner juice. Store the juice in an airtight container in the refrigerator to best preserve nutrients. Sip the juice throughout the day and finish it within 24 hours.

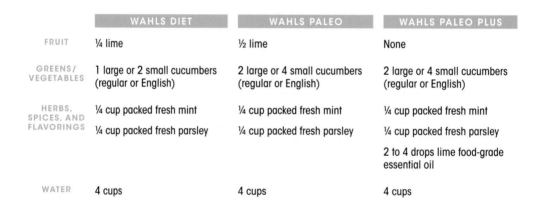

	WAHLS DIET	WAHLS PALEO	WAHLS PALEO PLUS
FRUIT	¼ lime	½ lime	None
GREENS/ VEGETABLES	1 large or 2 small cucumbers (regular or English)	2 large or 4 small cucumbers (regular or English)	2 large or 4 small cucumbers (regular or English)
HERBS, SPICES, AND FLAVORINGS	¼ cup packed fresh mint	¼ cup packed fresh mint	¼ cup packed fresh mint
	¼ cup packed fresh parsley	¼ cup packed fresh parsley	¼ cup packed fresh parsley
			2 to 4 drops lime food-grade essential oil
WATER	4 cups	4 cups	4 cups

Note for Wahls Paleo Plus: You can add 1 teaspoon to 2 tablespoons MCT oil as needed to stay in ketosis. For some, though, this juice will take you out of ketosis, even though it is a vegetable juice. Monitor your ketones to determine whether this juice works for you.

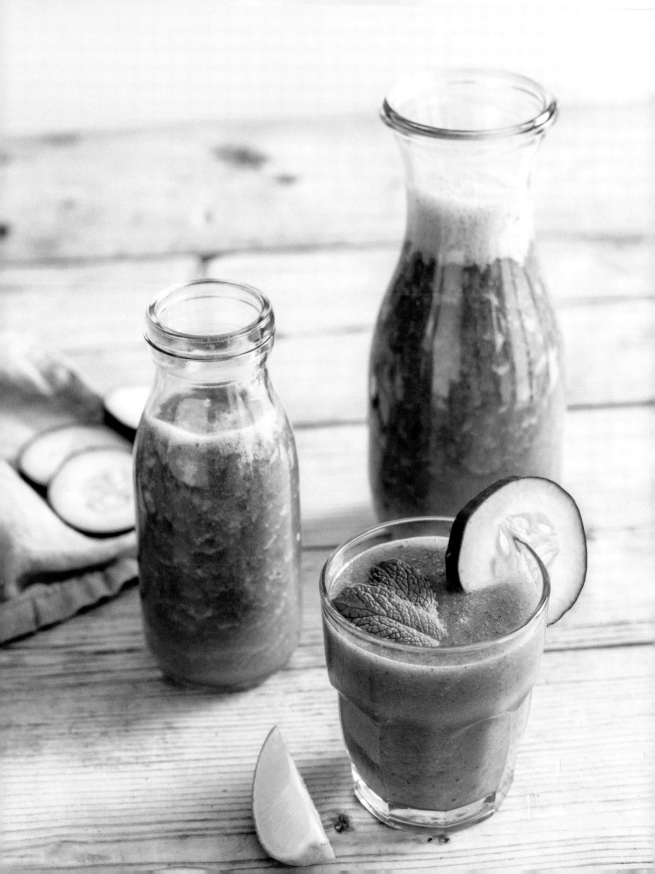

This recipe is perfect for hot summer days when melons are at their peak of ripeness. Try to find local ones, if they are available.

SUMMER MELON JUICE

MAKES 2 SERVINGS
1 serving = 1 Wahls and Wahls Paleo veg/fruit cup
Note: This recipe is not appropriate for Wahls Paleo Plus.

TO MAKE: Put all the ingredients in a Vitamix or other high-speed blender and blend until liquefied. Add water as needed if you prefer a thinner juice. Store the juice in an airtight container in the refrigerator to best preserve nutrients. Sip the juice throughout the day and finish it within 24 hours.

	WAHLS DIET	WAHLS PALEO
FRUIT	2 cups balled or cubed cantaloupe, honeydew, or watermelon	1 cup balled or cubed cantaloupe, honeydew, or watermelon
GREENS/ VEGETABLES	1 carrot, coarsely chopped	2 carrots, coarsely chopped
HERBS, SPICES, AND FLAVORINGS	4 fresh basil leaves (optional)	4 fresh basil leaves (optional)
WATER	4 cups	4 cups

WAHLS WARRIORS SPEAK

My name is Nina Sonovia Brown, and my husband is Brent Brown. My husband met and had lunch with Dr. Terry Wahls in the spring of 2015. That meeting with Dr. Terry Wahls transformed our lives. Brent has celiac disease, so eating clean is familiar to us. However, once Brent met and heard Dr. Wahls's story, he called and told me he wanted us to start following the Wahls Protocol. That day I ordered the book, and the journey and transformation began. For Brent, the biggest transformation was a healthier gut. After about one month of using the protocol, Brent told me that he doesn't worry about what to eat any longer. It was the first time since being diagnosed that he feels better than he has felt in years.

Meanwhile, while we were busy learning, reading, and applying the tips in the book *The Wahls Protocol*, I was researching options to treat a recently discovered fibroid tumor. During an annual visit to my doctor, I pointed out a fibroid. During that meeting, the doctor found a 17-cm fibroid, and because of a history of uterine cancer in my family, I elected to have a hysterectomy. Prior to surgery, I used the principles in *The Wahls Protocol* to prepare my body and cells. Six weeks prior to surgery, while using the protocol, I also increased my daily walking and running from four miles a day to six miles a day. I attribute the success of my operation and my recovery to the Wahls Protocol.

During my surgery, it was discovered that my nonsymptomatic fibroid had grown and attached to my colon. The doctor mentioned to me that she didn't know how I wasn't having problems with my bowel. I reminded her how I eat every day according to the Wahls Protocol.

Two hours after surgery I had stomach activity, eight hours after surgery I was walking—only five steps, but I was walking. After surgery, it was expected that I would stay in the hospital for four days, but I was home within twenty-four hours. Because of my stomach activity, I was able to have solid foods within sixteen hours after my surgery. My first hospital meal was an egg white omelet with *extra* spinach, mushrooms, and tomatoes.

During my in-home recovery, we continued to cook and eat according to the Wahls Protocol, but a modified version, to assist me with foods that would be easier on my digestive tract. We took out the three cups of sulfur-based vegetables until I could handle the gas. I am glad to report that we are back up to all vegetables and fruits. Recovery is continuing to go well, and I am looking forward to successfully participating and completing the Wahls Protocol Coaching Program and a great ski season with my Wahls Warrior husband!

—Wahls Warriors NINA AND BRENT

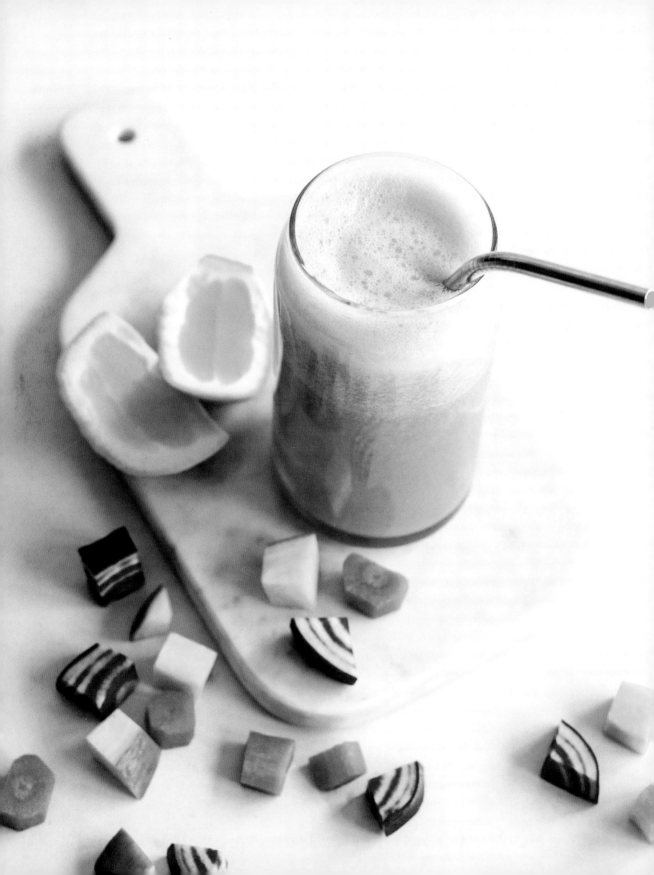

This juice is an excellent health tonic in addition to being delicious. The ginger, dandelion, and beet all help increase the production of digestive enzymes, bile, and enzymes involved in the liver's complex process of detoxification. This particular juice gives your cells terrific support for making enzymes that are very important to the detoxification processes in both the liver and kidneys, as well as better blood vessel health. If you are able to buy your beets with the greens attached, go ahead and substitute the beet greens for the dandelion greens in this recipe. Chop the beet stems and add those to the juice as well.

BEET-LICIOUS JUICE WITH GINGER AND ORANGE

MAKES 2 SERVINGS
1 serving = 1½ Wahls veg/fruit cups
1 serving = 1 Wahls Paleo veg/fruit cup
1 serving = ½ Wahls Paleo Plus veg/fruit cup

TO MAKE: Put the ginger in a Vitamix or other high-speed blender and blend until it is finely minced (you can grate it before adding, if you prefer). If the ginger is organic, no need to peel it first. Add the remaining ingredients and blend until liquefied. Add water as needed if you prefer a thinner juice. Store the juice in an airtight container in the refrigerator to best preserve nutrients. Sip the juice throughout the day and finish it within 24 hours.

RECIPE CONTINUES

	WAHLS DIET	**WAHLS PALEO**	**WAHLS PALEO PLUS**
FRUIT	2 oranges (peels may be included), seeds removed	1 orange (peel may be included if organic), seeds removed	2 tablespoon lemon or lime juice
GREENS/ VEGETABLES	½ cup chopped raw red or golden beets (peeling is optional)	¾ cup coarsely chopped raw red or golden beets (peeling is optional)	¾ cup coarsely chopped raw red or golden beets (peeling is optional)
	1 medium carrot, chopped	1 medium carrot, chopped	1 medium carrot, chopped
		(Alternatively, use 1 full cup chopped raw beets for an intense beet juice.)	(Alternatively, use 1 full cup chopped raw beets for an intense beet juice.)
HERBS, SPICES, AND FLAVORINGS	1 (¼-inch) piece fresh ginger	1 (¼-inch) piece fresh ginger	1 (¼-inch) piece fresh ginger
	Twist of black pepper	Twist of black pepper	Twist of black pepper
			4 drops orange food-grade essential oil and/or 1 tablespoon orange zest
WATER	4 cups	4 cups	4 cups

Note for Wahls Paleo Plus: You can add 1 teaspoon to 2 tablespoons MCT oil as needed to stay in ketosis.

People over the age of fifty often have more difficulty making enough acid in the stomach. The result can be a lot of belching, bloating, or even heartburn. Having a glass of ginger-lime (or -lemon) juice prior to your meals can be very helpful in combating this problem. This juice is also useful to combat bone loss. Some people experience bone loss due to excess acidity in the body, which causes the body to pull minerals from the skeleton to neutralize the acid and keep the blood pH in its necessary narrow range. This juice is an excellent way to help counteract this process. Adding sea salt to this recipe increases your mineral absorption.

ALKALINIZING GINGER LIME JUICE

MAKES 2 SERVINGS
1 serving = ½ Wahls veg/fruit cup
1 serving = 1 Wahls Paleo and Wahls Paleo Plus veg/fruit cup

TO MAKE: Put the ginger in a Vitamix or other high-speed blender and blend until it is finely minced (you can grate it separately before adding, if you prefer). Add the remaining ingredients and blend until liquefied. Fine-tune the flavor by reducing the lime or lemon or adding more water if the taste is too tart. If your lemon or lime is organic, you can include the peels. Taste your juice before adding the peel, and then add the peel and decide which way you prefer it. You can also include the cilantro stems to reduce food waste. Add water as needed if you prefer a thinner juice. Store the juice in an airtight container in the refrigerator to best preserve nutrients. Drink a cup or so before meals and finish it within 24 hours.

Note: This is *not a sweet juice!* It is tart, but although lemons and limes taste acidic, they have an alkalizing effect in the body, which is quite therapeutic. I recommend drinking 1 cup of this juice half an hour before a big meal.

RECIPE CONTINUES

	WAHLS DIET	WAHLS PALEO	WAHLS PALEO PLUS
FRUIT	½ lime, peeled and seeded (or use a citrus juicer to juice directly into Vitamix), or 1 tablespoon fresh lime or lemon juice	1 lime, peeled and seeded (or use a citrus juicer to juice directly into Vitamix), or 2 tablespoons fresh lime or lemon juice	2 tablespoons fresh lime or lemon juice
GREENS/ VEGETABLES	1 cup fresh cilantro or parsley leaves, or ½ cup stems	2 cups fresh cilantro or parsley leaves, or 1 cup stems	2 cups fresh cilantro or parsley leaves, or 1 cup stems
HERBS, SPICES, AND FLAVORINGS	1 (¼-inch) piece fresh ginger Twist of black pepper Pinch of sea salt	1 (¼-inch) piece fresh ginger Twist of black pepper Pinch of sea salt	1 (¼-inch) piece fresh ginger Twist of black pepper Pinch of sea salt 4 drops lemon or lime food-grade essential oil, or 1 to 2 teaspoons extract
WATER	4 cups	4 cups	4 cups

Note for Wahls Paleo Plus: You can add 1 teaspoon to 2 tablespoons MCT oil as needed to stay in ketosis.

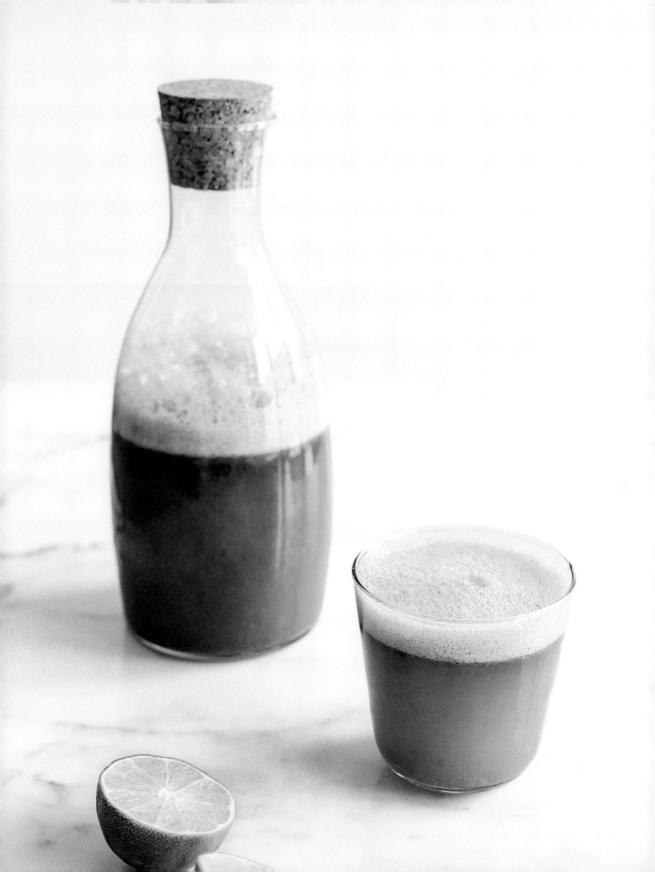

Wild foods have more vitamins, minerals, and antioxidants than foods grown on farms. The USDA has measured the vitamin and mineral content of our meat and vegetables and has found that the content has steadily reduced over time. Learning how to forage for edible wild greens abundant in locations that are not being sprayed with herbicides is a terrific way to get more nutrition. For more about foraging wild greens, see page 186.

DAILY DETOX JUICE WITH WILD GREENS

MAKES 2 SERVINGS
1 serving = 1½ Wahls and Wahls Paleo veg/fruit cups
1 serving = 1 cup Wahls Paleo Plus veg/fruit cup

TO MAKE: Put the ginger in a Vitamix or other high-speed blender and blend until it is finely minced (you can grate it before blending, if you prefer). If the ginger is organic, no need to peel it first. Add the remaining ingredients and blend until liquefied. Add water as needed if you prefer a thinner juice. Store the juice in an airtight container in the refrigerator to best preserve nutrients. Sip the juice throughout the day and finish it within 24 hours.

WAHLS KITCHEN TIP: GINGER AND TURMERIC

I am very fond of fresh ginger and turmeric, but some people are reluctant to use them over their dried, powdered forms, because they think they are more difficult to cook with. Not true! Fresh grated ginger and turmeric root are quite delicious and easy to prepare. If you can find organic ginger and turmeric roots, there is no need to peel them. You can simply grate the root with the fine section of your grater. If they are not organic, just slice off the portion you want, cut off the skin, and mince or grate. If I am adding ginger or turmeric root to a sauce, I mince it and then blend it with the other ingredients in my Vitamix until smooth. When I am sautéing with fresh ginger or turmeric, I find that sautéing the grated root with the vegetables gives my dish a delicious, vibrant taste. Don't be afraid to try it! You may never go back to the powdered stuff.

	WAHLS DIET	WAHLS PALEO	WAHLS PALEO PLUS
FRUIT	1 lime, peeled (you could keep the rind if organic) and seeded (or juiced directly into the Vitamix with a citrus juicer)	1 lime, peeled (you could keep the rind if organic) and seeded (or juiced directly into the Vitamix with a citrus juicer)	2 tablespoons fresh lime juice
	2 Granny Smith apples, cored	1 Granny Smith apple, cored	
GREENS/ VEGETABLES	1 cup any wild greens (dandelion, chicory, purslane, lamb's quarters, grape leaves, etc.)	2 cups any wild greens (dandelion, chicory, purslane, lamb's quarters, grape leaves, etc.)	2 cups any wild greens (dandelion, chicory, purslane, lamb's quarters, grape leaves, etc.)
HERBS, SPICES, AND FLAVORINGS	½ teaspoon ground turmeric	½ teaspoon ground turmeric	½ teaspoon ground turmeric
	1 (¼-inch) piece fresh ginger, chopped or grated	1 (¼-inch) piece fresh ginger, chopped or grated	1 (¼-inch) piece fresh ginger, chopped or grated
	Twist of black pepper	Twist of black pepper	Twist of black pepper
			2 to 4 drops citrus food-grade essential oil, or 1 teaspoon citrus extract
WATER	4 cups	4 cups	4 cups

Note for Wahls Paleo Plus: You can add 1 teaspoon to 2 tablespoons MCT oil as needed to stay in ketosis.

SPRITZERS

Spritzers are a fun way to dilute juice so you don't get the blood-sugar hit you would with straight juice. I mix a little bit of fruit juice with sparkling mineral water for an excellent snack, or even dessert. Try it in a champagne glass if you are feeling festive, instead of a daily happy hour cocktail. Spritzers taste special, even indulgent, but without the ill effects of sugar and/or alcohol. Remember to use only fresh juice. Spritzers are a great way to use up a batch of juice you made in the morning but haven't finished by early evening. Use this template to guide you.

BASIC SPRITZER TEMPLATE

| MAKES 1 SERVING

TO MAKE: Combine all the ingredients in a glass over ice, give it a quick stir, and enjoy immediately.

	WAHLS DIET	WAHLS PALEO	WAHLS PALEO PLUS
FRESH JUICE	¼ cup	1 tablespoon	1 tablespoon vegetable or herb juice, made in a Vitamix or other high-speed blender so the fiber is retained (see page 90), or no more than 1 tablespoon fresh lemon or lime juice (no other fruit juices)
FLAVORINGS (ESSENTIAL OILS)	2 or 3 drops food-grade essential oil, if desired	2 or 3 drops food-grade essential oil, if desired	2 or 3 drops food-grade essential oil, if desired
SPARKLING MINERAL WATER	1 cup	1 cup	1 cup

Note for Wahls Paleo Plus: Since I try to stay in ketosis, I often make my spritzers with nothing but food-grade essential oils. A couple drops of lime, lemon, orange, or grapefruit essential oil in my sparkling mineral water is absolutely delicious. Most important, essential oils are also loaded with polyphenols, which are antioxidants that support our cells' ability to do the chemistry of life more effectively. I highly recommend them, especially as a replacement for fruit in Wahls Paleo Plus beverages. (See page 61 for more on essential oils.)

This spritzer is refreshing at any time of year. Try it when you are overheated in summer (it's a better choice than sugary lemonade), or when you have a cold or virus in the winter.

CITRUS SPRITZER

| MAKES 1 SERVING

TO MAKE: Combine all the ingredients in a glass over ice, give it a quick stir, and enjoy immediately.

	WAHLS DIET	WAHLS PALEO	WAHLS PALEO PLUS
JUICE	¼ cup fresh lime, orange, or grapefruit juice, or a combination	1 tablespoon fresh lime, orange, or grapefruit juice, or a combination	None
FLAVORINGS (ESSENTIAL OILS)	None	1 or 2 drops lime, lemon, or grapefruit food-grade essential oil (optional)	2 or 3 drops lime, lemon, orange, or grapefruit food-grade essential oil
SPARKLING MINERAL WATER	1 cup	1 cup	1 cup

HAPPY HOUR OR TEETOTALER?

I am often asked about whether alcohol can be part of the Wahls Protocol. My answer? Sometimes, depending on the extent of your health issues and how well you tolerate it. While some people do fine occasionally adding a small amount of alcohol to a spritzer or drinking it in another preferred form (that does not include sugar or gluten), others will recover more quickly without it. If you want to maximize your healing, avoid it for now. If you are on a slower course to wellness and you get a lot of enjoyment out of the occasional cocktail, keep it to no more than one or two drinks per week. If you want to learn more about the health benefits of either no or limited alcohol intake, please see *The Wahls Protocol.*

This is a good spritzer for summer, when berries are in season. If you don't already have berry juice on hand, just juice a handful of berries or throw a handful into your Vitamix or other high-speed blender with a little water to make the juice. Try it with strawberries, raspberries, blackberries, blueberries, or a combination. You could also try some of the more nutrient-dense, rarer berries for a boost, like açaí, goji, or aronia berries.

If you grow berries in your yard, they will be even more nutrient-dense than what you can buy at the store. Aronia berries and raspberries are particularly easy to grow and you can freeze them as well. When they are in season, they'll stay fresh for 2 to 4 weeks. Eating more berries has been associated with lower rates of heart disease, strokes, and cognitive decline.

Another option that is even easier than breaking out the juicer or Vitamix is to throw a few berries into your glass, crush them up with a spoon, pour in your sparkling water, then eat them after you drink the water. I especially recommend this for Wahls Paleo Plus because consuming a small amount of whole fruit is a better option than juice for keeping you in ketosis.

BERRY SPRITZER

MAKES 1 SERVING

TO MAKE: Combine all the ingredients in a glass over ice, give it a quick stir, and enjoy immediately.

	WAHLS DIET	WAHLS PALEO	WAHLS PALEO PLUS
JUICE	¼ cup fresh berry juice, any type	2 tablespoons fresh berry juice, any type	1 tablespoon crushed berries, any type (optional)
FLAVORINGS (ESSENTIAL OILS)	None	None	1 to 3 drops berry food-grade essential oil, or ¼ to ½ teaspoon extract if you aren't using berries
SPARKLING MINERAL WATER	1 cup	1 cup	1 cup

THE POWER OF THE LIME

Lime juice is such a simple, easy-to-find ingredient that its healing properties are often overlooked. Yet it is very powerful for anyone working to combat a chronic disease because it increases bile production, which helps to prevent gallstones and makes the body's natural waste elimination system work more efficiently.

Tangy and herbaceous, this alcohol-free cocktail alternative will give any artisanal cocktail a run for its money. Plus, it contains nutrients and will not interfere with your healing, as alcohol could.

I really like using herbs in my spritzers and juices, because unlike other vegetables that have been bred to be sweeter, larger, and heavier, herbs are closer to their natural state and retain a higher level of antioxidants. Plus, adding herbs to your spritzers will give them a lovely zing and unique flavor that I have learned to enjoy very much. This spritzer is best with fresh herbs picked from your own garden or purchased from a farmers' market the same day they were picked.

GREEN HAPPY HOUR SPRITZER

MAKES 2 SERVINGS

Note: This recipe is appropriate for all levels of the Wahls Protocol.

1 tablespoon fresh lime juice

¼ cup fresh garden herbs (such as lemon balm, mint, or parsley)

2 cups sparkling water

TO MAKE: Put the lime juice, herbs, and ¼ cup tap water in a Vitamix or other high-speed blender and blend until smooth. Mix in the sparkling water and divide between two glasses.

Note: **If you want to make just one serving, use half the lime-herb mixture and freeze the rest for the next time you want to have a greener, healthier happy hour.**

This tasty spritzer is great for any time of year, but especially in the winter, when oranges are in season. You can use any kind of oranges—standard navel oranges, or something more exotic, like cara cara or blood oranges.

ORANGE SPRITZER

MAKES 1 SERVING

TO MAKE: Combine all the ingredients in a glass over ice, give it a quick stir, and enjoy immediately.

	WAHLS DIET	WAHLS PALEO	WAHLS PALEO PLUS
JUICE	¼ cup fresh orange juice	¼ cup fresh orange juice	1 tablespoon fresh lemon juice
FLAVORINGS (ESSENTIAL OILS)	1 or 2 drops mint, cinnamon, or orange food-grade essential oil (optional)	1 or 2 drops mint, cinnamon, or orange food-grade essential oil (optional)	1 or 2 drops mint, cinnamon, or orange food-grade essential oil (optional)
SPARKLING MINERAL WATER	1 cup	1 cup	1 cup

Note: If you don't have fresh orange juice on hand, blend 1 chopped orange (with the peel, if organic) with 1 cup water. Measure out the amount required for the recipe and refrigerate the rest to use later.

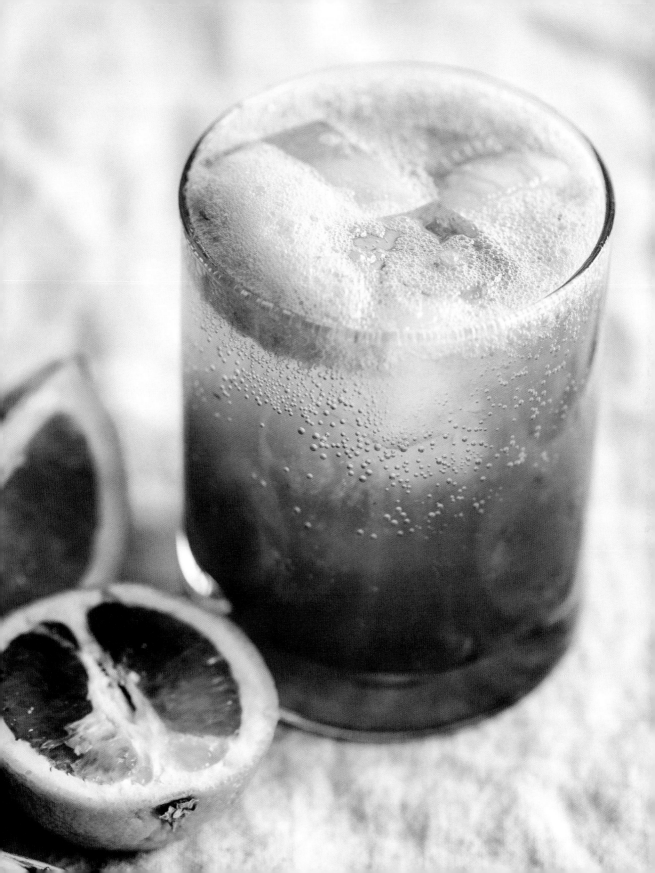

TEAS AND INFUSIONS

Sometimes a hot beverage is just the thing when you need to sip something comforting or calming. Tea, or infusions using other herbs or plants and hot water, fits the bill. Whether you use black tea, green tea, yerba mate (a caffeinated South American shrub whose leaves are used to make a stimulating but nutrient-rich infusion), or dried herbs or other plants, these drinks can be both soothing and medicinal. I recommend buying teas and dried herbs from your local health food market, or using herbs grown in your own garden.

Feel free to experiment with tea, herbs, roots, and leaves, or any combination—just tea, or just herbs, or just roots or leaves. Teas and infusions are highly flexible, so combinations often work beautifully. You can also serve any of the teas in this chapter over ice.

A special feature of my tea and infusion recipes is that you can always use full-fat coconut milk as part of the liquid. This creates a rich, creamy tea that feels extra indulgent but actually benefits your health. Do this especially if you are on Wahls Paleo Plus

BLACK TEA VS. GREEN TEA

Black tea is made from tea that has been oxidized under controlled conditions, which allows it to have a shelf life of several years. Green tea is more fragile and loses flavor by the end of a year. All tea has health-promoting antioxidants, but green tea has more antioxidants than black tea. There is caffeine in both black and green tea, but green tea has significantly less. If black tea makes you jittery, try green tea instead. If even that is too much for you, switch to herbal teas and infusions.

because this can help you get in your daily dose of coconut milk and keep you in ketosis. You don't have to use coconut milk in your tea, of course. Some people prefer their tea plain (but it's delicious with coconut milk!).

Use the following template to infuse your own hot beverages. The template makes two servings (1 serving is 1 cup of liquid). Have two cups if you like, share with someone, or save the second cup for later, covered, in the refrigerator. If you make a tea without any caffeine (caffeinated teas and infusions are marked with an asterisk), you can enjoy a second cup before bed. Other tea recipes in this section make up to four servings, so check the recipe.

Note: All teas and infusions in this chapter are appropriate for all levels of the Wahls Protocol.

WHAT ABOUT COFFEE?

Some people are extremely attached to their morning cup of coffee, and in some cases, that is fine. However, conventional coffee (and tea and cocoa) are grown using a lot of pesticides, which lowers the amount of antioxidants produced by the plant and also introduces that residue into your system, which we are trying to heal, so I much prefer you choose organic, shade-grown coffee for maximum antioxidant impact with minimum pesticide contamination. Also consider how coffee affects you. If it makes you feel wired or jittery, it is best to avoid it. If you feel fine on it, drink up to two cups per day. Full-fat coconut milk makes a tasty creamer. You may do better with yerba mate, which has a higher caffeine content than tea, but less than coffee. It seems to be energizing without the jittery aspect for many of my patients. There are also some interesting herbal "coffees" available, but if you try these, be sure they are gluten-free.

To make a basic tea or infusion, use green or black tea or yerba mate (these options contain caffeine), or fresh or dried herbs, spices, roots, or leaves.

BASIC TEA/INFUSION TEMPLATE

MAKES 2 SERVINGS

TO MAKE: Heat water in a kettle (on the stove or in an electric kettle) until it is boiling rapidly. Take it off the heat. Put about 1 teaspoon loose tea or alternative in a tea infuser and put the infuser in a cup. Pour the hot water over the infuser and steep the tea/infusion for 1 to 10 minutes, depending on how strong you like the flavor. (If you are using matcha [powdered green tea], you don't need an infuser. Just put it in your cup, add the hot water, and stir.) After the tea has steeped, stir in the coconut milk, prewarmed on the stove for a hotter beverage. For a latte-like, creamier beverage, pour the coconut milk and the steeped tea into a Vitamix or other high-speed blender and blend. (Be careful blending hot liquids—start slowly.)

	WAHLS DIET, WAHLS PALEO, AND WAHLS PALEO PLUS
GREEN TEA LEAVES,* MATCHA (GREEN TEA POWDER),* OR YERBA MATE*	1 teaspoon dried tea, or ¼ teaspoon matcha green tea powder
HERBS/SPICES	1 teaspoon
ROOTS/LEAVES	1 teaspoon
FLAVORINGS	As desired
LIQUID	2 cups water, or 1 cup water plus 1 cup canned full-fat coconut milk

*contains caffeine

Note: When using dried roots (such as dandelion root or burdock root) in any tea or infusion, steep them for longer than you would tea or dried herbs—at least 15 minutes will help to draw out more of the beneficial ingredients from dried roots.

This tea may sound unusual, and it is, but it has a savory taste and ingredients that are powerful detoxifiers. The turmeric and black pepper work together in this recipe—black pepper helps your body absorb the healing properties of turmeric. This tea also contains some caffeine, so it is a great way to start the morning, if you need a little jump-start.

DETOXIFYING TURMERIC PEPPER CREAM TEA

MAKES 2 SERVINGS

1 teaspoon green tea* or yerba mate*

½ teaspoon ground turmeric

3 or 4 twists black pepper

1 cup boiling water

1 cup canned full-fat coconut milk

TO MAKE: Steep the green tea or yerba mate, turmeric, and black pepper in the boiled water for 5 minutes, then add the coconut milk. You can warm the coconut milk on the stove first if you want a hotter beverage. For a creamier beverage, pour the coconut milk and the steeped tea into a Vitamix or other high-speed blender and blend.

*contains caffeine

This powerful tea has a detoxifying effect and, because of the ginger, can also help with nausea. The dandelion root or burdock root is optional but particular good for supporting liver function via the stimulation of bile production. (This is why dandelion and burdock roots are often included in commercially available "detox" teas.) Note that this recipe makes four servings. Make a batch and enjoy it in the morning or evening over the next few days. Just reheat or serve over ice.

ROSEMARY GINGER TEA

MAKES 4 SERVINGS

1 teaspoon green tea* or yerba mate*

1 teaspoon fresh rosemary

1 teaspoon dried dandelion root and/or 1 teaspoon dried burdock root

4 cups boiling water

TO MAKE: Steep the green tea, rosemary, and dandelion root and/or burdock root in the boiled water for a full 15 minutes. (Remember that whenever you make a tea from dried roots, you need to allow the tea to steep much longer—in this case, 15 minutes—to obtain all the benefits of the compounds in the dried roots.) This tea will keep in the refrigerator for up to 3 days.

*contains caffeine

WILD GREENS TEA

Most teas contain dried ingredients, but you don't have to dry wild greens to use them in tea. You can infuse fresh chopped greens in hot water for about 15 minutes and enjoy this caffeine-free green infusion without any other addition (I do this often), or you can add chopped wild greens to any other tea for added nutrition and flavor. Try purslane, dandelion leaves (or freshly picked dandelion roots, which are powerful liver detoxifiers), chicory, lamb's quarters, or any other wild green that is safe to eat. If you dry your wild greens in a dehydrator or in the oven (or under the sun) for cold-weather storage, or if you freeze them, they will also work great for tea. Weed your yard, freeze the greens, and enjoy Wild Greens Tea all winter long.

This is a great infusion for the morning. Even though it doesn't contain caffeine, the minty flavor and coconut milk will wake you up in a very pleasant way.

HERBAL RISE-AND-SHINE TEA

MAKES 2 SERVINGS

½ teaspoon dried oregano

½ teaspoon dried mint

1 cup boiling water

1 drop peppermint food-grade essential oil

1 cup canned full-fat coconut milk (at room temperature or warmed)

TO MAKE: Steep the oregano and mint in the boiled water for 5 minutes, then add the peppermint oil and coconut milk. For a frothy beverage, blend the steeped herbs, peppermint oil, and coconut milk in a Vitamix or other high-speed blender on high for up to 2 minutes.

A good digestive drink without any caffeine, Ginger Lemon Infusion has a lovely taste and is quite simple to make. You don't even have to steep it. Ginger has a long history of medicinal use to reduce nausea and improve gastric emptying, so you can use this infusion medicinally when you are having stomach issues.

GINGER LEMON INFUSION

MAKES 2 SERVINGS

1 (¼-inch) piece fresh ginger, peeled and grated

1 teaspoon fresh lemon or lime juice

2 cups boiling water, or 1 cup water and 1 cup canned full-fat coconut milk

TO MAKE: Stir the ginger and lemon or lime juice into the boiled water and enjoy. You can also blend it all in a Vitamix or other high-speed blender with or without the full-fat coconut milk.

Another excellent detoxifying and eye-opening drink, this recipe combines caffeinated yerba mate with the power of marigold, more often called calendula by herbalists. Like other herbs in other recipes in this chapter, calendula stimulates the production of bile. Herbalists also use calendula tea to help prevent the development of gallstones. Sometimes I like this tea made with just water, and sometimes I want the coconut milk version. Try both and see which you prefer.

YERBA MATE WITH CALENDULA

MAKES 2 SERVINGS

1 teaspoon yerba mate*

1 teaspoon dried calendula

Twist of black pepper

1 (¼-inch) piece fresh ginger, peeled and grated (optional)

1 cup boiling water

1 teaspoon fresh lime juice

1 cup canned full-fat coconut milk (at room temperature or warmed)

TO MAKE: Steep the yerba mate, calendula, black pepper, and ginger in the boiled water for 5 to 15 minutes, then stir in the lime juice and coconut milk. For a thicker, frothier drink, blend the tea, juice, and coconut milk in a Vitamix or high-speed blender for up to 2 minutes on high.

*contains caffeine

NOT YOUR GARDEN-VARIETY MARIGOLD

Calendula is made from wild marigold flowers that traditionally grow in the Mediterranean region—not the marigolds you might have in your garden. You can grow *Calendula officinalis,* but be sure you are using the right kind (common garden marigolds are in the genus *Tagetes,* and are the type people often use in the garden for pest control). If you do grow calendula, harvest the flowers (petals only) and dry them in your dehydrator overnight (or out in the sun on a clear, dry day). You can also purchase calendula "tea," which looks like dried yellow flower petals. It has a very mild flavor.

Chamomile tea is a gentle, calming herbal tea with a mild, pleasant flavor. Commonly used to help people relax before bedtime, chamomile is also good whenever you are feeling stressed. Herbalists use chamomile for its anti-inflammatory, antibacterial, and antispasmodic properties, as well as its very mild sedative properties. For this recipe, I like to add coconut milk for a creamier texture. The cardamom and vanilla are optional, but they add a lovely aroma and flavor. On occasion, I'll add a shot of rum to this tea, for a very pleasant nightcap. Note that I've added the option of freshly grated nutmeg—this is quite nice, but you could also use a sprinkle of ground nutmeg or eliminate this completely.

CHAMOMILE AND COCONUT MILK TEA

MAKES 2 SERVINGS

1 chamomile tea bag, or
1 teaspoon loose chamomile tea

1 cardamom pod (optional)

1 cup boiling water

¼ teaspoon vanilla extract

1 cup canned full-fat coconut milk

Freshly grated nutmeg (optional)

TO MAKE: Steep the chamomile tea bag (or loose chamomile tea in an infuser) with the cardamom pod (if using) in the boiled water for 5 minutes, then stir in the vanilla, coconut milk, and nutmeg (if using). For a frothier version, blend the steeped tea with the other ingredients in a Vitamix or other high-speed blender.

Another very simple recipe, this infusion uses dried red clover blossoms. Red clover includes isoflavones, which help stimulate the estrogen beta receptors. (The estrogen beta receptors are in the brain and bones but not in the breast, so clover is not risky for those with breast cancer.) Herbalists use it to help reduce hot flashes and assist with reducing the risk of osteoporosis. In addition, the isoflavones in red clover boost the level of HDL cholesterol (the "good" cholesterol). If red clover grows in your yard or in wild areas and you know it has not been sprayed with pesticides or herbicides, you can harvest it and dry the clover blossoms overnight to make your own tea. There is not as much research on the health benefits of white clover, so if you are doing this for health benefits, stick with red clover blossoms.

RED CLOVER TEA

MAKES 2 SERVINGS

1 teaspoon dried red clover flowers

2 cups boiling water, or 1 cup water and 1 cup canned full-fat coconut milk

TO MAKE: Put the red clover flowers into a tea infuser and steep in the boiled water for 15 minutes. You can also infuse the clover in 1 cup boiling water, then combine it with warmed coconut milk in a Vitamix or other high-speed blender.

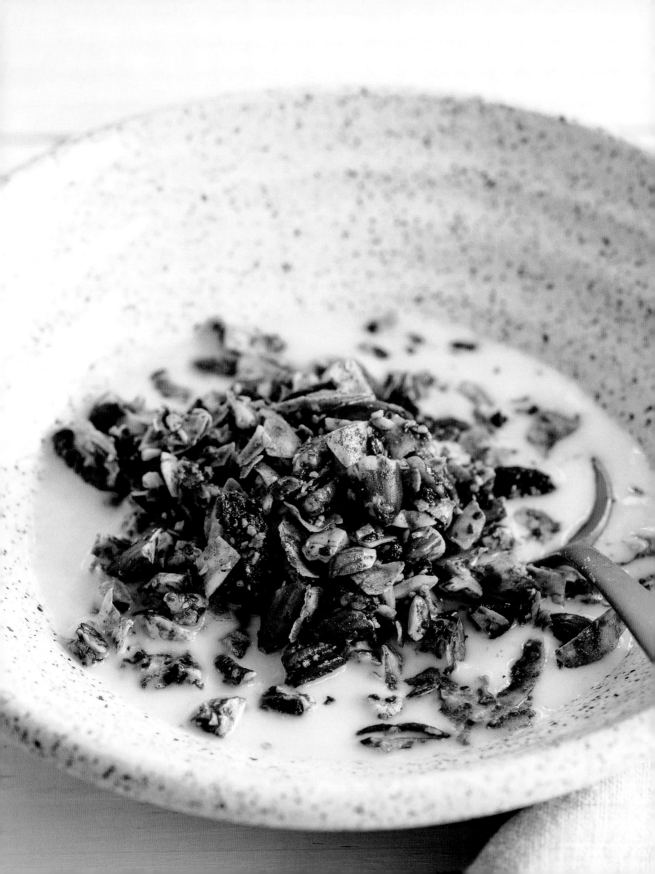

NUTS AND SEEDS: ROASTED, RAW, OR SOAKED?

There are pros and cons to eating nuts and seeds raw versus roasted. Nuts have a lot of healthy monounsaturated and polyunsaturated fats in them. In addition, they are good sources of vitamin E, which protects their natural fats from oxidation. When you eat nuts and seeds raw, you get all the benefit from those fats. Roasting can cause them to oxidize. However, some people prefer the taste of roasted nuts and seeds, and research shows that both roasted and raw nuts improve our cholesterol profiles. If you will only eat them roasted, that is probably better than not eating them at all.

However, the ideal way to eat nuts and seeds is to soak them when they are raw. This initiates the sprouting response and eliminates some of the potentially harmful compounds, like lectins and phytates. Lectins are compounds that increase inflammation in people who are genetically susceptible. Phytates can bind minerals, making them less available to your cells. Roasting reduces the phytates somewhat, but soaking raw nuts and seeds for 2 to 6 hours initiates the germination process, and soaking longer (such as for 12 hours, or overnight) can actually sprout them (even if you do not see little sprouts—they are inside the nut or seed). Sprouting significantly reduces the phytate and lectin content, makes minerals more available, reduces the inflammation risk, and increases the vitamin and enzyme content. Plus, I think soaked or sprouted nuts and seeds are tastier. You can still get that crispy, crunchy texture by drying soaked/sprouted nuts and seeds in a dehydrator or oven after soaking. This is also a prevention against mold, if you don't plan to use them immediately (wet nuts and seeds can become moldy quickly).

You can also make granola out of soaked/sprouted nuts and seeds, and then roast the granola after mixing. If you do this, pat everything dry as well as you can before roasting. Granola made from soaked nuts/seeds will take longer to dry than granola made from unsoaked nuts/seeds, but I think you will find that this method is the tastiest (not to mention the most healthful) way to prepare your granola.

This tasty granola has a warming, spicy quality I think you'll love. It's easy to make and will last you all week unless you decide to share.

CINNAMON ORANGE GRANOLA

MAKES 8 SERVINGS

TO MAKE: Soak the nuts and seeds for at least 2 hours or up to overnight, then drain, rinse, and pat dry. Pulse all or half the nuts and seeds in a food processor or blender. Mix in the remaining ingredients. Dry in a dehydrator or in the oven at the lowest possible temperature, stirring every 15 minutes, for 2 hours or until crisp.

	WAHLS DIET	WAHLS PALEO	WAHLS PALEO PLUS
NUTS AND SEEDS	2½ cups any combination of raw seeds and nuts	2½ cups any combination of raw seeds and nuts	2½ cups any combination of raw seeds and nuts
UNSWEETENED COCONUT FLAKES OR CHIPS	1 cup	1 cup	1 cup
FRUIT	1 medium Granny Smith apple, grated	1 medium Granny Smith apple, grated	½ medium Granny Smith apple, grated
	¼ cup snipped dried apricots (optional)	1 to 2 tablespoons snipped dried apricots (optional)	
FAT	⅓ cup ghee or coconut oil, melted	⅓ cup ghee or coconut oil, melted	⅓ cup ghee or coconut oil, melted
FLAVORINGS	Zest of 1 orange, or ¼ teaspoon orange food-grade essential oil	Zest of 1 orange, or ¼ teaspoon orange food-grade essential oil	Zest of 1 orange, or ¼ teaspoon orange food-grade essential oil
	2 tablespoons ground cinnamon	2 tablespoons ground cinnamon	2 tablespoons ground cinnamon
	¼ teaspoon ground nutmeg	¼ teaspoon ground nutmeg	¼ teaspoon ground nutmeg

Variation: For a stronger spice taste, add any of the following for any level of the plan: ¼ teaspoon ground cloves, ¼ teaspoon ground cardamom, ¼ teaspoon anise seeds.

Not only does this granola have a rich nutty taste, but it will keep you full all morning. It's also good for getting things moving if you are feeling a little bit constipated. You can thank the ground flaxseeds for both the taste and the action. Grind flaxseeds just before you use them for best results. This granola is a good one for anyone who is allergic to tree nuts, because it contains only seeds.

SEEDY FLAX GRANOLA

MAKES 8 SERVINGS

TO MAKE: Soak the seeds *except the flaxseeds* for at least 2 hours or up to overnight, then drain, rinse, and pat them dry. Pulse all or half the soaked seeds in a food processor or blender. Mix together everything except flaxseeds. Dry in a dehydrator or in the oven at the lowest possible temperature, stirring every 15 minutes, for 2 hours or until crisp.

	WAHLS DIET	WAHLS PALEO	WAHLS PALEO PLUS
NUTS AND SEEDS	2 cups any raw seeds (such as a mix of sunflower and pumpkin seeds)	2 cups any raw seeds (such as a mix of sunflower and pumpkin seeds)	2 cups any raw seeds (such as a mix of sunflower and pumpkin seeds)
	½ cup flaxseeds, ground in a blender or spice grinder	½ cup flaxseeds, ground in a blender or spice grinder	½ cup flaxseeds, ground in a blender or spice grinder
UNSWEETENED COCONUT FLAKES OR CHIPS	1 cup	1 cup	1 cup
FRUIT	¼ cup raisins or snipped prunes	1 Granny Smith apple, grated	½ Granny Smith apple, grated
FAT	⅓ cup ghee or coconut oil, melted	⅓ cup ghee or coconut oil, melted	⅓ cup ghee or coconut oil, melted
FLAVORINGS	1 teaspoon ground cinnamon (optional)	1 teaspoon ground cinnamon (optional)	1 teaspoon ground cinnamon (optional)
	¼ teaspoon ground nutmeg (optional)	¼ teaspoon ground nutmeg (optional)	¼ teaspoon ground nutmeg (optional)

Note: **Never roast flaxseeds, or you will oxidize the omega-3 fat. Add after heating.**

Chocolate and coconut for breakfast? I have quite a few clients who will sign up for this delicious combination. Add a teaspoon of cinnamon for a Mexican chocolate variation, or go with an amaretto, orange, or peppermint twist with extracts or essential oils (see the variation).

COCO-NUTTY GRANOLA

| MAKES 8 SERVINGS

TO MAKE: Soak the nuts and seeds for at least 2 hours or up to overnight, then drain, rinse, and pat them dry. Pulse all or half the nuts and seeds in a food processor or blender, depending on how chunky you like your granola. Mix together all the remaining ingredients with the nuts and seeds. Dry in a dehydrator or in the oven at the lowest possible temperature, stirring every 15 minutes or so, for 2 hours or until crisp.

	WAHLS DIET	WAHLS PALEO	WAHLS PALEO PLUS
NUTS AND SEEDS	2½ cups raw almonds and/or raw pecans	2½ cups raw almonds and/or raw pecans	2½ cups raw almonds and/or raw pecans
UNSWEETENED COCONUT FLAKES OR CHIPS	1 cup	1 cup	1 cup
FRUIT	¼ cup raw cacao nibs or dark chocolate chips (at least 70% cacao)	¼ cup raw cacao nibs or dark chocolate chips (at least 70% cacao)	¼ cup raw cacao nibs or dark chocolate chips (at least 70% cacao)
	¼ cup chopped unsweetened dates (optional)	1 to 2 tablespoons chopped unsweetened dates (optional)	
FAT	⅓ cup coconut oil, melted	⅓ cup coconut oil, melted	⅓ cup coconut oil, melted
FLAVORINGS	1 tablespoon unsweetened cocoa powder (not Dutch process)	1 tablespoon unsweetened cocoa powder (not Dutch process)	1 tablespoon unsweetened cocoa powder (not Dutch process)
	1 teaspoon ground cinnamon (optional)	1 teaspoon ground cinnamon (optional)	1 teaspoon ground cinnamon (optional)

Note: Cacao is technically a fruit, so that is why I have included it in the fruit column in this ingredient chart, but raw unsweetened cacao does not contain fruit sugar, so it is fine for Wahls Paleo Plus.

Variation: For all levels, you can add any of the following for a flavor twist: ¼ teaspoon almond extract, ¼ teaspoon orange food-grade essential oil, or ¼ teaspoon peppermint food-grade essential oil.

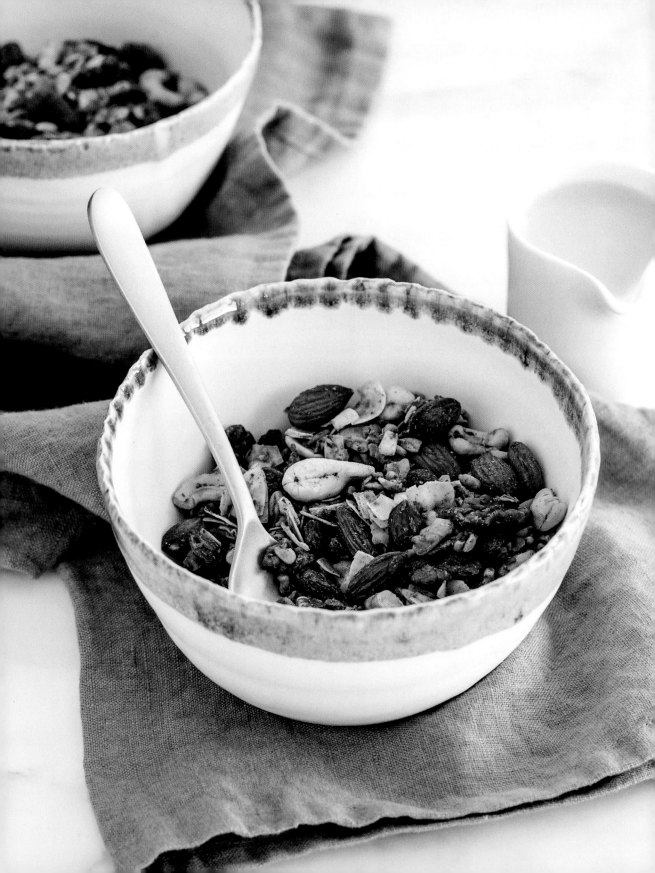

Perfect for a chilly fall morning when you are craving apple pie and cinnamon, this granola is better than any cereal you could buy at the store. You can vary the spices according to your taste, and you can even stir in some pumpkin puree (just not for Wahls Paleo Plus)—much better for you than a pumpkin spice latte! Add raisins or dried cranberries if you'd like.

HARVEST NUT AND SPICE GRANOLA

MAKES 8 SERVINGS

TO MAKE: Soak nuts and seeds for at least 2 hours or up to overnight; drain, rinse, and pat dry. Pulse all or half the nuts and seeds in a food processor or blender. Mix together with all the remaining ingredients. Dry in a dehydrator or in the oven at the lowest possible temperature, stirring every 15 minutes, for 2 hours or until crisp.

	WAHLS DIET	WAHLS PALEO	WAHLS PALEO PLUS
NUTS AND SEEDS	2½ cups any raw nuts and seeds	2½ cups any raw nuts and seeds	2½ cups any raw nuts and seeds
UNSWEETENED COCONUT FLAKES OR CHIPS	1 cup	1 cup	1 cup
FRUIT	1 medium Granny Smith apple, grated	1 medium Granny Smith apple, grated	1 medium Granny Smith apple, grated
	¼ cup dark or golden raisins or dried cranberries (optional)	¼ cup dark or golden raisins or dried cranberries (optional)	
	½ cup pumpkin puree (optional)	¼ cup pumpkin puree (optional)	
FAT	⅓ cup ghee or coconut oil, melted	⅓ cup ghee or coconut oil, melted	⅓ cup ghee or coconut oil, melted
FLAVORINGS	1 tablespoon pumpkin pie spice, or:	1 tablespoon pumpkin pie spice, or:	1 tablespoon pumpkin pie spice, or:
	2 tablespoons ground cinnamon	2 tablespoons ground cinnamon	2 tablespoons ground cinnamon
	¼ teaspoon ground nutmeg	¼ teaspoon ground nutmeg	¼ teaspoon ground nutmeg
	¼ teaspoon ground cloves	¼ teaspoon ground cloves	¼ teaspoon ground cloves
	¼ teaspoon ground cardamom	¼ teaspoon ground cardamom	¼ teaspoon ground cardamom

COOKED MORNING PORRIDGE

Porridge is an excellent breakfast, especially on cold mornings, but just like granola, conventional porridge usually has an oat base. One option is a porridge made with quinoa or brown rice. Most people on the Wahls Diet and Wahls Paleo can enjoy these porridges (though I do not recommend it for those following Wahls Paleo Plus).

But there's also another great way to make a delicious grain-free hot porridge. The secret is combining nuts and seeds with ground flaxseeds and/or chia seeds. Just like oats, which form a soluble fiber–rich paste when cooked, flaxseeds and chia seeds will bind all your ingredients together and leave you feeling full and satisfied.

Use the following template to create your own porridge recipes, or try the recipes on the following pages. Don't feel restricted by the ingredient list—for such a basic meal, there are hundreds of options. These are just a few.

Note: Porridge is best made fresh, so these recipes make 1 serving. You can easily double, triple, or quadruple the recipes to make enough servings for friends and family, too.

SUGAR ON THAT PORRIDGE?

"What sweetener can I have?" This is one of the most common questions I receive, especially when it comes to breakfast. People want to put brown sugar or maple syrup on their oatmeal, in their smoothies, or to sweeten their granolas. This is because our brains are programmed to like sweet flavors. Food companies know this and use sugars and artificial sugars to create sweet flavors to drive up consumption of their products. However, all added sugars are associated with health problems, which is why I limit added sweetener—whether that is sugar, honey, maple syrup, coconut sugar, or any other sweetening product—to no more than 1 teaspoon per day. Artificial sweeteners shift the gut microbiome and are associated with higher rates of fatty liver, heart disease, and diabetes, so I don't recommend those at all (including processed stevia extract—stevia leaves picked from a plant you grow yourself are fine).

Instead, my advice to patients is to stop the sweeteners altogether. This will create changes in your gut microbiome, and you will eventually stop craving that sweet taste. Use spices with a little heat and natural sweetness, such as cinnamon and cardamom. They make food taste sweeter without giving your brain that hit of sugar. It will take two weeks to two months to get past the sugar craving, but it will happen. The longer you abstain, the easier it gets, and you will find you'll be able to taste the natural sweetness in whole foods. Whole fruit will begin to satisfy your sweet craving, and you will be on your way to a healthier you.

For some people with stubborn and resistant sugar cravings, it is better to give up all sugar, including fruit, in order to get over sugar cravings. Typically, the cravings will steadily diminish after two weeks and will be mostly gone after two months. Then you can decide whether to reintroduce fruit and sweeteners. If you do, have no more than 2 or 3 servings of fruit per day, and no more than 1 teaspoon of any natural sweetener, such as honey, maple syrup, or coconut sugar. If you are following Wahls Paleo Plus, do not have any added sweetener at all, and eat no more than ¼ to ½ cup berries each day.

BASIC PORRIDGE TEMPLATE

MAKES 1 SERVING

TO MAKE: Blend all the dry ingredients (except the toppings) in a Vitamix or other high-speed blender until chopped to the texture you like. Heat the liquid on the stove until it is steaming, then turn off the heat. Stir in the dry ingredients, wait 5 minutes, and then top with your favorite chopped nuts or seeds or a few fresh berries.

	WAHLS DIET	WAHLS PALEO	WAHLS PALEO PLUS
FLAXSEEDS, CHIA SEEDS, OR GLUTEN-FREE GRAIN	¼ cup	¼ cup	¼ cup
HOT LIQUID (WATER, UNSWEETENED PLANT MILK, OR FULL-FAT COCONUT MILK)	1 cup	1 cup	1 cup
NUTS, SEEDS, AND/OR FRUITS	1 cup	1 cup	1 cup nuts or seeds only
FAT	Up to 1 tablespoon melted coconut oil or MCT oil	Up to 1 tablespoon melted coconut oil or MCT oil	2 tablespoons melted coconut oil or MCT oil
FLAVORINGS/ TOPPINGS	As desired	As desired	As desired, except no fruit or sweetener other than fresh berries

Note for Wahls Paleo Plus: Not everyone on Wahls Paleo Plus can stay in ketosis after eating porridge, even when it is nut-based. But for some, the occasional warm bowl of porridge works just fine. If you do choose to try porridge, note that the template and the recipes in this chapter always include more fat for your level of the diet. This will help keep you in ketosis.

Hemp hearts are rich in protein and essential fatty acids and add a pleasant nutty flavor to this nutritious porridge.

HEMP HEART PORRIDGE

MAKES 1 SERVING

TO MAKE: Blend all the dry ingredients (except the toppings) in a Vitamix or other high-speed blender until chopped to the texture you like. Heat the liquid on the stove until it is steaming, then turn off the heat. Stir in the dry ingredients, wait 5 minutes, and then top with the hemp hearts.

	WAHLS DIET, WAHLS PALEO	WAHLS PALEO PLUS
FLAXSEEDS, CHIA SEEDS, OR GLUTEN-FREE GRAIN	¼ cup freshly ground flaxseeds or chia seeds	¼ cup freshly ground flaxseeds or chia seeds
HOT LIQUID	1 cup steaming-hot boxed nut milk or canned full-fat coconut milk	1 cup steaming-hot boxed nut milk or canned full-fat coconut milk
NUTS, SEEDS, AND/OR FRUITS	1 small Granny Smith apple, cored and finely chopped (optional)	1 small Granny Smith apple, cored and finely chopped (optional)
FAT	1 tablespoon any nut or seed butter	2 tablespoons melted coconut oil or MCT oil
FLAVORINGS	1 teaspoon ground cinnamon	1 teaspoon ground cinnamon
	¼ teaspoon ground nutmeg	¼ teaspoon ground nutmeg
	⅛ teaspoon ground cloves	⅛ teaspoon ground cloves
TOPPINGS	2 tablespoons hemp hearts	2 tablespoons hemp hearts

If you love and miss those tasty "everything bagels," this porridge can fill that gap in your life.

EVERYTHING PORRIDGE

| MAKES 1 SERVING

TO MAKE: Chop all the dry ingredients (except the toppings) in a Vitamix or other high-speed blender. Heat the liquid on the stove until it is steaming, then turn off the heat. Stir in the dry ingredients, wait 5 minutes, and then add the toppings.

	WAHLS DIET	WAHLS PALEO	WAHLS PALEO PLUS
FLAXSEEDS, CHIA SEEDS, OR GLUTEN-FREE GRAIN	¼ cup freshly ground flaxseeds	¼ cup freshly ground flaxseeds	¼ cup freshly ground flaxseeds
HOT LIQUID	1 cup steaming-hot boxed or homemade nut milk or canned full-fat coconut milk	1 cup steaming-hot boxed or homemade nut milk or canned full-fat coconut milk	1 cup steaming-hot boxed or homemade nut milk or canned full-fat coconut milk
NUTS, SEEDS, AND/OR FRUITS	1 teaspoon chia seeds	1 teaspoon sesame seeds	1 teaspoon sesame seeds
	1 small Granny Smith apple, cored and chopped	1 teaspoon poppy seeds	1 teaspoon poppy seeds
		1 teaspoon chia seeds	1 teaspoon chia seeds
		1 small Granny Smith apple, cored and chopped	
FAT	None	None	2 tablespoons melted coconut oil or MCT oil
FLAVORINGS	¼ teaspoon ground cardamom	¼ teaspoon ground cardamom	¼ teaspoon ground cardamom
TOPPINGS	1 teaspoon sesame seeds	1 teaspoon sesame seeds	1 teaspoon sesame seeds
	1 teaspoon poppy seeds	1 teaspoon poppy seeds	1 teaspoon poppy seeds
	1 tablespoon coarsely chopped walnuts	1 tablespoon coarsely chopped walnuts	1 tablespoon coarsely chopped walnuts
	1 tablespoon dark or golden raisins		

Variation: For Wahls Paleo, add up to 1 tablespoon dark or golden raisins, but no more than once or twice a week. For Wahls Paleo Plus, you can add up to ¼ cup berries, but then limit your fruit intake for the rest of the day.

I am very fond of almonds, so I love sprinkling them on this porridge, but you can use any combination of chopped nuts as a topping. This rich and tasty porridge will keep you full for hours.

COCONUT ALMOND PORRIDGE

MAKES 1 SERVING

TO MAKE: Blend all the dry ingredients (except the toppings) in a Vitamix or other high-speed blender until they are chopped to the texture you like. Heat the liquid on the stove until it is steaming, then turn off the heat. Stir in the dry ingredients, wait 5 minutes, and then add the toppings.

	WAHLS DIET, WAHLS PALEO	WAHLS PALEO PLUS
FLAXSEEDS, CHIA SEEDS, OR GLUTEN-FREE GRAIN	¼ cup chia seeds or freshly ground flaxseeds	¼ cup chia seeds or freshly ground flaxseeds
HOT LIQUID	1 cup steaming-hot canned full-fat coconut milk	1 cup steaming-hot canned full-fat coconut milk
NUTS, SEEDS, AND/OR FRUITS	1 pitted date	1 small Granny Smith apple, cored and coarsely chopped
FAT	1 tablespoon almond butter	1 tablespoon almond butter
		2 tablespoons melted coconut oil or MCT oil
FLAVORINGS	1 teaspoon ground cinnamon	1 teaspoon ground cinnamon
	¼ teaspoon ground cardamom	¼ teaspoon ground cardamom
TOPPINGS	2 tablespoons unsweetened coconut flakes or chips	2 tablespoons unsweetened coconut flakes or chips
	1 tablespoon chopped or sliced almonds	1 tablespoon chopped or sliced almonds

I like this porridge during the summer, when peaches are at their peak ripeness. You can also use fresh nectarines or apricots in this recipe.

SUNNY PEACH PORRIDGE

MAKES 1 SERVING
1 serving = 1 Wahls and Wahls Paleo veg/fruit cup

TO MAKE: Combine all the ingredients (except the toppings) in a Vitamix or other high-speed blender and blend until smooth. Transfer to a small saucepan and heat on the stovetop, if desired. Top with more plant or coconut milk if you like, and sprinkle on the toppings.

	WAHLS DIET	WAHLS PALEO	WAHLS PALEO PLUS
FLAXSEEDS, CHIA SEEDS, OR GLUTEN-FREE GRAIN	¼ cup freshly ground flaxseeds or chia seeds	¼ cup freshly ground flaxseeds or chia seeds	¼ cup freshly ground flaxseeds or chia seeds
HOT LIQUID	1 cup steaming-hot boxed or homemade nut milk	1 cup steaming-hot boxed or homemade nut milk	1 cup steaming-hot canned coconut milk or homemade nut milk
NUTS, SEEDS, AND/OR FRUITS	1 ripe peach or nectarine, or 2 ripe apricots, pitted and coarsely chopped	1 ripe peach or nectarine, or 2 ripe apricots, pitted and coarsely chopped	None
FAT	1 tablespoon melted ghee or almond butter	1 tablespoon melted ghee or almond butter	2 tablespoons coconut oil or MCT oil
FLAVORINGS	1 sliver fresh ginger, minced	1 sliver fresh ginger, minced	1 sliver fresh ginger, minced
	¼ teaspoon vanilla extract	¼ teaspoon vanilla extract	¼ teaspoon vanilla extract
			¼ teaspoon peach extract
TOPPINGS	1 tablespoon unsweetened coconut flakes or chips, lightly toasted in a skillet	1 tablespoon unsweetened coconut flakes or chips, lightly toasted in a skillet	1 tablespoon unsweetened coconut flakes or chips, lightly toasted in a skillet

Note for Wahls Paleo Plus: Peaches are not appropriate for your level of the plan. Use a peach extract for a peach flavor.

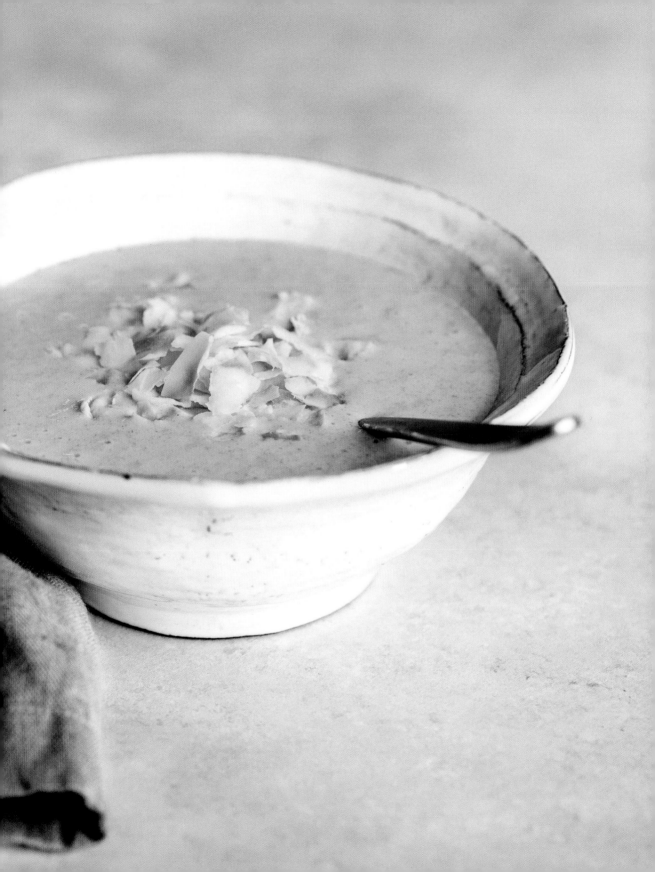

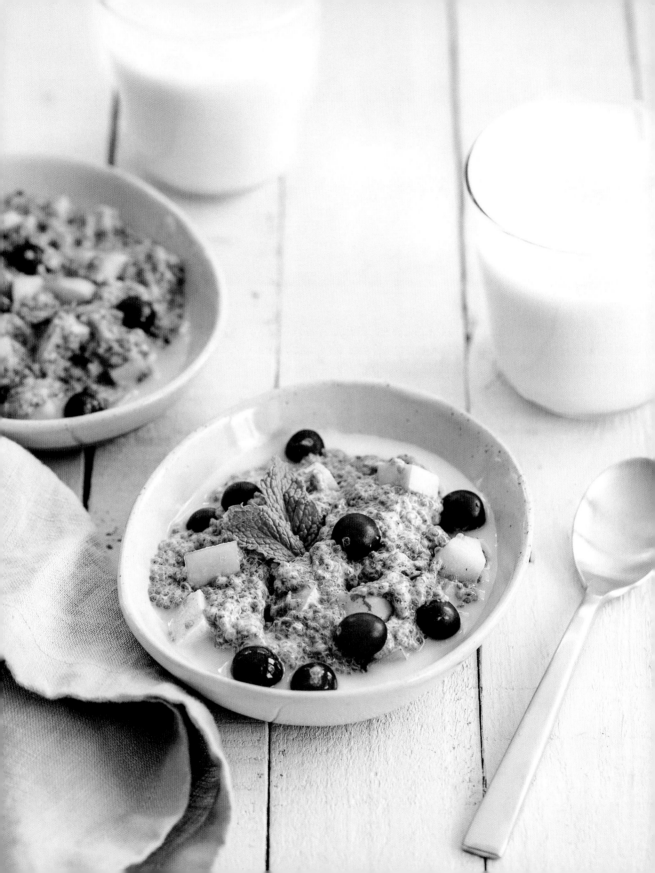

This porridge has a holiday hue and is a good breakfast for winter, when fresh cranberries hit the stores. The cinnamon gives it a wintry flavor as well. It is also rich in soluble fiber and vitamin C.

CHIA-ALMOND PORRIDGE WITH CRANBERRIES

| MAKES 1 SERVING

TO MAKE: Heat the nut milk or coconut milk until steaming. Transfer to a bowl, add the remaining ingredients (except the toppings), and mix by hand until smooth. Pour into bowls and let sit for 5 minutes. Top with more plant or coconut milk if you like, and sprinkle on the toppings.

	WAHLS DIET	WAHLS PALEO	WAHLS PALEO PLUS
FLAXSEEDS, CHIA SEEDS, OR GLUTEN-FREE GRAIN	¼ cup chia seeds	¼ cup chia seeds	¼ cup chia seeds
HOT LIQUID	1 cup steaming-hot boxed or homemade nut milk	1 cup steaming-hot boxed or homemade nut milk	1 cup steaming-hot canned full-fat coconut milk
NUTS, SEEDS, AND/OR FRUITS	¼ cup fresh or thawed frozen cranberries	¼ cup fresh or thawed frozen cranberries	¼ cup fresh or thawed frozen cranberries
	1 small Granny Smith apple, cored and coarsely chopped	1 small Granny Smith apple, cored and coarsely chopped	
FAT	1 tablespoon almond butter	1 tablespoon almond butter	1 tablespoon almond butter
			2 tablespoons melted coconut oil or MCT oil
FLAVORINGS	½ teaspoon ground cinnamon	½ teaspoon ground cinnamon	½ teaspoon ground cinnamon
TOPPINGS	1 tablespoon sliced almonds	1 tablespoon sliced almonds	1 tablespoon sliced almonds
	Fresh mint or basil leaf, for garnish	Fresh mint or basil leaf, for garnish	Fresh mint or basil leaf, for garnish

This porridge has a sunny golden color and is the only porridge recipe in this chapter made with grain—sort of. Quinoa is an ancient seed, not a true grain, from South America with a high protein content, which makes it popular with vegetarians. It is grainlike, however, so if you are trying to stay in ketosis, you may not be able to consume it.

GOLDEN QUINOA PORRIDGE

MAKES 1 SERVING

TO MAKE: Soak the quinoa in water to cover for 2 to 6 hours or up to overnight, then drain and rinse. Combine all the ingredients (except the toppings) in a small saucepan and simmer over medium heat until the quinoa is soft, about 15 minutes if unsoaked, about 5 minutes if soaked. Top with more coconut milk if you like, and sprinkle on the toppings. (Wahls Paleo Plus, see page 150 for your directions.)

	WAHLS DIET	WAHLS PALEO	WAHLS PALEO PLUS
FLAXSEEDS, CHIA SEEDS, OR GLUTEN-FREE GRAIN	¼ cup quinoa	¼ cup quinoa	¼ cup freshly ground golden flaxseeds
HOT LIQUID	1 cup canned full-fat coconut milk	1 cup canned full-fat coconut milk	1 cup canned full-fat coconut milk
NUTS, SEEDS, AND/OR FRUITS	2 tablespoons unsweetened coconut flakes or chips	2 tablespoons unsweetened coconut flakes or chips	2 tablespoons unsweetened coconut flakes or chips
FAT	1 tablespoon almond butter	1 tablespoon almond butter	1 tablespoon almond butter
			2 tablespoons melted coconut oil or MCT oil
FLAVORINGS	½ teaspoon ground cinnamon	½ teaspoon ground cinnamon	½ teaspoon ground cinnamon
	Pinch of saffron, or ¼ teaspoon ground turmeric	Pinch of saffron, or ¼ teaspoon ground turmeric	Pinch of saffron, or ¼ teaspoon ground turmeric
TOPPINGS	1 tablespoon chopped walnuts	1 tablespoon chopped walnuts	1 tablespoon chopped walnuts
	¼ cup golden raisins or white or golden raspberries	¼ cup golden raisins or white or golden raspberries	¼ cup white or golden raspberries (optional)

RECIPE CONTINUES

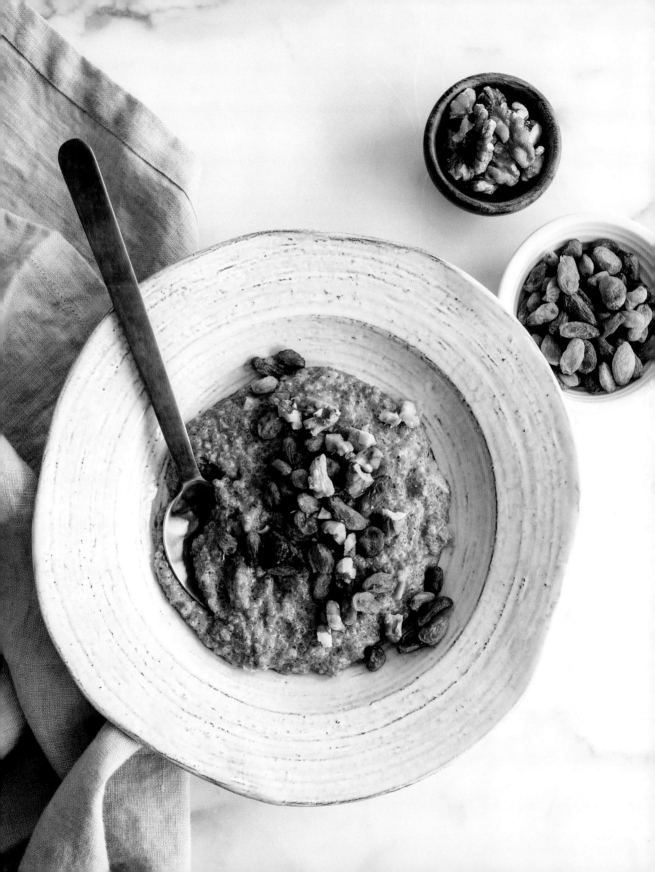

Note for Wahls Paleo Plus: Your instructions for this recipe are slightly different because quinoa is not an acceptable food for your level of the diet. Instead, substitute ground golden flaxseeds for the quinoa. Instead of soaking, grind the flaxseeds and blend them with the other ingredients by hand or in a blender on low speed, along with heated coconut milk. The flax will thicken into porridge and still be quite good without the quinoa.

Variation: If you are on the Wahls Diet, you could substitute any gluten-free grain, such as millet, buckwheat, amaranth, wild rice, brown rice, or even cornmeal, for the quinoa in this recipe. However, I do recommend that you use only organic gluten-free grains so that there is no pesticide or herbicide residue in your breakfast. Note that this option is only safe for the Wahls Diet level and for only very occasional use on Wahls Paleo, and that it must be cooked on the stove, not just mixed or blended.

WAHLS WARRIORS SPEAK

I am thankful for life because of you, Dr. Wahls. I learned how to truly appreciate life after struggling with pain for eight years. Your diet has given me back my health for the last three years, and because of you, I was able to spend the day snow-sledding with my daughter. I am inspired to tell the whole world that the Wahls Paleo diet really works!

—Wahls Warrior BETH

This hearty porridge is filling and sweet (it is also grain-free and nut-free). Use raisins in this recipe if you are following the Wahls Diet or Wahls Paleo, and use berries if you are following Wahls Paleo Plus.

FLAX RAISIN OR BERRY PORRIDGE

| MAKES 1 SERVING

TO MAKE: Heat the nut milk or coconut milk until steaming. Transfer to a blender, add the remaining ingredients (except the toppings), and blend on low speed until smooth. (Alternatively, mix all the ingredients in a bowl by hand until smooth.) Pour into bowls and let sit for 5 minutes. Top with more plant or coconut milk if you like, and sprinkle on the toppings.

	WAHLS DIET	WAHLS PALEO	WAHLS PALEO PLUS
FLAXSEEDS, CHIA SEEDS, OR GLUTEN-FREE GRAIN	¼ cup freshly ground flaxseeds	¼ cup freshly ground flaxseeds	¼ cup freshly ground flaxseeds
HOT LIQUID	1 cup steaming-hot boxed or homemade nut milk	1 cup steaming-hot boxed or homemade nut milk	1 cup steaming-hot canned full-fat coconut milk
NUTS, SEEDS, AND/OR FRUITS	2 tablespoons unsweetened coconut flakes or chips	2 tablespoons unsweetened coconut flakes or chips	2 tablespoons unsweetened coconut flakes or chips
			¼ cup fresh blueberries or any other fresh berry
			2 tablespoons pumpkin or sunflower seeds
FAT	1 tablespoon melted coconut oil or ghee	1 tablespoon melted coconut oil or ghee	2 tablespoons melted coconut oil or MCT oil
FLAVORINGS	½ teaspoon ground cinnamon	½ teaspoon ground cinnamon	½ teaspoon ground cinnamon
TOPPINGS	¼ cup raisins	2 tablespoons raisins	1 tablespoon pumpkin or sunflower seeds
	1 tablespoon pumpkin or sunflower seeds (optional)	1 tablespoon pumpkin or sunflower seeds (optional)	

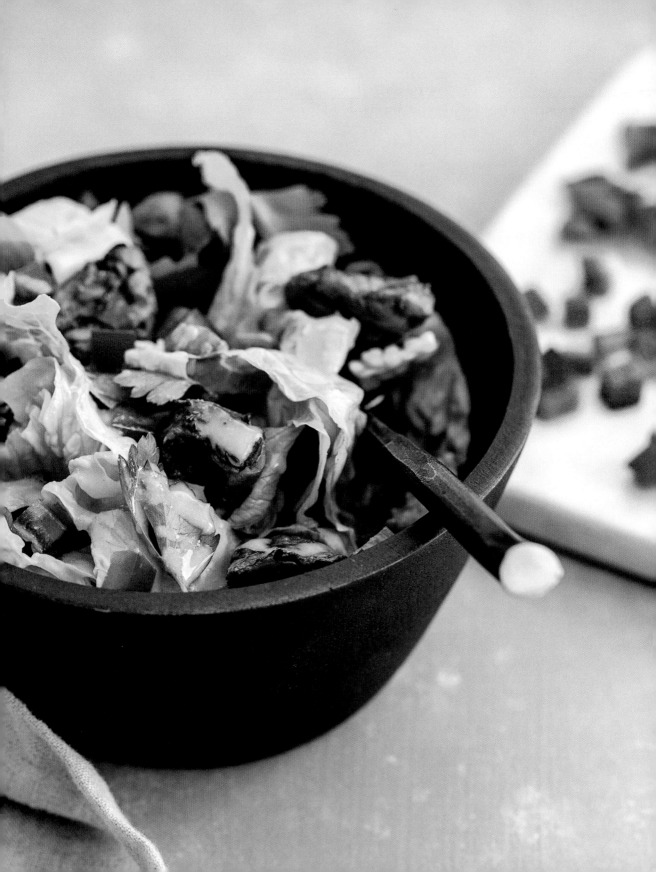

MAIN COURSE SALADS, SIDE SALADS, AND WRAPS

SALADS ARE THE EASIEST WAY TO GET MORE FIBER to feed the health-promoting bacteria in your gut and meet your Wahls Protocol daily dose of leafy greens, sulfur-rich vegetables, and brightly colored vegetables and fruits. Most salads prominently feature greens, and there are many reasons to get a lot of greens in your diet: Greens are a rich source of magnesium, calcium, antioxidants, and vitamin K, and they also provide key nutrients that your retinas and the lenses in your eyes need. Studies have shown that daily consumption of leafy greens lowers your risk of developing cataracts and macular degeneration. If you are worried about a family history of these eye diseases, eat your greens. Lots of them.

I often make a huge salad with some meat for a meal, or enjoy a side salad along with a main course meat dish (such as one of my skillet recipes—see chapter 8). Salads are also economical because you can use up whatever greens, vegetables, and meats you have left over to make them. The taste combinations are endless, and I encourage you to experiment and vary your salad ingredients often. Remember that the more you vary your diet, the more micronutrients you will take in to feed your cells.

Personally, I love to pick greens and other vegetables from my garden and eat them within the hour. Salads are one of the best reasons to garden! I also like foraging, and some of my patients have made foraging a hobby. There are many delicious greens available in lawns, or growing as weeds in gardens, abandoned city lots, and in other wild areas. As long as you know they haven't been sprayed with pesticides or other chemicals, I recommend including foraged greens in your salads whenever you can. (The Wild Salad recipe on page 184 is specifically designed to celebrate foraged greens, and I will give you more information about foraging later in this chapter.)

LEAFY GREENS AND KIDNEY STONES

If your medical team has recommended a specific dietary plan to reduce the risk of recurrent kidney stones, you may think you can't enjoy leafy greens. However, there are different types of kidney stones, and each one requires a specific type of diet to reduce the risk of reoccurrence. Work with your physician and a nutrition professional to customize your greens and learn what is safe for you. This website contains more information to help you select greens that are low in oxalates, if that is an issue for you: http://lowoxalateinfo.com/guide-to-low-oxalate-greens.

Salad dressing not only makes salads richer and more interesting, it also adds fat, which significantly increases your body's ability to absorb and use the nutrients in raw vegetables. However, not all fats are appropriate for healing. Stick with cold-pressed extra-virgin olive oil, which you can also flavor with sesame or cold-pressed nut oils. Other industrially produced oils that are not cold-pressed tend to be inflammatory, and I strongly advise against them.

For acids, use a high-quality apple cider vinegar or wine vinegar, or any fresh citrus juice.

BASIC SALAD DRESSING TEMPLATE

MAKES 6 SERVINGS
Note: These salad dressings are appropriate for all levels of the Wahls Protocol.

TO MAKE: Put all the ingredients in a glass jar or bottle and shake to combine, or whisk all the ingredients together in a bowl until well combined. Shake or whisk again before each use. Dressings without creamy or vegetable ingredients will keep at room temperature for up to 1 week. Dressings containing coconut milk, nut or seed butters, or any vegetable ingredients will keep in the refrigerator for up to 5 days.

	WAHLS DIET, WAHLS PALEO, AND WAHLS PALEO PLUS
COLD-PRESSED EXTRA-VIRGIN OLIVE OIL	6 tablespoons
ACIDS (VINEGAR OR CITRUS JUICE)	2 tablespoons
OPTIONAL THICKENERS (COCONUT MILK, NUT BUTTER, EGG-FREE MAYONNAISE, OR AVOCADO, TO MAKE A CREAMY DRESSING)	Up to ½ cup
FLAVORINGS (HERBS, SPICES, NUT OR SEED OILS, ETC.)	Up to 2 tablespoons

MIXED GREENS SALAD DRESSING

MAKES 6 SERVINGS

¼ cup extra-virgin olive oil

2 tablespoons flaxseed oil

2 tablespoons fresh lemon or lime juice

2 tablespoons tahini (sesame butter)

1 tablespoon coconut aminos

1 tablespoon nutritional yeast

TO MAKE: Put all the ingredients in a glass jar or bottle and shake to combine, or whisk all the ingredients together in a bowl until well combined. Shake or whisk again before each use. Store in the refrigerator for up to 5 days.

SIMPLE OLIVE LEMON VINAIGRETTE

MAKES 6 SERVINGS

6 tablespoons extra-virgin olive oil

2 tablespoons fresh lemon juice or apple cider vinegar

½ teaspoon sea salt

Freshly ground black pepper

TO MAKE: Put all the ingredients in a glass jar or bottle and shake to combine, or whisk all the ingredients together in a bowl until well combined. Shake or whisk again before each use. Store at room temperature for up to 1 week.

BALSAMIC VINAIGRETTE

MAKES 6 SERVINGS

6 tablespoons extra-virgin olive oil

2 tablespoons balsamic vinegar

1 teaspoon minced garlic

½ teaspoon sea salt

Freshly ground black pepper

TO MAKE: Put all the ingredients in a glass jar or bottle and shake to combine, or whisk all the ingredients together in a bowl until well combined. Shake or whisk again before each use. Store in the refrigerator for up to 5 days.

WAHLS RANCH-STYLE DRESSING

MAKES 8 SERVINGS

3 tablespoons extra-virgin olive oil

3 tablespoons hemp oil (or use all extra-virgin olive oil)

2 tablespoons fresh lemon juice or apple cider vinegar

½ cup canned full-fat coconut milk

¼ cup egg-free mayonnaise (such as Vegenaise)

2 teaspoons dried dill (or 2 tablespoons fresh)

2 garlic cloves, minced

1 teaspoon garlic powder

1 teaspoon dried mustard/mustard powder (I prefer dehydrated Dijon mustard powder, which you can find online)

½ teaspoon sea salt

½ teaspoon onion powder

⅛ teaspoon freshly ground black pepper

TO MAKE: Put all the ingredients in a glass jar or bottle and shake to combine, or whisk all the ingredients together in a bowl until well combined. Shake or whisk again before each use. Store in the refrigerator for up to 5 days.

Variation: **Add 2 teaspoons poppy seeds.**

WAHLS ITALIAN DRESSING

| MAKES 6 SERVINGS

¼ cup extra-virgin olive oil

2 tablespoons flaxseed oil or hemp oil

2 tablespoons apple cider vinegar

1 teaspoon minced garlic

1 teaspoon fresh or dried oregano

½ teaspoon fresh or dried thyme

½ teaspoon sea salt

Freshly ground black pepper

TO MAKE: Put all the ingredients in a glass jar or bottle and shake to combine, or whisk all the ingredients together in a bowl until well combined. Shake or whisk again before each use. Store in the refrigerator for up to 5 days.

Note: You can use 2 teaspoons of premixed Italian seasoning instead of the garlic, oregano, and thyme. If your Italian seasoning contains salt and pepper, omit those as well.

WAHLS CAESAR-STYLE DRESSING

| MAKES 8 SERVINGS

½ cup egg-free mayonnaise (such as Vegenaise)

5 garlic cloves, minced

3 tablespoons extra-virgin olive oil

2 tablespoons fresh lemon juice

1½ tablespoons Dijon mustard

½ teaspoon sea salt

½ teaspoon freshly ground black pepper

TO MAKE: Put all the ingredients in a glass jar or bottle and shake to combine, or whisk all the ingredients together in a bowl until well combined. Shake or whisk again before each use. Store in the refrigerator for up to 5 days.

Variation: You can add minced anchovy fillets or anchovy paste for a more authentic Caesar taste, or add 1 teaspoon nutritional yeast for a cheesier taste.

I have been a Wahls Warrior for two years, and I go back and forth between Wahls Paleo and Wahls Paleo Plus. I was diagnosed with multiple sclerosis and Lyme disease ten years ago. I tried two different MS drugs and eight years of antibiotics on and off for Lyme disease. I had constant symptoms and was miserable. Two years ago I saw Dr. Wahls's TED Talk and I changed my diet and lifestyle. I lost one hundred pounds and got my life back! I had eighteen months with no symptoms. I recently got an accidental bite of gluten in a restaurant and that caused my first flare in almost two years. I am recovering and feeling great. Three years ago, I could not read a book and remember what it said; this year, I am back in school to become an NTP (nutritional therapy practitioner) and I just started training with Dr. Wahls to become a Wahls Certified Coach. I am so grateful for Dr. Wahls and her diet. My husband and children are also very happy to have their wife and mother back! This is a recipe for what I call "My Sauce," from my blog, *realfoodinspiredme* (https://choosehealthntp.com).

MY SAUCE

1 cup apple cider vinegar

½ cup coconut aminos

2 garlic cloves, or more to taste

1 cup extra-virgin olive oil or avocado oil

1 cup tahini (sesame butter)

Juice of 1 lemon

1 tablespoon honey

1 teaspoon Himalayan salt

3 tablespoons parsley (fresh is best, but dried works)

To make: Put the apple cider vinegar, coconut aminos, garlic, and 1 cup water in a Vitamix or other high-speed blender. Blend until the garlic is pureed. Add the oil, tahini, lemon, honey, salt, and parsley; blend and serve. This fills two 16-ounce jars plus enough for a salad or two right away. I am always working on new variations of "My Sauce" and I will share them in the future. Try adding dill to make it taste like ranch, or a bit of hot sauce to get the fires burning!

—Wahls Warrior BETH (and family)

MAIN COURSE SALADS

Meet the main course salad. A hearty and filling meal can be as simple as a big bowl of leafy greens with added vegetables, a portion of meat, and a savory dressing to tie it all together.

Use this template to create your own salads out of the leftover meat you have on hand (whenever I cook meat, I always like to make some extra for this purpose), some greens, and any other vegetables you have in your refrigerator (or in your garden). Drizzle with dressing, and you've got an amazing lunch or dinner. In fact, all a main course salad needs to be is meat with salad greens. Throw in some garden herbs, an extra-virgin olive oil–flaxseed oil blend, and some apple cider vinegar and lemon or lime juice (at about a 3:1 ratio). Season with sea salt and freshly ground black pepper. It's as simple as that.

And don't feel like you need to stick to tiny salad bowls for these main course salads. A great big bowl, even a mixing bowl, is a fine serving vessel, and the high sides make it better than a plate for tossing. The recipes in this chapter make one serving, but you can easily double, triple, or quadruple them to serve family or friends. Just toss everything together in a big bowl, then distribute into individual serving bowls. Top with the protein last, after you toss the greens and vegetables with the dressing. Garnish with fresh herbs, if you have them.

Use this template to invent your own main course salads. The possibilities are endless! You can double, triple, or quadruple this recipe to serve more people.

BASIC MAIN COURSE SALAD TEMPLATE

MAKES 1 SERVING
1 serving = 4 Wahls and Wahls Paleo veg/fruit cups
1 serving = 3 Wahls Paleo Plus veg/fruit cups

TO MAKE: Put the greens and vegetables in a large bowl and drizzle with the dressing. Toss to coat. Arrange your meat, poultry, or seafood on top. Garnish with toppings as desired.

	WAHLS DIET	WAHLS PALEO	WAHLS PALEO PLUS
GREENS	3 cups	3 cups	3 cups
OTHER VEGETABLES AND FRUITS	1 cup	1 cup	1 cup vegetables only
DRESSING	2 tablespoons	2 tablespoons	2 tablespoons
ANIMAL PROTEIN	3 to 4 ounces	3 to 4 ounces	3 to 4 ounces
GARNISHES (FRESH HERBS, NUTS, SEEDS, ETC.)	1 to 2 tablespoons	1 to 2 tablespoons	1 to 2 tablespoons

Note for Wahls Paleo Plus: **You may add up to ½ cup berries to a main course salad, but don't have any other fruit during the day.**

This elegant salad is easy to throw together with canned smoked oysters, which you should be able to find in most grocery stores (look near the canned tuna). (See photo on page 152.)

SMOKED OYSTER SALAD

MAKES 1 SERVING
1 serving = 4 Wahls veg/fruit cups

3 cups chopped romaine lettuce or other sturdy lettuce

1 cup thinly sliced red bell pepper

1 tablespoon extra-virgin olive oil

1 tablespoon fresh lime juice

Sea salt and freshly ground black pepper

3 to 4 ounces canned smoked oysters

2 tablespoons chopped fresh herbs (such as flat-leaf parsley, thyme, basil, and/or rosemary)

TO MAKE: Put the lettuce and bell pepper in a large bowl and drizzle with the olive oil and lime juice. Season with sea salt and black pepper. Toss to coat. Arrange the oysters on top and garnish with chopped fresh herbs.

This delicious Mexican-inspired salad has a surprise twist: halibut! It's a fresh, lighter salad that satisfies a craving for Mexican flavors without the heaviness. This is a warm salad, so prepare the halibut and sautéed vegetables fresh.

FAJITA HALIBUT SALAD

MAKES 1 SERVING
1 serving = 4 Wahls veg/fruit cups

1 tablespoon ghee, plus more as needed

3 to 4 ounces halibut

½ cup thinly sliced white onion (cut into rings)

½ cup thinly sliced bell pepper or mildly spicy pepper (such as Anaheim or poblano)

½ teaspoon ground cumin

½ teaspoon chili powder

½ teaspoon sea salt

½ teaspoon freshly ground black pepper

3 cups chopped mixed greens

2 tablespoons Wahls Ranch-Style Dressing (page 157) or other Wahls-appropriate dressing

2 tablespoons Wahls Guacamole (page 48)

2 tablespoons Fresh Salsa (page 45)

Chopped fresh cilantro leaves

Lime wedge

TO MAKE: Heat the ghee in a skillet. Add the halibut and sauté until it easily flakes with a fork. Transfer the fish to a plate. Add the onion, bell pepper, cumin, chili powder, sea salt, black pepper, and ¼ cup water to the pan and sauté until the onions are translucent and the bell peppers are tender, about 15 minutes. (Add more ghee if necessary.)

Put the greens in a large bowl and drizzle with the dressing. Toss to coat. Arrange the halibut on top, breaking it into bite-size pieces or leaving it whole. Top with the guacamole, salsa, and cilantro, and serve with a wedge of lime to squeeze over the salad.

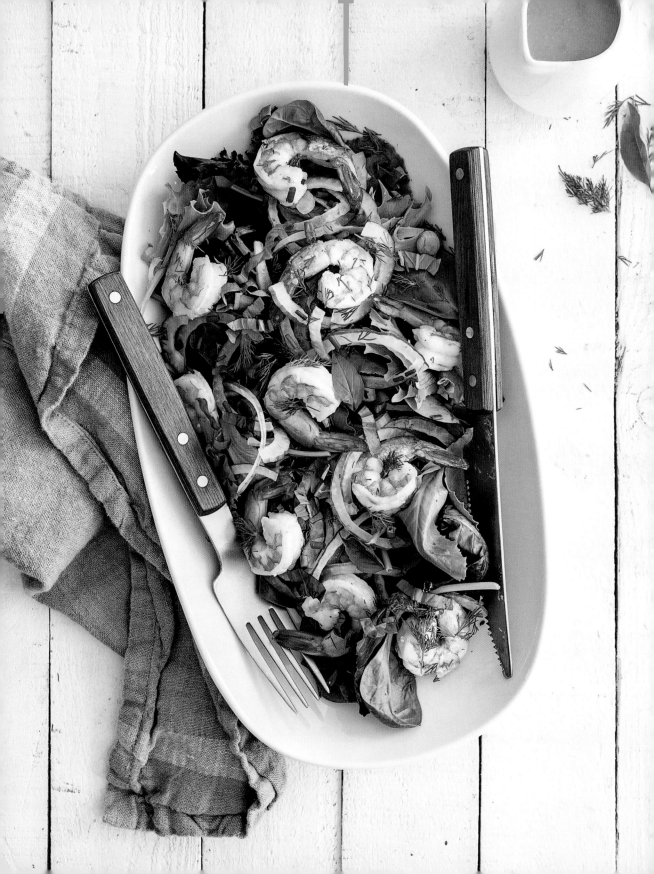

You can use leftover shrimp (or scallops) for this salad, or just buy wild-caught precooked frozen shrimp, rinse them until they have thawed, and use those. You could also quickly sauté the shrimp first in a little coconut oil, if you prefer a warm salad.

SPRING HERB SALAD WITH SHRIMP, ONIONS, AND CHIVES

MAKES 1 SERVING
1 serving = 3 Wahls veg/fruit cups

3 cups spring greens or a mix of greens and fresh herbs

2 tablespoons Mixed Greens Salad Dressing (page 156) or other Wahls-appropriate dressing

3 to 4 ounces cooked shrimp

1 tablespoon thinly sliced fresh basil

1 tablespoon fresh tarragon, dill, parsley, cilantro, or other fresh herbs

TO MAKE: Put the greens in a large bowl and drizzle with the dressing. Toss to coat. Arrange the shrimp on top and garnish with the basil and other fresh herbs of your choice.

This salad also features a potato that is still a novelty to many people: purple potatoes! Purple potatoes make this otherwise basic chicken salad unique and beautiful. If you can't find purple potatoes, you can substitute heirloom red or blue potatoes, or sweet potatoes or yams. All options are delicious.

GRILLED CHICKEN AND PURPLE POTATO SALAD

MAKES 1 SERVING
1 serving = 4 Wahls veg/fruit cups

TO MAKE: Put the greens and vegetables in a large bowl and drizzle with the dressing. Toss to coat. Arrange the grilled chicken on top and garnish with the toppings as desired.

	WAHLS DIET AND WAHLS PALEO	WAHLS PALEO PLUS
GREENS	3 cups mixed greens	3 cups mixed greens
OTHER VEGETABLES AND FRUITS	½ cup bite-size pieces cooked purple potatoes	½ cup bite-size pieces leftover cooked cauliflower stems and/or boiled turnips
	¼ cup thinly sliced red onion	¼ cup thinly sliced red onion
	¼ cup thinly sliced radishes	¼ cup thinly sliced radishes
DRESSING	2 tablespoons Wahls Italian Dressing (page 158) or any other Wahls-appropriate freshly made dressing	2 tablespoons Wahls Italian Dressing (page 158) or any other Wahls-appropriate freshly made dressing
ANIMAL PROTEIN	3 to 4 ounces cooked chicken, sliced	3 to 4 ounces cooked chicken, sliced
GARNISHES	A few sprigs fresh parsley or cilantro	A few sprigs fresh parsley or cilantro

Note: I often make this salad with leftover grilled chicken, but you could also make the chicken fresh before assembling the salad, if you are up for that. Just marinate the chicken in ½ cup apple cider vinegar, 1 tablespoon sea salt, and any fresh herbs you have on hand for a few hours, then grill or broil it until just cooked through, with no pink left in the middle. Slice it for the salad.

Note for Wahls Paleo Plus: Potatoes are too starchy for this level of the diet. Substitute boiled turnips or cauliflower stems in place of the potatoes for a similar texture and satisfying taste.

POTATOES AND RESISTANT STARCH

White and yellow potatoes are generally too high in starch for me, especially since I mostly follow Wahls Paleo Plus. However, I have learned that when you boil a potato and eat it cold the next day with coconut oil, it has a greatly increased resistant starch content. This means that the starch in the potato is more resistant to digestion—it passes right through you, without having such a large impact on blood sugar, and moves on down to your colon, where it becomes food for your good gut bacteria. Likewise, if you gently boil other root vegetables and tubers, then let them cool and eat them cold, they are much less likely to spike your blood sugar. I like to mix cold, boiled potatoes in a salad along with onions and garlic. Delicious!

If you are following Wahls Paleo Plus, keep in mind that we all have a unique tolerance for how many carbohydrates we can eat and remain in ketosis. Some of you will be able to have ½ cup of the cold potato salad made with potatoes or yams and remain in ketosis. Some will find that this takes you out of ketosis. If that happens, try making the potato salad with boiled turnips. If that doesn't work, use boiled chopped cauliflower stem. Pay attention to how you respond. For me, I can still occasionally add a small amount of cold boiled potato, yam, or turnip to my salads and stay in ketosis.

This salad is a good one for using up leftover grilled chicken, or you can grill or broil it and slice it before serving.

ARUGULA CHICKEN SALAD WITH BERRIES AND LEMON

MAKES 1 SERVING
1 serving = 3 Wahls veg/fruit cups

3 cups arugula

½ cup fresh berries

2 tablespoons Simple Olive Lemon Vinaigrette (page 156) or other Wahls-appropriate dressing

3 to 4 ounces grilled chicken, sliced

1 tablespoon sunflower or pumpkin seeds

TO MAKE: Combine the arugula and berries. Drizzle with the dressing and toss to coat. Arrange the grilled chicken on top, then sprinkle with the sunflower or pumpkin seeds.

This is another salad in which I often use leftover chicken. However, you can prepare the chicken for this salad first by sautéing it in 1 tablespoon coconut oil and then adding 1 tablespoon minced garlic just as the chicken is beginning to brown. Cut the chicken into bite-size pieces for this salad, and add any garlic left in the pan. If your chicken was not prepared with garlic, add 1 tablespoon minced garlic to the asparagus before cooking.

GARLIC CHICKEN SALAD

MAKES 1 SERVING
1 serving = 4 Wahls veg/fruit cups

3 cups chopped romaine lettuce

1 cup chopped steamed, sautéed, or grilled asparagus

½ cup thinly sliced red onion

2 tablespoons Simple Olive Lemon Vinaigrette (page 156) or other Wahls-appropriate dressing

3 to 4 ounces cooked chicken, cut into bite-size pieces

Fresh parsley, cilantro, or other fresh herbs, for garnish (optional)

TO MAKE: Put the lettuce, asparagus, and onion in a large bowl. Drizzle with the dressing. Toss to coat. Arrange the chicken on top. Garnish with fresh herbs, if desired.

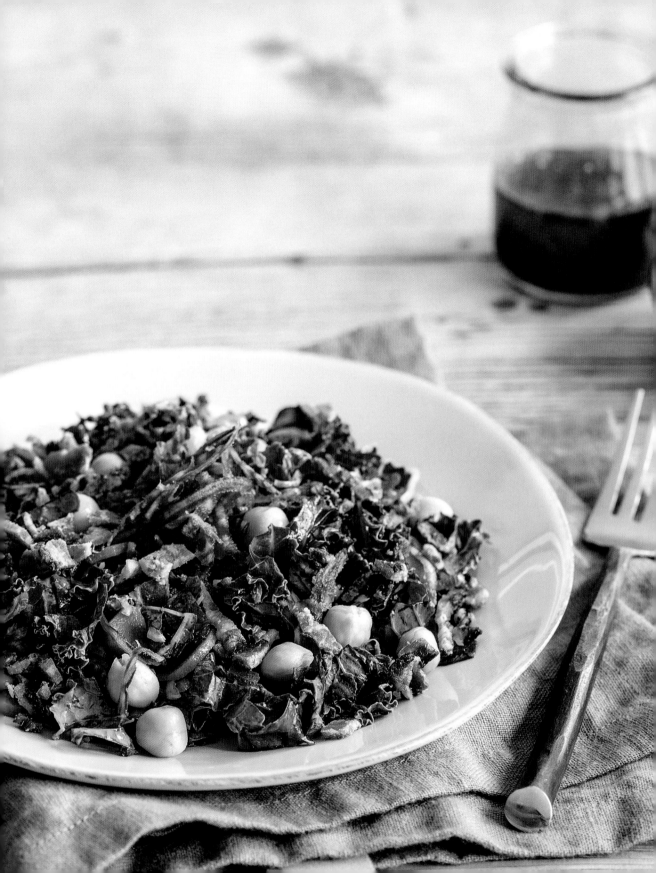

An extremely hearty and filling warm salad with Brussels sprouts, beets, kale, and smoky, salty bacon! Look for nitrate-free bacon, preferably from a local processor. (This is easy to find in Iowa, where I live, but there are more and more brands producing high-quality nitrate-free bacon, so it is more widely available than ever before.)

BACON SALAD

MAKES 1 SERVING
1 serving = 4 Wahls veg/fruit cups

1 bunch curly or lacinato kale

1 or 2 bacon slices

½ cup thinly sliced Brussels sprouts

½ cup grated or sliced raw carrots

2 tablespoons Balsamic Vinaigrette (page 157)

¼ cup grated raw beets

TO MAKE: Cut the kale leaves from the thick stems and save the stems for another use. Roll up the leaves and thinly slice them crosswise. Steam them using a steamer basket and a sauce pan, or cook in a skillet with 1 tablespoon of water, and set them aside to cool. Alternatively, you can massage them with ¼ cup apple cider vinegar or lime juice and then let them sit for 30 minutes to an hour. (Both steaming and massaging with acid reduce the natural bitterness in kale.) This should yield approximately 3 cups of chopped kale leaves.

Meanwhile, cook 1 or 2 slices of bacon on low for 10 to 12 minutes until desired level of crispness. Remove the bacon from the pan, and drain on paper towels. Add the Brussels sprouts and carrots to the bacon grease and cook for 3 to 5 minutes or until tender. Put the kale into a large bowl and drizzle with the dressing. Add the Brussels sprouts–carrot mixture and beets. Toss everything to coat. Crumble the bacon over the top of the salad.

Variation: For a meatier salad, you can add ½ cup cubed ham or Canadian bacon to the cooked vegetable mixture in the last minute of cooking, just to warm it up.

Variation for Wahls Diet and Wahls Paleo: Add 2 tablespoons cooked or canned rinsed chickpeas to this salad.

In my opinion, cubed avocados make an excellent upgrade from the boring croutons in a classic Caesar salad. To make this salad even more interesting, if you haven't put anchovies in your Wahls Caesar-Style Dressing, consider adding these little fishes directly to this salad.

WAHLS CHICKEN CAESAR SALAD

MAKES 1 SERVING
1 serving = 3½ Wahls veg/fruit cups

3 cups chopped romaine lettuce

½ cup cubed avocado

2 tablespoons Wahls Caesar-Style Dressing (page 158)

3 to 4 ounces cooked chicken, sliced or cut into bite-size pieces

2 tablespoons Rawmesan (page 42)

TO MAKE: Combine the lettuce and avocado. Drizzle with the dressing and toss to coat. Arrange the chicken on top. Garnish with the Rawmesan.

This salad is an excellent way to use up leftover cooked salmon, and it would also work with other firm-fleshed fish.

POACHED (OR GRILLED) SALMON SALAD

MAKES 1 SERVING
1 serving = 4 Wahls veg/fruit cups

3 cups mixed greens

½ cup chopped cucumber

½ cup finely chopped celery

¼ cup scallions (white and green parts)

2 tablespoons Simple Olive Lemon Vinaigrette (page 156)

3 to 4 ounces cooked salmon

2 tablespoons chopped fresh dill

1 tablespoon capers

1 teaspoon fresh thyme

Squeeze of fresh lemon or lime juice

TO MAKE: Toss together the greens, cucumber, celery, and scallions in a large bowl. Drizzle with the dressing and toss to coat. Arrange the salmon on top. Garnish with the dill, capers, thyme, and lemon or lime juice.

Variation: You could also add good-quality olives to this salad, for a Mediterranean twist.

This salad tastes very gourmet because of the duck, which is an excellent and underutilized animal protein. I make this salad whenever I have leftover roasted duck. The preparation is simple!

WILTED KALE AND DUCK SALAD WITH BEETS, WALNUTS, AND SOFT CHEEZ

MAKES 1 SERVING
1 serving = 3½ Wahls veg/fruit cups

3 cups chopped kale leaves

2 tablespoons Wahls Italian Dressing (page 158)

3 to 4 ounces cooked duck, sliced

½ cup grated raw beet

1 tablespoon raw walnuts

1 tablespoon Soft Cheez (page 43)

TO MAKE: Wilt the kale by steaming for 2 minutes, or massaging vigorously with a tablespoon of apple cider vinegar or citrus juice and letting it sit for about 30 minutes to an hour, to tenderize (both steaming and massaging with acid reduce the natural bitterness in kale).

Put the wilted kale on a plate. Drizzle with the dressing, and toss to coat. Top with the duck. Arrange the beets, walnuts, and Soft Cheez (in dabs) over the top.

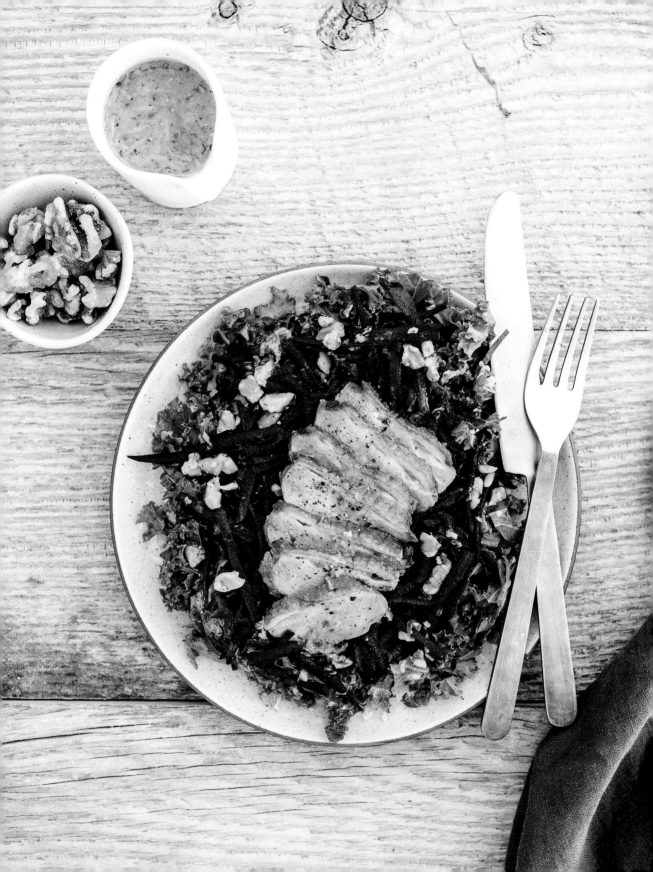

SIDE SALADS

Just about any dinner can benefit from more vegetables, and a side salad is the perfect way to boost your veggie intake. Side salads are simple to compose with whatever vegetables (and fruits) you have left over. They don't even need to contain greens, although most of them do. Just throw some veggies together in a bowl with some homemade dressing, and feel fuller after dinner. You don't really need a template for a side salad, but if you feel better using one, the one on the following page works great.

Note: Some of the Side Salad recipes in this chapter serve one, but can be easily multiplied for more people.

Use this template to create your own salads. Don't be afraid to try new and novel greens, vegetables, and herbs. The more you vary your vegetables, the more diverse your nutrient intake.

BASIC SIDE SALAD TEMPLATE

MAKES 1 SERVING

TO MAKE: Put the greens and vegetables in a large bowl and drizzle with the dressing. Toss to coat and garnish with toppings as desired.

	WAHLS DIET	WAHLS PALEO	WAHLS PALEO PLUS
GREENS	Up to 3 cups	Up to 3 cups	Up to 3 cups
OTHER VEGETABLES, HERBS, FRUITS	Up to 2 cups	Up to 2 cups	1 cup, no fruit
DRESSING	2 tablespoons	2 tablespoons	2 tablespoons
GARNISHES (FRESH HERBS, NUTS, SEEDS, ETC.)	1 to 2 tablespoons	1 to 2 tablespoons	1 to 2 tablespoons

Variation for Wahls Paleo Plus: You can add ½ cup berries to a side salad, but don't have any other fruit during the day.

This simple salad is special because it includes a tasty homemade pesto.

LIGHT ALMOND TOMATO SALAD

MAKES 1 SERVING
1 serving = 3 Wahls veg/fruit cups (if using only half of the pesto)

2 cups tender greens (fresh oregano, basil, baby kale, or a combination)

1 cup extra-virgin olive oil

⅓ cup vinegar or fresh lime juice

4 garlic cloves

1 tablespoon almond butter, or 2 tablespoons shelled pumpkin seeds or other seed/nut of your choice

½ teaspoon sea salt

2 medium tomatoes, sliced

1 to 2 tablespoons slivered or sliced almonds

TO MAKE: Put the greens, olive oil, vinegar, garlic, almond butter, and salt in a Vitamix or other high-speed blender and blend until smooth.

Arrange the tomatoes on a plate. Drizzle with half the pesto and sprinkle with the almonds.

Note: You will only need half the pesto in this pesto recipe for this particular salad, so store the remaining pesto in an airtight container in the refrigerator for up to 3 days and use it as a sauce over meat or as a dip for vegetables.

Peppery arugula is a nice foil for mild cucumbers and bell peppers. The Simple Olive Lemon Vinaigrette tastes great on this easy side salad. This makes enough for a big family.

ARUGULA SALAD WITH FRESH LEMON VINAIGRETTE

MAKES 6 SERVINGS
1 serving = ¾ Wahls veg/fruit cup

3 cups arugula

1 cup chopped cucumber

½ cup chopped bell pepper

2 tablespoons Simple Olive Lemon Vinaigrette (page 156)

2 tablespoons chopped scallions (white and green parts), for garnish

TO MAKE: Combine all the ingredients except the scallions in a bowl and toss to coat. Garnish with the scallions.

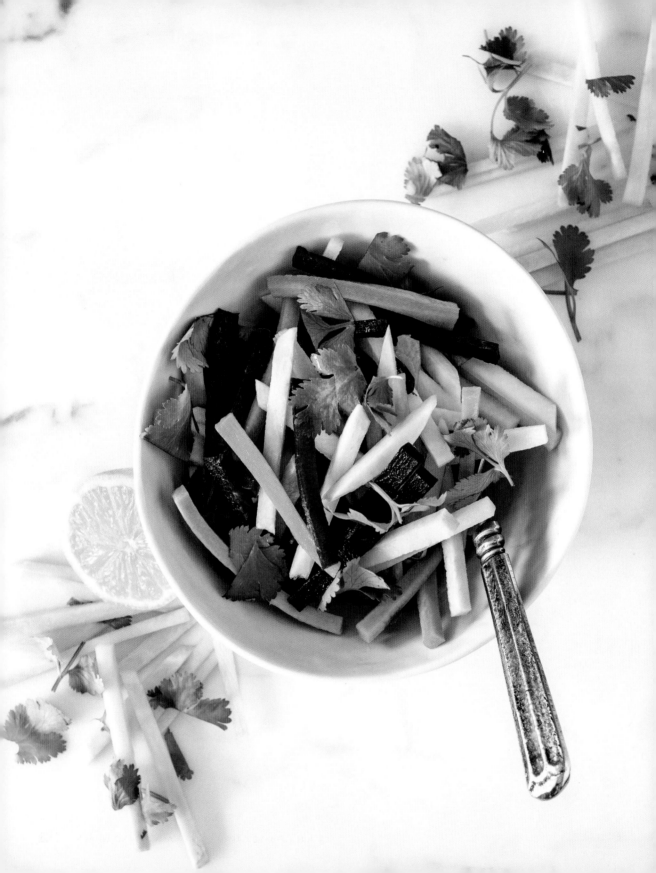

This recipe is a great dish to bring to a picnic, barbecue, or potluck, or to serve a lot of guests. The only challenge in making this beautiful, colorful salad is that you need to chill each of the vegetables separately in ice water. This keeps the beets from leaching their color into the salad and turning the whole thing red. If you have a matchstick slicing blade for your food processor, cutting the vegetables is a breeze!

BEET, CARROT, AND RUTABAGA MATCHSTICK SALAD WITH FRESH CILANTRO

MAKES 8 SERVINGS
1 serving = ½ Wahls veg/fruit cup

1 medium beet (peeling optional), cut into matchsticks

1 large or 2 medium carrots, cut into matchsticks

1 medium rutabaga, peeled and cut into matchsticks

½ cup Simple Olive Lemon Vinaigrette (page 156), or more as desired

½ cup chopped fresh cilantro leaves

½ cup chopped fresh flat-leaf parsley leaves

TO MAKE: Put each vegetable in its own bowl of ice water and let them sit for about 1 hour. Drain and rinse, then combine the vegetables in a large bowl with the dressing. Top with the cilantro and parsley and serve.

The cucumber and orange in this salad make it refreshing, but the avocado and Wahls Ranch-Style Dressing give it a rich taste, too. This salad has it all!

WATERCRESS CUCUMBER SALAD WITH AVOCADO AND ORANGE SLICES

MAKES 6 SERVINGS
1 serving = 1 Wahls veg/fruit cup

3 cups watercress

1 cup thinly sliced cucumber

¼ cup Wahls Ranch-Style Dressing (page 157), or more as desired

1 avocado, pitted, peeled, and sliced

1 orange, sliced

TO MAKE: Toss the watercress and cucumber with the dressing, then arrange the avocado and orange slices decoratively on top.

Note for Wahls Paleo Plus: Omit the orange. You could substitute 1 cup berries, but then limit any other fruit for the day.

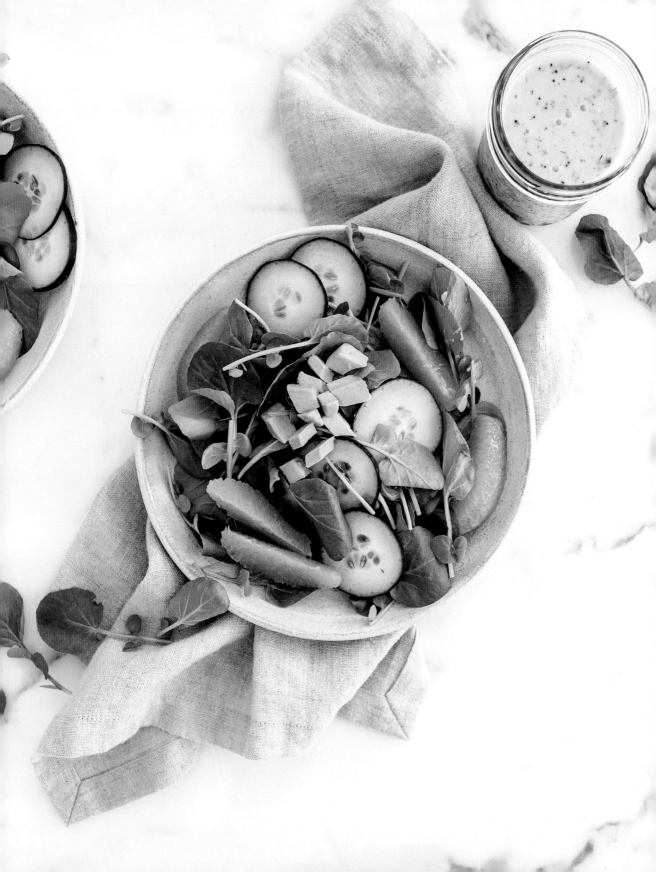

Wild Salad is probably the most nutrient-dense salad in this book, simply because wild greens and other plants tend to have a much higher nutrient and antioxidant content than any cultivated vegetables. You can add whatever you want to your Wild Salad. If you can't find the quantity of wild greens called for, supplement with spring mix, baby kale, arugula, watercress, or a combination. I like Wahls Italian Dressing (page 158) with my Wild Salad because it holds up to the more robust taste of wild greens.

WILD SALAD

MAKES 6 SERVINGS
1 serving = 2 Wahls veg/fruit cups

About 12 cups wild greens, rinsed well and dried

Thinly sliced fresh vegetables (such as cucumbers, radishes, carrots, and celery)

¼ cup dressing of your choice

TO MAKE: Toss together the greens and vegetables. Add the dressing and toss to coat.

WAHLS WARRIORS SPEAK

At fourteen, my daughter Romy was a great student and mature for her age, but by the end of eighth grade, she had begun to struggle in math and her grades had begun to fall. I hired a tutor, but she suddenly seemed unable to absorb the concepts and put them into practice. Then at the end of the summer, I noticed that Romy's right eye was not moving in conjunction with her left when she looked to the left. I videotaped this unusual phenomenon and set up a series of appointments, starting with an optometrist, then an ophthalmologist, and finally a neurologist. By the time we were able to see the doctors, her eye had corrected itself, but because I had videotaped it, the neurologist admitted Romy to the Hospital for Sick Children in Toronto. One week and a battery of tests later, the team of specialists informed the family that Romy had eight lesions on her brain and one located on her cervical spine. The diagnosis was shattering: multiple sclerosis. We were told that the condition would progress, and that there was no cure. The hospital team handed me pamphlets from the MS Society and a list of available drugs to choose from. We were sent home with instructions to return for a follow-up after having made a decision about which drug we would like to start with.

Backtrack two years, while I was on my own journey healing from IBS. I had spent a week in Austin, Texas, at a Paleo conference, where I heard Dr. Terry Wahls speak about her own healing path from progressive MS mostly by adopting a nourishing, plant-based Paleo diet. I was deeply impressed with her healing story and I remember feeling compelled to go up, meet her, and have her autograph my Paleo Toronto T-shirt. Little did I know that two years later, my own teenage daughter would be diagnosed with the very same disorder!

Both Romy and I knew we didn't want to experiment with the MS drugs suggested by the neurologist. We studied the research on the drugs offered and believed that not only would those medications not heal the multiple sclerosis, but they might even exacerbate the condition. Even so, we were riddled with fear that we might be making the wrong decision. Fear is dangerous, and we had to deal with that first. I was afraid for Romy to take the drugs, and afraid of what would happen if she didn't.

For support, we turned to the Wahls website community and a functional medicine nutritionist, with whom I had already been working. Both were instrumental in putting our fears to rest. We recognized that any decisions we made involved risks, so we decided to risk the natural healing path—instead of the greater risks of the potentially ineffective prescription medications and their likely side effects.

I believe that every disease can be reversed, and that the starting point must always be to find and fix the root causes. So we began to hunt for root causes, and discovered that Romy's blood work showed some interesting things: two strains of the Epstein-Barr virus, herpes, cytomegalovirus, strep A and B, and high levels of mercury and aluminum. Any of these infections, or the high levels of heavy metals, or a combination, might have served as the primary triggers for the multiple sclerosis. Additionally, our nutritionist found that Romy had a leaky gut, was not absorbing B vitamins, had very low stomach acid, and had a congested liver—the list seemed to go on and on.

The day after Romy arrived home from the hospital with her new diagnosis, we started her on the Wahls Protocol. The transition from her prior diet was fairly easy. I made a food pyramid based on the Wahls Protocol, highlighted all of Romy's favorite foods, and put the list on the fridge. Romy has dedicated herself completely to the protocol and has even become a good cook!

Romy said to me recently, "Mom, MS is the best thing that has ever happened to me. Just look at the way we eat, how well I am sleeping, and how we changed things in our house to make everything healthier. We are better off now!" When asked if she suffers from MS, Romy now replies, "No, MS suffers from me!" I think what she means is that she is making it very hard for MS to exist in her life or in her body!

According to the Hospital for Sick Children in Toronto, the average age of MS symptom onset is fifteen, but the average diagnosis doesn't happen until people are in their thirties. We were fortunate enough to catch the first symptoms with her optic nerve, so I figure we are at least fifteen years ahead of the game in healing!

—Wahls Warriors SHANNON AND ROMY
(adapted from Shannon's blog, www.healingisfreedom.com)

FORAGING FOR EDIBLE WEEDS
AND WILD PLANTS

My clinical practice is within the veterans' administration medical center where I teach therapeutic lifestyle classes. This means that the majority of the men and women I see have limited financial resources. Often, however, they are open to gardening, hunting, fishing and/or foraging for food. It's a fun hobby that gets my patients outdoors and learning new things, so I'm all for it. Foraging is something potentially anyone can do. In the wild places that have not been sprayed with pesticides and herbicides, there are many plants with edible and delicious greens for your salads. You may also be able to find many edible weeds in your own yard, if you don't use any lawn chemicals. Especially in the spring, the tender shoots of a wide variety of plants can be used in salads or as a base for cooked greens. These include violet leaves and their flowers, young clover leaves, purslane, plantain, chickweed, chicory, dandelion, wild garlic, wild onion, wild leeks, curly dock, lamb's quarters, amaranth (also called pigweed), watercress, winter cress, wood sorrel, and fiddleheads (the curly new shoots of ferns). Mustard garlic is an invasive plant that is actually an escaped potherb. The tender leaves can be added to a salad, and more mature leaves can be used as a cooked green. The tender shoots from wild asparagus and cattails are also excellent additions to your salad or cooked greens. There is simply no better way to afford the leafy green prescription in the Wahls Protocol than to learn

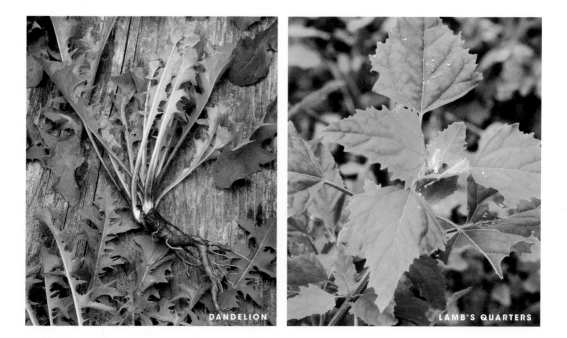

DANDELION

LAMB'S QUARTERS

which weeds are edible in your garden, yard, or nearby wild spaces. Just be sure you know what plant you are eating, as some can be poisonous. Check with your local library or bookstore for books on foraging safely for wild foods native to your area, or look on reputable websites. Sites dedicated to hunting and foraging for wild plants often have a lot of information and provide classes. Here are a few sites to get you started:

- www.wildmanstevebrill.com

- www.wildedible.com

- www.superfoods-for-superhealth.com/wild edible-greens.html

- http://wildfoodgirl.com

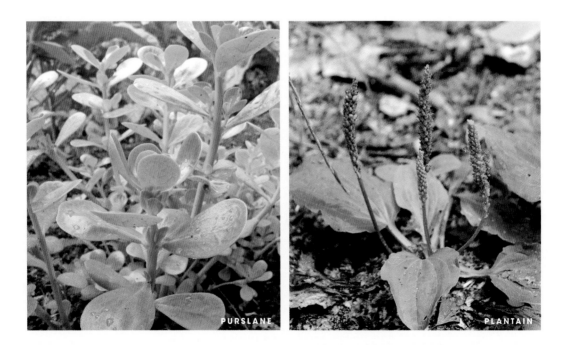

PURSLANE

PLANTAIN

WRAPS

Wraps are simply handheld salads and may be the quickest and easiest way to get some greens and a nutritious meal. They are practically fast food. All you have to do is fill a large green leaf or two with any leftover meat and/or cooked vegetables you happen to have on hand, wrap up the leaf, and eat it. Lunch is done!

BASIC WRAP TEMPLATE

MAKES 1 SERVING

Lay out one or two large green leaves. Put meat, vegetables, dressing, and other fillings in the middle, fold over the ends, and roll up. Eat immediately.

	WAHLS DIET, WAHLS PALEO, AND WAHLS PALEO PLUS
LEAFY GREEN WRAPS	1 or 2 large raw lettuce leaves, such as Boston or butter lettuces, romaine, or tender kale leaves
OTHER VEGETABLES AND HERBS	About 1 cup, or a little less, depending on size and number of leaf wraps
ANIMAL PROTEIN	3 to 4 ounces
GARNISHES (FRESH HERBS, NUTS, SEEDS, ETC.)	1 to 2 tablespoons (optional)

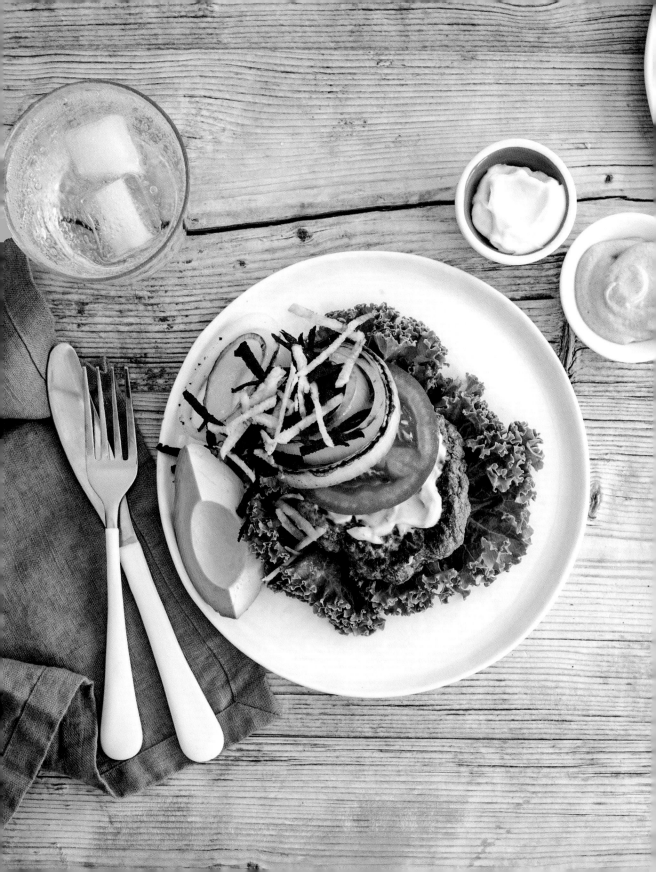

Enjoy a burger (preferably made with grass-fed beef or bison, or a gluten-free burger made from turkey, pork, or lamb) or a gluten-free sausage or brat (preferably nitrate-free) without the nutritional liability in this easy wrap. Just wrap your cooked burger or brat in kale leaves, add the toppings you like, roll up, and enjoy.

DRIVE-THROUGH WRAP

MAKES 1 SERVING
1 serving = 1½ Wahls veg/fruit cups

TO MAKE: Lay out 1 or 2 large lettuce or curly kale leaves. Top with 1 cooked burger or bratwurst and the toppings of your choice, such as 1 or 2 tomato slices, a few avocado slices, ¼ cup raw shredded beets, or onion slices fried in ghee. Add mustard or egg-free mayonnaise to taste, if desired.

Note: I have learned not to use ketchup on my burgers. Even the natural varieties have too much sugar. Instead, egg-free mayonnaise and a tomato slice or two or some good spicy mustard make excellent condiments for this wrap.

If you used to love deli or submarine sandwiches, you can still enjoy a similar experience with a wrap. Put all your favorite sandwich ingredients into large butter lettuce leaves and enjoy a filling lunch without the gluten or carbohydrate load. I don't include amounts here because you can fill up your leaves with as much or as little as you like, and all suggestions are optional. Make it your way! A kale or collard leaf is sturdier than the lettuce leaf if you prefer a more durable wrap.

DELI SANDWICH WRAP

MAKES 1 SERVING
1 serving = 1½ Wahls veg/fruit cups

TO MAKE: Lay out 1 or 2 large butter or Boston lettuce leaves. Add any nitrate-free deli meat, with or without 1 or 2 cooked slices of bacon. Add any toppings, such as fresh basil leaves, tomato slices, fermented pickle slices, and guacamole (page 48). Add condiments as desired, such as Dijon mustard, egg-free mayonnaise (such as Vegenaise), pesto (see page 178), or salad dressing.

WAHLS WARRIORS SPEAK

I'm a healthy person and I have always had an interest in natural health. I'm grateful that I happened to see Dr. Wahls on Facebook, and then on her TED Talk, as this spurred me on to learn more, and motivated me to greatly increase my organic fruit and veggie consumption. I have since referred many people to Dr. Terry Wahls and others. I'm so glad holistic health practices are gaining momentum and becoming more mainstream. Thank you, Dr. Wahls! You are a big part of this change.

—Wahls Warrior AMY

BASIC SOUP TEMPLATE

MAKES 4 SERVINGS

On some days, you may prefer a long, slow-cooked soup, and on other days, you may prefer a soup that is brighter and has more texture. Here are the two easy methods I use to make my soups:

FROM-SCRATCH METHOD: Put all the ingredients except young, tender green leaves into a slow cooker or a large stockpot or soup pot. (If using ground meat, brown it first. Other meat can be put into the pot raw.) Cook on low in the slow cooker for 8 to 10 hours, or over medium-low heat on the stovetop for up to 2 hours, watching to prevent boiling over. Turn off the heat and stir in any tender green leaves and fresh herbs. Serve immediately. Transfer to storage containers and refrigerate for up to 4 days, or freeze individual servings for quick meals when you need them.

QUICK-COOK METHOD: You can make a fresher-tasting soup if you have leftover cooked meat. Combine the broth and vegetables in a soup pot or stockpot and bring to a boil. Cook for 5 minutes. Stir in the cooked meat, remove from the heat, and let sit for 2 to 5 minutes for the meat to warm, then serve. Alternatively, you can serve immediately, depending on the size of the meat pieces. This method keeps the vegetables crisper and brighter in color.

RECIPE CONTINUES

	WAHLS DIET AND WAHLS PALEO	WAHLS PALEO PLUS
BROTH	1 quart (4 cups) Basic Bone Broth (page 29)	1 quart (4 cups) Basic Bone Broth (page 29)
MEAT, POULTRY, OR SEAFOOD	1 pound	1 pound
GREEN LEAVES (KALE, COLLARDS, CHARD, ASIAN GREENS, SPINACH, OR HERBS)	2 to 4 cups (2 cups chopped mature greens, such as kale or collards, or up to 4 cups tender, young greens, such as young spinach or chopped parsley, or a combination)	2 to 4 cups (2 cups chopped mature greens, such as kale or collards, or up to 4 cups tender, young greens, such as young spinach or chopped parsley, or a combination)
VEGGIES/FRUITS	4 cups, cut into bite-size pieces	2 to 4 cups, cut into bite-size pieces
FAT	1 (14-ounce) can full-fat coconut milk (optional, to make a creamy soup)	2 (14-ounce) cans full-fat coconut milk
FLAVORINGS (HERBS, SPICES, SAUCES)	As desired	As desired

Note: The coconut milk is optional for Wahls Diet and Wahls Paleo levels but will turn any soup into a lovely cream soup.

Note for Wahls Paleo Plus: Stick with non-starchy vegetables like leafy greens, onions, and mushrooms. Also, for this level, coconut milk is a requirement, not an option. Use 2 (14-ounce) cans of coconut milk in all soup recipes to help you stay in ketosis.

Some people (myself included) love to eat bone marrow roasted, straight out of the bone, but if this is too intense for you, try this super-rich and extremely nourishing soup. Beef marrow bones are typically available at a low price from your grocery store meat counter. Usually, the nutrient-dense marrow just goes to waste! You can sip this as a therapeutic and comforting broth, or use it as a bone broth base for any other soup. Unlike other bone broths, this one contains coconut milk, which helps to emulsify the marrow fats into the broth.

BEEF MARROW BROTH

MAKES 4 SERVINGS
1 serving = ½ Wahls veg/fruit cup

TO MAKE: Put all the ingredients in a slow cooker and cook on low for 8 hours. Alternatively, put all the ingredients in a soup pot and simmer on the stovetop over low heat for up to 8 hours.

	WAHLS DIET AND WAHLS PALEO	WAHLS PALEO PLUS
BROTH	1 quart (4 cups) Basic Bone Broth (page 29)	1 quart (4 cups) Basic Bone Broth (page 29)
MEAT, POULTRY, OR SEAFOOD	2 pounds beef marrow bones	2 pounds beef marrow bones
GREEN LEAVES	None	None
VEGGIES/FRUITS	4 garlic cloves, crushed	4 garlic cloves, crushed
FAT	1 cup canned full-fat coconut milk	1½ to 2 cups canned full-fat coconut milk
FLAVORINGS	2 tablespoons apple cider vinegar	2 tablespoons apple cider vinegar

Italian Variation: **Add 1 tablespoon chopped fresh oregano, 1 tablespoon chopped fresh basil, and 1 bay leaf. Remove and discard the bay leaf before serving.**

Indian Variation: **Add 2 teaspoons ground turmeric, ½ teaspoon ground cumin, ½ teaspoon ground coriander, and freshly ground black pepper to taste.**

Many of us do not get enough potassium in our diet, which increases our risk of developing high blood pressure. Potassium helps our blood vessels stay young and flexible, and potassium broth also helps with gastrointestinal issues. When we have a GI bug and have vomiting or diarrhea, we often lose a lot of potassium in the process, along with a lot of glutamine. Our intestinal cells use glutamine, not sugar, as their primary fuel. When our bodies are short on glutamine, we pull the glutamine and potassium from our muscles, which contributes to the achiness we feel. Drinking a lot of potassium broth replaces lost minerals and glutamine and helps your bowels heal.

POTASSIUM BROTH

MAKES 4 SERVINGS
1 serving = 2 Wahls veg/fruit cups
Note: This recipe is appropriate for all levels of the Wahls Protocol.

6 celery stalks, quartered

6 garlic cloves, minced

1 bunch watercress, parsley, or cilantro

4 kale, collard, or chard leaves, sliced into thick ribbons

1 teaspoon dulse or kelp flakes

½ to 1 teaspoon sea salt

2 to 4 quarts Basic Bone Broth (page 29) or water

TO MAKE: Put all the ingredients in a slow cooker and cook on low for 6 to 12 hours. Alternatively, put all the ingredients in a soup pot and simmer on the stovetop over low heat for about 2 hours, watching to prevent boiling over. Strain the broth and discard the solids for a clear broth (this is preferable when ill), or transfer to a Vitamix or other high-speed blender and puree (be careful when blending hot liquids).

Variation (Wahls Diet and Wahls Paleo only): For a red Potassium Broth, add 2 chopped beets (peeling optional) and replace the kale, collard, or chard leaves with ¼ small head red cabbage, coarsely chopped.

This is another special healing broth that is so deeply nourishing and easy to make. Try it when you can't stomach a full meal but want something comforting and warm.

MUSHROOM BROTH

MAKES 4 SERVINGS
1 serving = 2 Wahls veg/fruit cups
Note: This recipe is appropriate for all levels of the Wahls Protocol.

4 cups Basic Bone Broth (page 29) or water

1 pound shiitake or maitake mushrooms, sliced or chopped

1 to 4 garlic cloves, crushed

1 small onion, chopped

½ to 1 teaspoon dulse or kelp flakes

¼ to 1 teaspoon sea salt

TO MAKE: Put all the ingredients into a slow cooker and cook on low for 6 to 8 hours or on high for 4 hours. Alternatively, put all the ingredients in a soup pot or stockpot and simmer over medium-low heat until the mushrooms are tender, 30 to 45 minutes. Eat as is, or transfer to a Vitamix or other high-speed blender and puree to the desired level of smoothness (be careful when blending hot liquids).

I like to make this recipe every time we have a roast chicken for dinner. I pull all the remaining meat off the carcass (save the carcass to make another batch of stock later, using the recipe for chicken bone broth on page 30). This meat, combined with bone broth you already have in your freezer, fresh veggies, and the surprise pop of cranberries, is a comforting and nourishing meal any time of year, whether you are feeling under the weather or feeling great.

OLD-FASHIONED CHICKEN SOUP

MAKES 4 SERVINGS
1 serving = 1¾ Wahls and Wahls Paleo veg/fruit cups
1 serving = 1½ Wahls Paleo Plus veg/fruit cups

TO MAKE: This soup is best cooked on the stove. Put all the ingredients except the young tender greens and herbs, and the carrots if you are following Wahls Paleo Plus (for that level, the carrots should remain raw), in a soup pot or stockpot, bring to a boil, then reduce the heat to medium-low and cook until the vegetables are tender, 20 to 45 minutes, depending on what kind of vegetables you use and how large you cut the pieces. Turn off the heat and stir in any tender green leaves and fresh herbs, and the carrots if you are following Wahls Paleo Plus. Serve immediately. Store in an airtight container in the refrigerator for up to 4 days, or freeze individual servings for quick meals when you need them.

QUICK CHICKEN BROTH

You can make chicken broth the slow-simmer way (see page 30), but you can also make broth much more quickly using a cut-up chicken. Put the chicken pieces in a soup pot, add water to cover them, 2 tablespoons apple cider vinegar, and a handful of fresh garden herbs and simmer for 20 minutes. Pull out the chicken, let it cool enough to handle, and take the meat off the bones. Cut up the meat for later use and strain the broth, discarding the solids. You now have chicken broth on hand. I like to make broth over a couple of days using the method on page 30 when I can, but this recipe is great in a pinch. Fresh broth in 30 minutes!

Note: Coconut milk is optional for Wahls Diet and Wahls Paleo levels, but if you use it, you'll have a thicker, richer, "cream of chicken" soup. For Wahls Paleo Plus, coconut milk is required.

Cooking Tip: If you want to make this recipe and you don't have leftover roast chicken, using a slow cooker is the easiest method. Put raw chicken pieces, on the bone or boneless, into the slow cooker with the broth. Cook for a full 8 hours on low or 4 hours on high, then remove the chicken from the soup, remove any bones, and shred the meat before returning it to the slow cooker. After that, add your vegetables. You can also do this on the stovetop: Simmer the chicken in the broth until cooked through, about 20 minutes for boneless or 45 minutes for chicken on the bone.

	WAHLS DIET AND WAHLS PALEO	WAHLS PALEO PLUS
BROTH	1 quart (4 cups) chicken bone broth (page 30)	1 quart (4 cups) chicken bone broth (page 30)
MEAT, POULTRY, OR SEAFOOD	1 pound cooked chicken	1 pound cooked chicken
GREEN LEAVES	2 cups tender baby spinach or baby kale leaves	2 cups tender baby spinach or baby kale leaves
VEGGIES/FRUITS	1 cup chopped onion	½ cup chopped onion
	1 cup chopped celery	½ cup chopped celery
	1 cup chopped zucchini	½ cup chopped zucchini
	½ cup chopped carrots	½ cup fresh or frozen (not dried) cranberries
	½ cup fresh, frozen, or dried unsweetened cranberries	4 garlic cloves, minced or crushed
	4 garlic cloves, minced or crushed	
FAT	1 (14-ounce) can full-fat coconut milk (optional, to make a creamy soup)	2 (14-ounce) cans full-fat coconut milk
FLAVORINGS	¼ cup fresh parsley or cilantro leaves, chopped (add at the end)	¼ cup fresh parsley or cilantro leaves, chopped (add at the end)
	½ teaspoon fresh or dried thyme	½ teaspoon fresh or dried thyme
		1 teaspoon dried rosemary, or 2 or 3 springs fresh rosemary
		1 bay leaf

THE WAHLS PROTOCOL, BLENDERIZED

Some of my patients, and many people suffering with neurological issues or other chronic diseases, have trouble eating solid food because of an inability to swallow or persistent trouble with gagging or retching. This can be due to disease or damage to the nervous system, mouth, or esophagus. Both children and adults can be afflicted, and the danger of this condition is, of course, malnutrition. A diet of blenderized or pureed food is essential. Some people can't even swallow pureed food and require a feeding tube in their stomach or small bowel.

The official stance of the medical and nutrition establishment is to use commercial enteral nutrition products for those who require a feeding tube. However, if you check the ingredient label of these products, you will see that the main ingredient for calories is typically high-fructose corn syrup, with added vitamins, minerals, amino acids, and essential fats. This is far from whole, real food, and completely lacks the complex array and diversity of phytochemicals that exist in vegetables, fruits, nuts, and seeds, not to mention animal protein.

The concern that the medical establishment has with blenderized tube feedings is that the diet will lack sufficient nutrition to provide health, which is why they add the supplemental vitamins, minerals, etc. My concern is that those on this type of diet do not have the nutrition they need for optimal (not just minimal) health, and anyone who requires tube feeding is likely in great need of restored health.

I understand where the medical community is coming from. If people simply consumed a blenderized version of the standard American diet, it would likely be inferior to the nutrient profile in enteral nutrition products. However, blenderizing a diet that is rich in vegetables, berries, and high-quality protein and fats provides many more nutrients, including phytochemicals and fiber, accelerates healing, builds a healthier microbiome, and restores overall health.

Many of my patients who require a liquid diet or tube feeding use the Wahls Protocol instead of a commercial formula, and the results are dramatic. First I heard from people with ALS and traumatic brain injury who switched to blenderized whole-food diets and reported marked improvement in their energy, mood, mental clarity, and health. Then parents of children suffering from neurological disorders began contacting me about their experiences using the Wahls Protocol via G tube with their children. A family whose son has Krabbe disease, a rare neurological disorder that affects the ability of the brain to make vital brain structures, wrote to describe the dramatic positive impact the Wahls Diet had on their child. With Krabbe disease, the brain is unable to make the proper insulation on the wiring in the brain. Infants have difficulty feeding within three months of life and begin to require a feeding tube because of their problems swallowing. They usually begin to deteriorate neurologically and rarely live past age two. However, the family who contacted me worked with their medical team to feed their son the Wahls Paleo Plus diet via a G tube. He is now three years old and doing very well neurologically!

Working with a dietitian is very important, and I'd even say it's an absolute requirement if you are feeding an infant or a child. Determining a child's ideal number of calories, protein, carbohydrates, and fat, along with the many essential micronutrients, is something pediatric dietitians do well. Plus, the dietitian can track the child's growth and help you make adjustments as the child grows, or fails to grow. For adults, involving a dietitian as you make the transition from formula to a blenderized whole-food diet helps ensure a smooth transition. You can also use resources on the Internet to find a community and the support you need.

A good place to start with a blenderized diet is with soups and stews. You can blend with sufficient water to keep the mixture thin enough to pass through the feeding tubes. I encourage including organ meats in these blends because they are so nutrient dense. If your bowels are working well (no diarrhea), you can add smoothies with greens and berries to the feedings. Include some nuts and some hemp oil, flaxseed oil, or fish oil to ensure a good supply of essential oils in the smoothies as well. For family meals, I suggest simply blenderizing what the rest of the family is eating as opposed to making a special meal. It's much easier to maintain the blenderized diet when everyone is eating the same thing.

WAHLS WARRIORS SPEAK

I am a severe traumatic brain injury survivor, speaker, and educator. In 2011, I fell twenty feet from a rooftop water tower scaffolding. My head struck a steel beam on the way down before I crashed onto the concrete rooftop below. I was rushed to the hospital and put on life support. While in a coma, an MRI revealed a severe diffuse axonal injury (DAI), which is one of the most devastating types of brain injury.

I couldn't eat, walk, or talk for months, and my left hand was completely flexed inward. Statistically, more than 90 percent of patients with this injury never regain consciousness, and those who do wake up will often remain in a persistent vegetative state. However, I have recovered beyond all expectations, and nutrition has been paramount in my successful recovery. I required tube feeding for some time, but instead of using the processed hospital liquid formula containing ingredients like corn syrup, canola oil, and soy protein isolate, I thrived on a blenderized diet of whole foods.

I have since been working with doctors, professors, therapists, and nutritionists to improve the health of my brain for my own recovery, and to show others how to do the same. Through my extensive research, I have found the dietary guidelines of the Wahls Paleo and Wahls Paleo Plus diets to be the most supportive for neurological health and recovery. I am often contacted by loved ones of survivors who are using blenderized formula and who see their loved ones deteriorating each and every day. It breaks my heart, and so I hope to continue to spread the word that whole-food diets, especially the Wahls Diet, when blenderized make a superior formula to the processed types so often used in hospitals. I am living proof.

—Wahls Warrior CAVIN

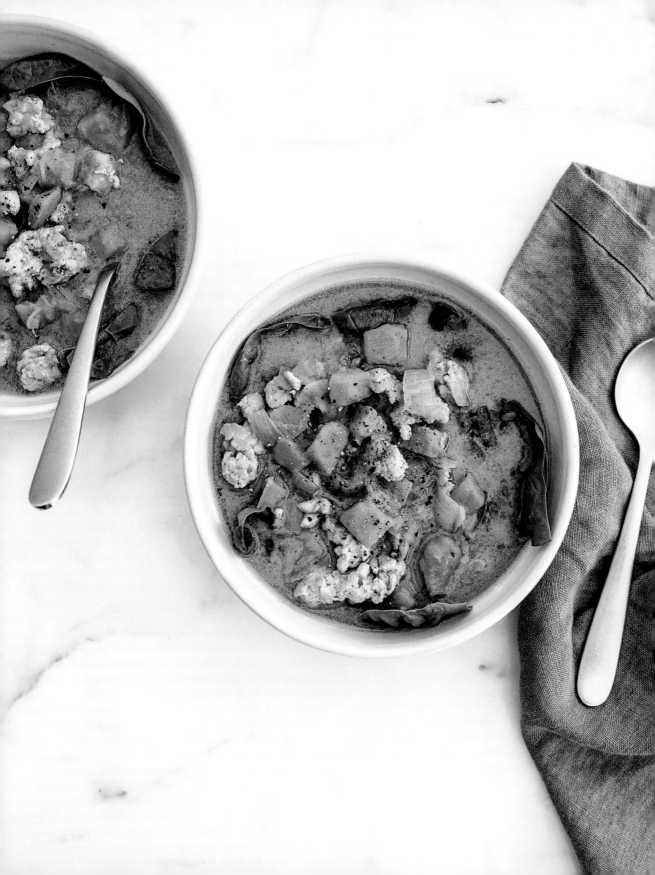

This is an easy recipe with an African-inspired flavor that yields impressive results.

KALE, SAUSAGE, AND YAM SOUP WITH COCONUT MILK

MAKES 4 SERVINGS
1 serving = 2 Wahls and Wahls Paleo veg/fruit cups
1 serving = 1½ Wahls Paleo Plus veg/fruit cups

TO MAKE: Put all the ingredients into a slow cooker and cook on low for 8 hours or on high for 4 hours. Or put all the ingredients in a soup pot or stockpot and simmer over medium-low heat for up to 2 hours.

	WAHLS DIET AND WAHLS PALEO	WAHLS PALEO PLUS
BROTH	1 quart (4 cups) Basic Bone Broth (page 29)	1 quart (4 cups) Basic Bone Broth (page 29)
MEAT, POULTRY, OR SEAFOOD	1 pound pork, turkey, or game-meat sausage, browned	1 pound pork, turkey, or game-meat sausage, browned
GREEN LEAVES	2 cups tender baby spinach or baby kale leaves	2 cups tender baby spinach or baby kale leaves
VEGGIES/FRUITS	3 cups cubed yams or sweet potatoes	1 cup shredded raw yams, stirred in just before serving
	1 cup chopped onion	1 cup chopped onion
	4 garlic cloves, minced or crushed	4 garlic cloves, minced or crushed
FAT	1 (14-ounce) can full-fat coconut milk	2 (14-ounce) cans full-fat coconut milk
FLAVORINGS	1 teaspoon sea salt	1 teaspoon sea salt
	Optional:	Optional:
	1 teaspoon minced fresh ginger	1 teaspoon minced fresh ginger
	1 teaspoon ground turmeric	1 teaspoon ground turmeric
	½ teaspoon ground cinnamon	½ teaspoon ground cinnamon
	½ teaspoon ground cumin	½ teaspoon ground cumin
	½ teaspoon coriander seeds	½ teaspoon coriander seeds
	Pinch of ground allspice	Pinch of ground allspice

This is a highly flavorful, deeply healing, meat-free soup I hope you will try. You will use an entire cauliflower for this soup—no waste! Try this when you want a lighter dinner that still has lots of exotic flavor. If you use the slow cooker, this recipe takes very little effort.

CAULIFLOWER CARROT GARLIC HEALING SOUP

MAKES 4 SERVINGS

1 serving = 2¾ Wahls and Wahls Paleo veg/fruit cups

Note: This recipe is not appropriate for Wahls Paleo Plus.

1 quart (4 cups) Basic Bone Broth (page 29)

1 whole cauliflower, cut into chunks (all of it, including the leaves and core)

3 to 5 large carrots, chopped

4 to 6 garlic cloves, crushed or minced

1 (¼- to ½-inch) piece fresh ginger, chopped

½ to 1 teaspoon coriander seeds or ground coriander

½ to 1 teaspoon cumin seeds or ground cumin

½ to 1 teaspoon ground turmeric

½ to 1 teaspoon dulse or kelp flakes

¼ teaspoon freshly ground black pepper (helps absorb the turmeric more effectively)

1 to 2 tablespoons coconut oil

TO MAKE: Place all the ingredients in a pot or a slow cooker and cook on low for 8 to 12 hours. If you need to make it more quickly, you can cut the vegetables smaller and simmer them until they are tender, 1 to 2 hours depending on how large the vegetables pieces are. Transfer the soup to a Vitamix or other high-speed blender and blend to the desired level of smoothness (be careful when blending hot liquids). This soup is wonderful hot or cold.

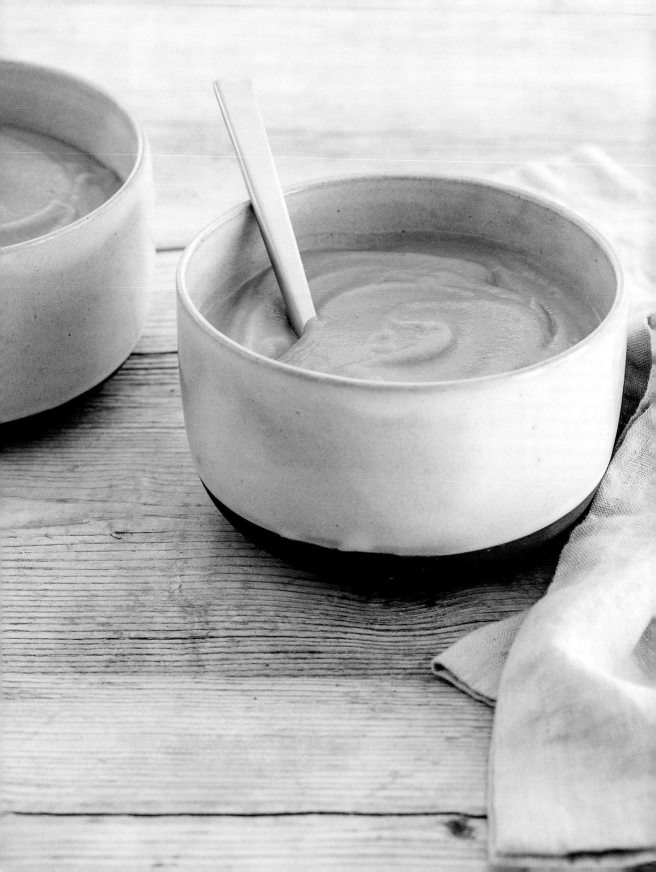

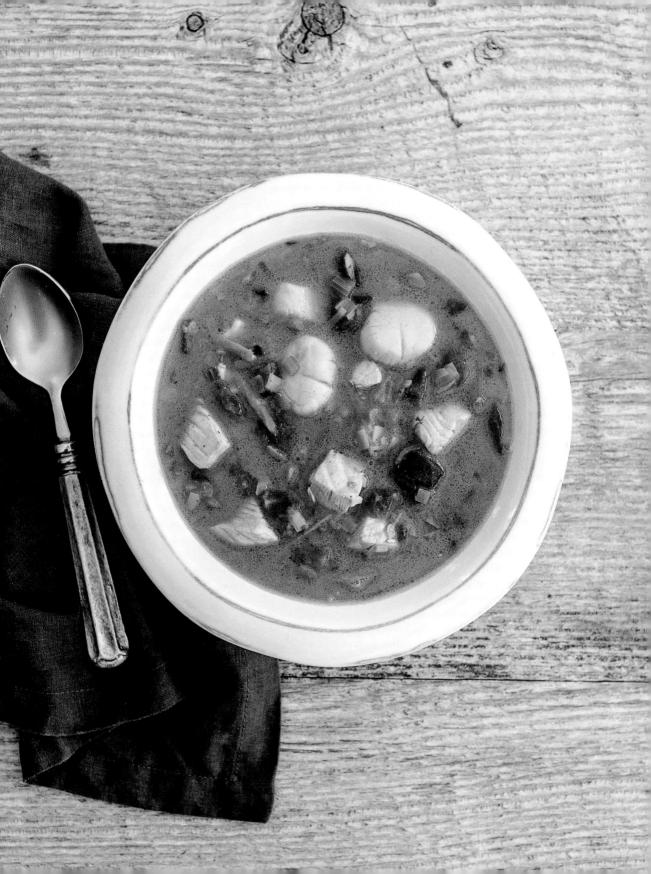

Bouillabaisse sounds fancy, but it's actually quite easy to prepare if you have good-quality, fresh ingredients. For this recipe, I use prepared fish or chicken stock.

BOUILLABAISSE WITH LEEKS, MUSHROOMS, AND SAFFRON

MAKES 4 SERVINGS
1 serving = 1½ Wahls veg/fruit cup
Note: This recipe is appropriate for all levels of the Wahls Protocol.

4 cups store-bought or homemade seafood stock or chicken stock

1 onion, chopped

1 celery stalk, finely chopped

2 carrots, grated

4 cups chopped tomatoes (fresh or canned)

1 pound scallops

1 pound salmon, cut into bite-size pieces

1 (¼-inch) piece fresh ginger, peeled and grated

¼ teaspoon saffron or ground turmeric

TO MAKE: Put the stock, onion, celery, carrots, and tomatoes in a soup pot. Simmer over medium-low heat until the vegetables are tender, about 30 minutes.

Add the scallops, salmon, ginger, and saffron. Bring the soup back to a simmer, cover, and turn off the heat. Wait 10 minutes, then stir and serve.

Note for Wahls Paleo Plus: **Add the grated carrots just before serving, instead of cooking them with the rest of the vegetables, so they are warm but remain raw.**

Variation: **Add 1 tablespoon crumbled dulse flakes to the broth along with the vegetables, to give the broth a richer, deeper briny flavor.**

Fava beans contain nutrients that help your body manufacture dopamine, which is important for conditions that tend to involve low dopamine levels, such as Parkinson's, anxiety, and attention deficit disorders. Use fresh, dried, or canned fava beans. Each has a different character and texture; soak and drain dried beans overnight, and rinse and drain canned beans. Fresh is always best, if you can find it. By the way, this is one of my daughter's favorite soups.

FAVA BEAN AND BACON SOUP

MAKES 4 SERVINGS
1 serving = 1¾ Wahls veg/fruit cup

1 quart (4 cups) Basic Bone Broth (page 29)

2 cups fresh or canned (drained and rinsed) fava beans, or 1 cup dried fava beans, soaked overnight and drained

2 onions, chopped

1 (14-ounce) can full-fat coconut milk (optional)

1 tablespoon dulse flakes

1 tablespoon minced garlic

1 teaspoon sea salt

½ teaspoon celery seed

Freshly ground black pepper

½ pound bacon, chopped and cooked until desired level of crispness

2 cups leafy greens

Minced fresh chives or parsley, for garnish

1 avocado, pitted, peeled, and cubed, for garnish

TO MAKE: Put the bone broth, fava beans, onions, coconut milk (if using), dulse flakes, garlic, sea salt, celery seed, and black pepper to taste in a big soup pot, bring to a boil, then reduce the heat to maintain a simmer and cook until the fava beans are tender and the vegetables are soft. Mash everything together or whirl gently in a Vitamix or other high-speed blender and return to the warm pot. Stir in the bacon and leafy greens. Garnish with the chives or parsley and/or fresh avocado, and serve.

Note for Wahls Paleo and Wahls Paleo Plus: This soup is not appropriate for those on Wahls Paleo Plus, and it is only appropriate for those on Wahls Paleo if the fava beans are soaked overnight before cooking.

Organ meats cost very little compared to muscle meats, and yet they are far superior in nutrition. There are also delicious ways to cook with them. It's easy to pulse heart, liver, and gizzards in a food processor and mix into dishes with other ground meat. This method eliminates what some people feel is an unpleasant, chewy texture. Another organ my family enjoys is cow tongue. This may sound unpleasant, but it is actually quite delicious and inexpensive. We like to make a tongue soup—I simmer the tongue all day in the slow cooker with spices (I often use 3 bay leaves, 1 star anise pod, 1 teaspoon sea salt, and a few twists of black pepper). When I get home at the end of the day, I take the tongue out, remove and discard the membrane, and cut the tongue meat into bite-size pieces. Then I remove the bay leaves and star anise from the broth and return the tongue pieces to the broth, along with any cut-up vegetables I have in my refrigerator or garden for a simple soup. You can also save some of the tongue for slicing and enjoy it warm or cold. It is quite tasty with mustard or horseradish. Even my kids like it a lot. This soup is appropriate for all levels of the Wahls Protocol.

ALL ABOUT SEAWEED

Seaweed comes in three categories: green, brown, and red. The main pigment of the seaweed determines at what depth it can grow—green grows in the shallowest water and red grows in the deepest. The mix of minerals and antioxidants in seaweed varies according to the species. All seaweeds are a good source of minerals. They all absorb heavy metals, plastics, solvents, and toxins and can increase the amount of toxins your body can eliminate each day. This is why I am also very careful about where I get my seaweed. I prefer to purchase seaweed from companies that test their seaweed for the presence of radiation, heavy metals, and other contaminants. (Here is a good source: www.seaveg.com/shop.)

You can get seaweed in several forms: dried whole leaf, flakes, or powder. I like to use the flakes as an added "spice" when I'm cooking. I also like to use a mix of seaweeds. Sometimes I use the red dulse flakes, sometimes the kelp flakes, and sometimes the mixed flakes. Kelp has more iodine than the other types of seaweed. Dulse has less iodine than kelp. When you are starting to add seaweed to your recipes, add it very gradually. Begin by adding just ¼ teaspoon of flakes per serving (for example, if your soup serves four, add 1 teaspoon). Do this just once a week initially, and work up gradually. Use dulse half the time because it is lower in iodine, to keep your iodine from jumping up too suddenly.

In my clinics, I tell people to consume seaweed once a week for a month before moving up to twice a week. After a month of doing that, if everything is going well, you can try adding seaweed to three meals a week.

A note of caution: If you take thyroid medication, you must check with your personal physician prior to adding seaweed to your diet, as eating seaweed could change the amount or dose of your thyroid medication. Also check with your physician prior to going any higher than three servings per week, even if you are not on any thyroid medication.

I love the delicious little lamb meatballs in this soup. This is also a great recipe to experiment with your garden herbs. I pick herbs from my garden, pull out the coarse stems, and pulse them in the food processor until they are minced. Or you can use dried herbs if you do not have fresh herbs. If I pick a large bowl of herbs, I might use some for the meatballs and leave the rest on a dinner plate to dry over the next several days. This is an easy way to make dried herbs without a dehydrator. Whether you are using herbs or pesto, you can use a food processor to mix the flavorings with the meat. There's no need to brown the meatballs first, although you can if you prefer to do so.

LAMB MEATBALL SOUP

MAKES 4 SERVINGS
1 serving = 1¼ Wahls veg/fruit cups

TO MAKE: Put the lamb and herbs in a large bowl. Mix thoroughly to combine. Form the meat mixture into meatballs about 1 inch in diameter. Put the meatballs and all the other ingredients except the greens into a slow cooker and cook on low for 8 to 10 hours. Alternatively, put the meatballs and all the other ingredients except the greens in a large stockpot or soup pot and simmer over medium-low heat on the stovetop for up to 2 hours (watch the pot on the stove to prevent it from boiling over). Turn off the heat and stir in the tender green leaves and any additional minced fresh herbs. Serve immediately. The soup will keep in the refrigerator for up to 4 days, or freeze individual servings for quick meals when you need them.

RECIPE CONTINUES

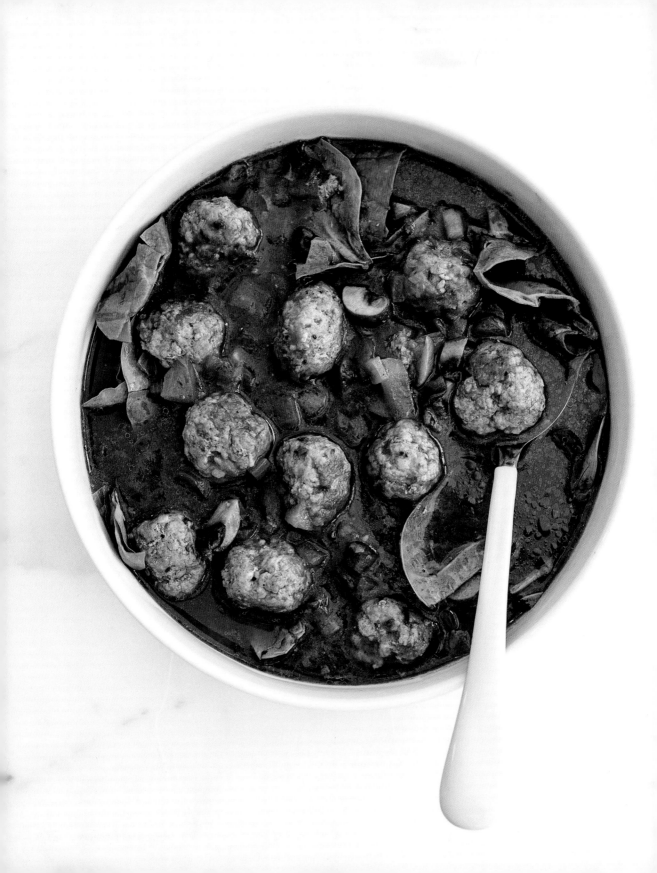

	WAHLS DIET AND WAHLS PALEO	WAHLS PALEO PLUS
BROTH	1 quart (4 cups) Basic Bone Broth (page 29)	1 quart (4 cups) Basic Bone Broth (page 29)
MEAT, POULTRY, OR SEAFOOD	1 pound lamb	1 pound lamb
GREEN LEAVES	2 cups tender greens	2 cups tender greens
VEGGIES/FRUITS	2 cups green beans, trimmed and cut into 1-inch pieces	2 cups green beans, trimmed and cut into 1-inch pieces
	1 cup sliced mushrooms	1 cup sliced mushrooms
	½ cup sliced carrots	½ cup grated carrots (added just before serving so that they are still raw)
FAT	1 (14-ounce) can full-fat coconut milk (optional, to make this a creamy soup)	2 (14-ounce) cans full-fat coconut milk
FLAVORINGS	Herbs for meatballs: 2 tablespoons minced fresh rosemary 1 tablespoon minced fresh savory 1 tablespoon minced fresh parsley or any other garden herbs you have	Herbs for meatballs: 1 tablespoon fresh rosemary 1 tablespoon fresh savory or any other garden herbs you have

Variation: Instead of the herbs, mix 1 to 2 tablespoons fresh pesto (page 178) into the meat.

TOMATO SAUCE FOR FREEZING

MAKES ABOUT 6 CUPS

Note: This recipe is appropriate for all levels of the Wahls Protocol.

4 cups chopped tomatoes (fresh or canned)

2 cups fresh garden herb leaves, such as basil, oregano, savory, chives, and/or parsley

1 cup chopped onions

1 teaspoon minced garlic

1 or more hot peppers (such as poblano or jalapeño), cored, seeded, and chopped, if you like a spicier sauce

TO MAKE: Put all the ingredients in a food processor and pulse until combined. There is no need to peel the tomatoes first. You could also simmer this after processing, to reach a desired level of thickness. This tomato sauce will taste more like a marinara. Let cool before transferring to quart-size freezer bags (for easy portions) and freezing.

Sometimes an Italian-inspired tomato soup is just what I want. For a delicious base, I like to use a homemade tomato sauce I make from the tomatoes in my own garden. I make the sauce in large quantities when tomatoes are ripe and keep it in the freezer. It's a great way to be sure no garden tomato (or tomato from that box you got on sale at the farmers' market) goes to waste. I rarely make this soup using canned tomatoes, but you certainly can if you don't have access to fresh tomatoes. This is a quick, easy, and very popular meal in my household.

BASIC TOMATO SOUP TEMPLATE

MAKES 4 SERVINGS
1 serving = 1¾ Wahls and Wahls Paleo veg/fruit cups
1 serving = 1½ Wahls Paleo Plus veg/fruit cups

	WAHLS DIET AND WAHLS PALEO	WAHLS PALEO PLUS
TOMATO SAUCE	1½ cups Tomato Sauce for Freezing (page 218)	1½ cups Tomato Sauce for Freezing (page 218)
BASIC BONE BROTH (PAGE 29)	1 quart (4 cups)	3 cups
GROUND MEAT	1 pound (ground beef, bison, elk, or turkey are all good in this soup)	1 pound (ground beef, bison, elk, or turkey are all good in this soup)
GREEN LEAVES	4 cups young, tender greens (such as baby spinach or kale, or fresh parsley)	4 cups young, tender greens (such as baby spinach or kale, or fresh parsley)
VEGETABLES	1 cup chopped onions 1 cup chopped mushrooms (optional)	2 cups chopped mushrooms (optional)
FAT	1 tablespoon coconut oil, for browning meatballs 1 cup canned full-fat coconut milk (optional, to make a creamy soup)	1 tablespoon coconut oil, for browning meatballs 2 cups canned full-fat coconut milk
FLAVORINGS (HERBS, SPICES, SAUCES)	1 tablespoon fresh basil, or 1 teaspoon dried 1 tablespoon fresh oregano, or 1 teaspoon dried ½ teaspoon fresh or dried thyme	1 tablespoon fresh basil, or 1 teaspoon dried 1 tablespoon fresh oregano, or 1 teaspoon dried ½ teaspoon fresh or dried thyme
GARNISH	1 avocado, pitted, peeled, and cubed, or 1 cup Wahls Guacamole (page 48)	1 avocado, pitted, peeled, and cubed, or 1 cup Wahls Guacamole (page 48)

RECIPE CONTINUES

Form the ground meat into very small meatballs. Heat the coconut oil in a pot, then brown the meatballs, stirring frequently, for about 10 minutes. Add all the other ingredients except the leafy greens. Cook over medium-high heat until the soup comes to a simmer. Simmer for about 5 minutes, turn off the heat, and stir in the tender green leaves. Ladle the soup into bowls, then garnish with cubed avocado or a scoop of guacamole for a beautiful red and green contrast. Serve immediately. Store in the refrigerator for up to 4 days, or freeze individual servings for quick meals when you need them (but whenever I make it, we don't have anything left).

Note for Wahls Paleo Plus: For Wahls Paleo Plus, coconut milk is a required ingredient for any tomato-based soup. Tomatoes have more carbs than many other vegetables, so the coconut milk will help keep you in ketosis. Also, stick with a 1 cup serving size if you are watching your ketones.

NIGHTSHADE-FREE "TOMATO" SOUP

Some people find they are bothered by vegetables in the nightshade family. These include tomatoes, peppers, white potatoes, and eggplants, which can increase joint pain and cause digestive discomfort. While many people are just fine with nightshades, those who avoid them can still have a "tomato soup" experience, simply by substituting one 15-ounce can pumpkin puree with ¼ cup chopped or grated cooked beets for one 15-ounce can (or about 1½ cups) tomato sauce in any soup recipe. If you do not like beets, you could try adding 2 tablespoons aronia berries to provide the deep red color. Note that this recipe will not work for Wahls Paleo Plus, as cooked pumpkins and beets have too many carbs and will likely take you out of ketosis. For more about nightshade-free substitutions, see page 46.

THREE CHILLED SOUPS

Chilled soups are perfect in the summer because they are easy to make, don't heat up the kitchen, and utilize ingredients at their peak of freshness. Some people enjoy them all year round (especially those suffering from hot flashes for hormonal reasons). These are three of my favorites.

Note: Tomato Gazpacho and Carrot Gazpacho have too many carbs for Wahls Paleo Plus. Avocado, Dill, and Nutmeg Chilled Cream Soup is appropriate for all levels of the Wahls Protocol.

AVOCADO, DILL, AND NUT MILK CHILLED CREAM SOUP

MAKES 4 SERVINGS

1 serving = ½ Wahls veg/fruit cup

Note: This soup is appropriate for all levels of the Wahls Protocol.

2 ripe avocados, pitted and peeled

4 cups nut milk (almond, hazelnut, cashew, etc.), from a carton or homemade, or 1 (14-ounce) can full-fat coconut milk for Wahls Paleo Plus

1 tablespoon fresh dill

1 teaspoon sea salt

TO MAKE: Put all the ingredients in a Vitamix or other high-speed blender (if using coconut milk for Wahls Paleo Plus, fill the can with water and add it to the blender). Puree on high for 3 to 4 minutes until the texture is as smooth as you wish, then chill in the refrigerator until very cold.

WAHLS WARRIORS SPEAK

I find your book very inspiring. After seeing you in an online video, I began to follow your diet gradually and take the supplements you recommend. Believe it or not, after only several weeks (and I have not always been rigorous), my belly fat has gone down and my stamina has increased. I can't wait to see what happens when I begin the diet full-force!

—Wahls Warrior TINA

CARROT GAZPACHO

MAKES 4 SERVINGS

1 serving = ¾ Wahls veg/fruit cup

Note: This recipe is not appropriate for Wahls Paleo Plus.

5 large carrots, coarsely chopped

1½ cups fresh orange juice

1 tablespoon chopped fresh parsley, including stems

1 teaspoon minced fresh ginger

1 teaspoon sea salt

Freshly ground black pepper

Optional garnishes: 1 cup each of diced cucumber, zucchini, and jicama

Hot sauce (optional, for serving)

TO MAKE: Puree all ingredients in your high-speed blender for 3 to 4 minutes until smooth, then chill. Just before serving, stir in the optional garnishes and hot sauce.

TOMATO GAZPACHO

MAKES 4 SERVINGS

1 serving = ¾ Wahls veg/fruit cup

Note: This recipe is not appropriate for Wahls Paleo Plus.

1 pound tomatoes (or carrots, for a nightshade-free version), coarsely chopped

1 (14-ounce) can full-fat coconut milk

1 cup fresh orange juice (*only if using carrots*)

1 tablespoon chopped fresh chives

1 tablespoon chopped fresh parsley, including stems

1 teaspoon minced fresh ginger

1 teaspoon sea salt

Freshly ground black pepper

Optional garnishes: 1 cup each of diced cucumber, zucchini, and jicama

Hot sauce (optional), for serving

TO MAKE: Puree all ingredients in your high-speed blender for 3 to 4 minutes until smooth, then chill. Just before serving, stir in the optional garnishes and hot sauce.

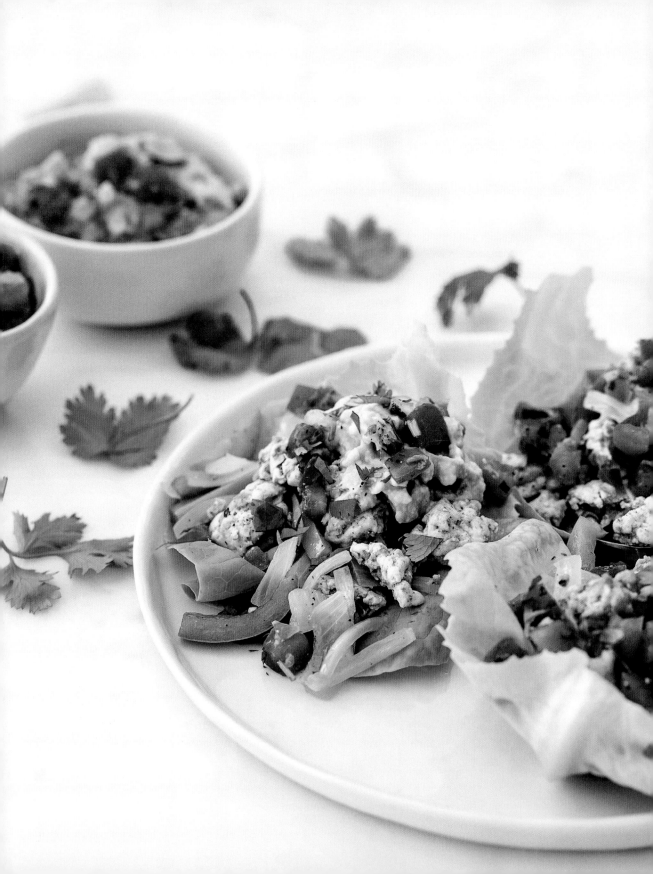

8 SAVORY SKILLETS

WHAT DO I EAT FOR DINNER ON MOST NIGHTS? A skillet. Skillets are simple to make and perfect for people who don't have the time or energy to spend cooking complicated things. Just brown some meat, add vegetables and greens (I aim for about 3 cups total vegetables per person), season, and serve. So easy. Skillets are also an easy way to get your Wahls-required veggies for the day. They are easy to adapt to whatever you have, and you can always add more veggies to make your meal more filling.

Ironically, I don't usually cook skillets in a skillet. If you have a really big skillet with high sides, it can work, but because I usually add so many vegetables, I find that a big soup pot or stockpot or Dutch oven works better. That way, I don't end up spilling vegetables all over my stove if I get too exuberant with my stirring.

Use the template in this chapter to make skillets out of whatever ingredients you have. These recipes serve four, but if you are cooking for fewer people, you can cut any of them in half, or save the leftovers for the next day (skillets don't keep much longer in the refrigerator, but many of them freeze nicely).

Try different things to find your favorites, or invent skillets based on the meat and vegetables you like best. Here are also some of my favorite skillet recipes—the ones I make again and again, that my children request, or that just make me feel good.

SKILLET VARIATION

You can cook any skillet recipe created from this template or in this book in the oven instead of in a skillet on the stove, if you prefer. Lightly grease a baking pan with coconut oil, arrange the meat and vegetables in the pan, and bake at 350°F for about 40 minutes. Some recipes may need slightly longer or shorter time than this, and you may have to experiment a bit to be sure the vegetables and meat are cooked but not overcooked. In the interest of simplicity, I do cook everything at the same time even though the result might be slightly better if I cooked meats and different vegetables for different lengths of time. For me, and perhaps for you, the "improvement" in doing this isn't really worth the effort when I want dinner to be simple. Most of the time, the pan version (and indeed, cooking everything at the same time in the pan) is just fine, and perfectly delicious.

GARLIC GOODNESS

Garlic is part of the sulfur category of vegetables. As you seek to meet your 9 cups of vegetables and fruits each day, as required on the Wahls Diet or Wahls Paleo (or 6 cups for Wahls Paleo Plus), you might be happy to learn that garlic gives you a lot of bang for your buck. Two garlic cloves equal 1 cup sulfur-rich vegetables, whether you are using them in a soup or a skillet or any other cooked dish. That means if your skillet serving contains just 2 garlic cloves, you have already fulfilled one of your required cups of vegetables for the day. Garlic has such strong benefits because it is a potent source of organic sulfur. The sulfur is what gives it its bite. Garlic improves detoxification efficiency, blood fluidity, and health of blood vessels, and it also reduces the risk of clogging of the arteries. It is a staple in my household, both for its flavor and its health benefits.

Garlic is also easy to prepare. Break apart a head of garlic by knocking it with the side of a large knife or just putting it on a cutting board and pressing on it with the heel of your hand. To peel individual cloves, put them on a cutting board, lay the side of a wide chef's knife or wooden spoon over them, and press on it with your hand to crush the clove. The peel will then slide right off. You can also put them through a sturdy garlic press without peeling them. Ideally, let the garlic rest for 5 to 15 minutes after you crush or chop the cloves to allow the sulfur compounds to complete their reaction prior to cooking.

BASIC SKILLET TEMPLATE

| MAKES 4 SERVINGS

TO MAKE: Heat the fat and a couple tablespoons of water, broth, or wine in a skillet over medium-high heat. (Adding water reduces the cooking temperature and cooks the food more gently than browning in fat, so it retains more of its micronutrients. You will see I do this frequently in skillet recipes.) Add the meat (ground, cut into bite-size pieces, or a whole piece) and seasonings, then cook to the desired level of doneness. Personally, I like my meat very rare, so that usually means just 1 to 2 minutes per side. My family likes their meat more done than I do, so I usually remove my meat first and cook theirs for 3 to 5 minutes per side. Of course, this depends on how thick the slice of meat is or how large the pieces are. Ground meat should always be cooked until no more pink remains.

Just a few minutes before the meat is done to your liking (the more you cook skillets, the better you will get at estimating when this is), add the vegetables. Because the vitamin C and antioxidants degrade after you cook vegetables longer than 5 minutes, I prefer to cook mine for just 2 minutes, no matter what kind of vegetables they are. If you

RECIPE CONTINUES

WAHLS WARRIORS SPEAK

I was diagnosed with aplastic anemia in 2010 and given three to six months to live. I decided to walk away from mainstream medicine and to research natural therapies. (I write about this on my blog, revivor.net, and in my book, *Beyond Terminal*.) I had read a lot of research from the cancer folks because they were the largest category of natural healers, and they were mainly recommending raw food, green food, and vegan diet. Well, I knew I couldn't do that. I was already having a hard time keeping food in me. When I read Dr. Wahls's book, I found that it was almost exactly the diet I was already doing. I was thrilled.... Dr. Wahls (and a few others) were recommending bone broth, fermented foods, and raw or barely cooked meat, along with lots of well-cooked vegetables and no sugar or gluten. I stand by that. Everybody is different, it's true, and each of us has to figure out for ourselves what works, but I believe that this is the best way to go for chronic illness. The raw movement includes a lot of fruit, and I don't support that. I had been including raw milk and kefir in my diet until recently, when I found they weren't working for me anymore, and now I have been off milk for a while, too. In general, I do lots of veggies for breakfast, lunch, and dinner, with some organic meat and fish, and either bitters or raw sauerkraut juice before each meal. I have just a small amount of carbs in the form of quinoa, sweet potatoes, and the like. I use coconut oil a lot, and also extra-virgin olive oil. I stay at around 147 pounds and I am sixty-four years old and doing well.

—Wahls Warrior CHRIS

only cook the vegetables for less than 5 minutes, they will still be a bit crisp, rather than mushy, which I also find enjoyable. If you prefer to cook your vegetables longer because you like them softer or your digestion is still adjusting to greater vegetable intake, that is fine. Cook them until they are suitable for you (up to 10 minutes or even a little longer), but consider gradually cooking them for a shorter time as your palate and digestion adjusts.

As soon as the vegetables start to look brightly colored and just begin to tenderize, add the garlic. If the greens have tender leaves (like spinach or mixed greens or baby kale), turn off the heat, stir them in, and allow them to wilt in the pan for 2 to 3 minutes. If they are tougher, like collard greens or kale, add them along with the other vegetables. I sometimes add whole mature kale leaves with my other vegetables and cook them so they remain quite firm. They are fun to eat with meat using steak knives. You can also chop the kale before cooking, if you prefer.

Serve immediately. Skillet meals also warm up nicely for lunch the next day. Store leftovers in individual serving containers in the refrigerator for up to 2 days or in the freezer for up to 2 months.

	WAHLS DIET	WAHLS PALEO	WAHLS PALEO PLUS
MEAT	1 pound any meat, ground, cut into bite-size pieces, or whole fillets, burgers, or brats (or equivalent in cooked legumes or quinoa)	1½ pounds	1 pound
VEGETABLES/ GREENS	12 cups	12 cups	8 cups
FAT	2 tablespoons ghee, extra-virgin olive oil, or coconut oil	2 tablespoons ghee, extra-virgin olive oil, or coconut oil	¼ cup coconut oil
SEASONINGS	As desired—stir garlic (if using) in at the end	As desired—stir garlic (if using) in at the end	As desired—stir garlic (if using) in at the end

CHICKEN-POTATO SKILLET

MAKES 4 SERVINGS

1 serving = 3 Wahls veg/fruit cups
1 serving = 2½ Wahls Paleo veg/fruit cups
1 serving = 2 Wahls Paleo Plus veg/fruit cups

TO MAKE: Heat half the coconut oil in a stockpot or large skillet over medium-high heat. Add the meat and cook until browned. Add the remaining oil plus two tablespoons water (or broth if you have it) to keep the cooking temperature lower. Add the potatoes, seasonings, and any thick leafy greens like collards or kale. Cook until the potatoes are fork-tender, 20 to 30 minutes. Add the vegetables, except tender leafy greens (young kale, chard, spinach). Cook for about 5 minutes more, until they are crisp-tender and brightly colored. Turn off the heat, stir in the tender greens, and serve.

	WAHLS DIET	WAHLS PALEO	WAHLS PALEO PLUS
MEAT	1 pound chicken breast, cut into strips or bite-size pieces	1½ pounds chicken breast, cut into strips or bite-size pieces	1 pound chicken breast, cut into strips or bite-size pieces
VEGETABLES/ GREENS	4 cups diced blue potatoes (or sweet potatoes or yams, if avoiding nightshades)	2 cups diced blue potatoes (or sweet potatoes or yams, if avoiding nightshades)	4 cups mature kale, coarsely chopped, or tender greens such as young kale, chard, or spinach
	4 cups mature kale, coarsely chopped, or tender greens such as young kale, chard, or spinach	4 cups mature kale, coarsely chopped, or tender greens such as young kale, chard, or spinach	2 cups chopped asparagus, cut into 1-inch pieces
	2 cups chopped asparagus, cut into 1-inch pieces	2 cups chopped asparagus, cut into 1-inch pieces	1 cup chopped onions
	1 cup chopped onions	1 cup chopped onions	1 cup sliced radishes
	1 cup sliced radishes	1 cup sliced radishes	
FAT	2 tablespoons coconut oil	2 tablespoons coconut oil	¼ cup coconut oil
SEASONINGS	1 teaspoon dried sage, or 1 tablespoon fresh	1 teaspoon dried sage, or 1 tablespoon fresh	1 teaspoon dried sage, or 1 tablespoon fresh
	1 teaspoon dried rosemary, or 1 tablespoon fresh	1 teaspoon dried rosemary, or 1 tablespoon fresh	1 teaspoon dried rosemary, or 1 tablespoon fresh
	1 teaspoon parsley, or 1 tablespoon gluten-free poultry seasoning	1 teaspoon fresh parsley, or 1 tablespoon gluten-free poultry seasoning	1 teaspoon fresh parsley, or 1 tablespoon gluten-free poultry seasoning
	½ teaspoon sea salt	½ teaspoon sea salt	½ teaspoon sea salt
	Freshly ground black pepper	Freshly ground black pepper	Freshly ground black pepper

STEAK AND MUSHROOM SKILLET

MAKES 4 SERVINGS
1 serving = 4 Wahls and Wahls Paleo veg/fruit cups
1 serving = 2½ Wahls Paleo Plus veg/fruit cups

TO MAKE: Quarter the turnips and boil for 20 minutes or until tender, then mash them with a tablespoon or two of the cooking water or run them through a food processor. Meanwhile, heat the fat plus two tablespoons water (or broth if you have it) in a skillet. Add the mushrooms and sauté for 2 to 5 minutes, then remove them from the pan and set aside. Add the steak strips to the skillet and cook until browned. Stir in the mustard greens (omitted for Wahls Paleo Plus), tarragon, and chili powder, and cook for 5 minutes more. Return the cooked mushrooms to the skillet, season with the salt and pepper to taste, and serve over the mashed turnips.

	WAHLS DIET	WAHLS PALEO	WAHLS PALEO PLUS
MEAT	1 pound steak, cut into strips	1½ pounds steak, cut into strips	1 pound steak, cut into strips
VEGETABLES/ GREENS	4 large turnips, trimmed	4 large turnips, trimmed	1 cup shiitake mushrooms, coarsely chopped
	1 cup shiitake mushrooms, coarsely chopped	1 cup shiitake mushrooms, coarsely chopped	1 cup fresh tarragon, chopped
	6 cups mustard greens	6 cups mustard greens	
	1 cup fresh tarragon, chopped	1 cup fresh tarragon, chopped	
FAT	1 tablespoon ghee	1 tablespoon ghee	1 tablespoon ghee
	2 tablespoons coconut oil		¼ cup coconut oil
SEASONINGS	1 tablespoon chili powder	1 tablespoon chili powder	1 tablespoon chili powder
	½ teaspoon sea salt	½ teaspoon sea salt	½ teaspoon sea salt
	Freshly ground black pepper	Freshly ground black pepper	Freshly ground black pepper

Note for Wahls Paleo Plus: If eating boiled turnips takes you out of ketosis, skip the turnip cooking instructions and instead, add grated raw turnips to the skillet right before removing from the heat.

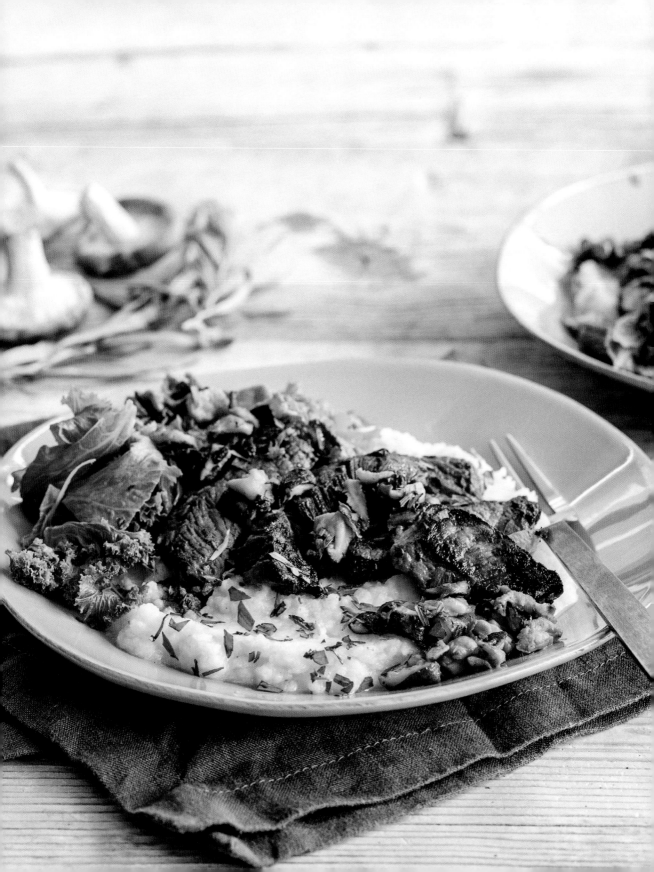

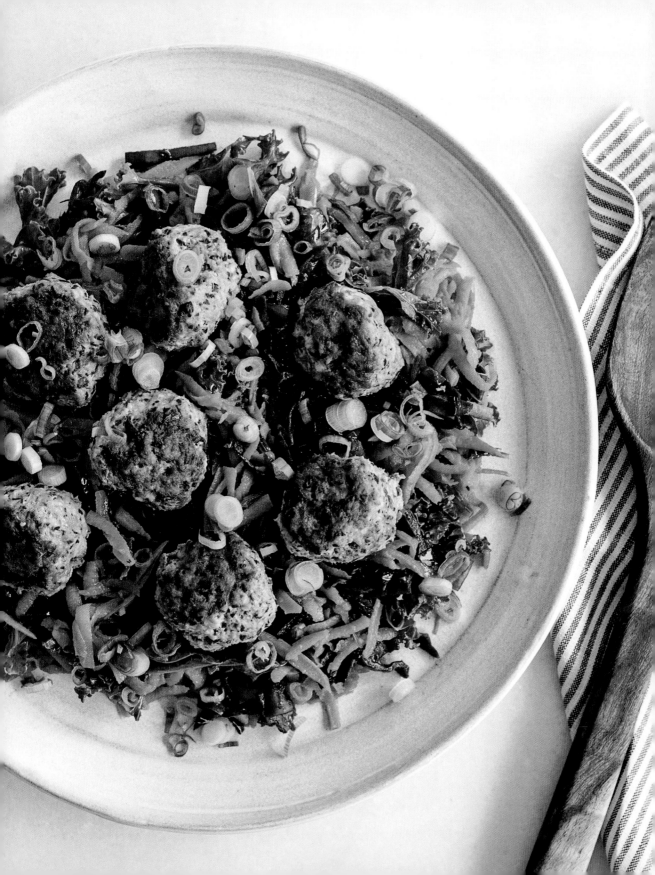

TURKEY MEATBALL SKILLET

MAKES 4 SERVINGS

1 serving = 3½ Wahls and Wahls Paleo veg/fruit cups

1 serving = 3¼ Wahls Paleo Plus veg/fruit cups

TO MAKE: Put the oregano, savory, and parsley in a food processor and pulse until minced. Remove half of the minced herbs and set aside. Add the ground turkey, salt, and pepper to the minced herbs in the food processor and process until the herbs are well mixed into the meat. Form the turkey mixture into meatballs.

Heat the fat, plus two tablespoons water (or broth if you have it) to keep the cooking temperature lower, in a stockpot or large skillet over medium heat. Add the meatballs. Add the reserved herb mixture, scallions, garlic, yams, cabbage, and kale to the skillet. Cook until the meat is done and the veggies are tender, 10 to 15 minutes.

RECIPE CONTINUES

WAHLS WARRIORS SPEAK

I would like to share my experience with my retina specialist at UC Davis today. I have been seeing this person for years for my intermediate uveitis, which led to a diagnosis of MS years ago. When I first told this person I did not want to take Methotrexate after steroid injections for my eye disease, he told me that I would not be able to bring down the inflammation without it. I told him about your protocol, and although he said very little, he agreed that we could try it and see what happens. Today, he told me that my progress is "really very remarkable." The nurses asked me for your name, and they said they had two other patients on your protocol. They are very impressed with how I am doing. I am so thankful for this information you share! Thank you!

—Wahls Warrior DONNA

	WAHLS DIET	WAHLS PALEO	WAHLS PALEO PLUS
MEAT	1 pound ground turkey	1½ pounds ground turkey	1 pound ground turkey
VEGETABLES/ GREENS	3 cups grated orange yams or sweet potatoes	4 cups chopped kale	4 cups chopped kale
	3 cups chopped red cabbage	3 cups grated orange yams or sweet potatoes	3 cups grated orange yams or sweet potatoes (stir in the grated raw yams or sweet potatoes just prior to serving so that they remain raw)
	4 cups chopped kale	3 cups chopped red cabbage	
	½ cup minced scallion (white and green parts)	½ cup minced scallion (white and green parts)	2 cups chopped red cabbage
	3 garlic cloves, minced	3 garlic cloves, minced	½ cup minced scallion (white and green parts)
			3 garlic cloves, minced
FAT	2 tablespoons ghee	2 tablespoons ghee	¼ cup coconut oil
SEASONINGS	1 cup fresh oregano	1 cup fresh oregano	1 cup fresh oregano
	½ cup fresh savory	½ cup fresh savory	½ cup fresh savory
	½ cup fresh parsley	½ cup fresh parsley	½ cup fresh parsley
	½ teaspoon sea salt	½ teaspoon sea salt	½ teaspoon sea salt
	Freshly ground black pepper	Freshly ground black pepper	Freshly ground black pepper

Note for Wahls Paleo Plus: Do not cook the yams. Instead, serve the meal on a bed of raw grated yams, which will warm up nicely and soak up the juices from the skillet without actually cooking and developing too much starch.

GROUND BISON SKILLET

MAKES 4 SERVINGS
1 serving = 3 Wahls and Wahls Paleo veg/fruit cups
1 serving = 2¼ Wahls Paleo Plus veg/fruit cups

TO MAKE: Put the oregano leaves in a food processor and pulse until minced. Add the bison meat and process until the herbs are thoroughly mixed into the meat. Form the mixture into four patties. Add the coconut oil, plus two tablespoons water (or broth if you have it) to keep the cooking temperature lower, to a stockpot or large skillet and heat over medium-high heat. Add the bison patties, fresh minced herbs of your choice, and the remaining vegetables except the salad greens to the skillet. Cook the patties for 8 to 10 minutes, flipping them once or twice, until cooked through, while stirring the vegetables around the patties until they are crisp-tender. Serve on a bed of salad greens.

	WAHLS DIET	WAHLS PALEO	WAHLS PALEO PLUS
MEAT	1 pound ground bison	1½ pounds ground bison	1 pound ground bison
VEGETABLES/GREENS	6 cups mixed salad greens	6 cups mixed salad greens	4 cups mixed salad greens
	2 cups chopped asparagus, cut into 1-inch pieces	2 cups chopped asparagus, cut into 1-inch pieces	1½ cups chopped asparagus cut into 1-inch pieces
	2 cups broccoli, cut into bite-size pieces	2 cups broccoli, cut into bite-size pieces	1½ cups broccoli, cut into bite-size pieces
	1 cup coarsely chopped onion	1 cup coarsely chopped onion	1 cup coarsely chopped onion
	1 cup fresh oregano leaves	1 cup fresh oregano leaves	1 cup fresh oregano leaves
FAT	2 tablespoons coconut oil or ghee	2 tablespoons coconut oil or ghee	¼ cup coconut oil
SEASONINGS	2 cups fresh minced herbs (such as garlic, chives, savory, parsley, and oregano)	2 cup fresh minced herbs (such as garlic, chives, savory, parsley and oregano)	¼ cup fresh minced herbs (such as garlic, chives, savory, parsley and oregano)

LAMB BURGER SKILLET

MAKES 4 SERVINGS

1 serving = 3½ Wahls and Wahls Paleo veg/fruit cups

1 serving = 2½ Wahls Paleo Plus veg/fruit cups

TO MAKE: Place the parsley and rosemary in a food processor and pulse until minced. Add the ground lamb and process until the herbs are well mixed into the meat. Form the lamb into small patties. Add the ghee (or coconut oil, for Wahls Paleo Plus), plus two tablespoons water (or broth if you have it) to keep the cooking temperature lower, to a stockpot or large skillet and heat over medium-high heat. Add the patties and cook to the desired level of doneness, 2 minutes per side for rare, 3 to 5 minutes per side for well-done. Add the remaining vegetables when you have about 5 minutes left for the meat to cook to the desired level of doneness. Sauté the vegetables for 5 minutes. Remove the skillet from the heat. Finally, combine the olive oil and Fermented Garlic Ginger Sauce in a small bowl and whisk to make a sauce. Plate the skillet meal and drizzle the sauce over the top of each serving.

	WAHLS DIET	WAHLS PALEO	WAHLS PALEO PLUS
MEAT	1 pound ground lamb	1½ pounds ground lamb	1 pound ground lamb
VEGETABLES/ GREENS	6 cups chopped curly kale	6 cups chopped curly kale	4 cups chopped curly kale
	4 cups chopped red cabbage	4 cups chopped red cabbage	3 cups chopped red cabbage
	2 cups coarsely chopped onion	2 cups coarsely chopped onion	1 cup coarsely chopped onion
FAT	1 tablespoon ghee	1 tablespoon ghee	¼ cup coconut oil
	1 tablespoon extra-virgin olive oil	1 tablespoon extra-virgin olive oil	1 tablespoon extra-virgin olive oil
SEASONINGS	2 cups fresh parsley and rosemary leaves	2 cups fresh parsley and rosemary leaves	2 cups fresh parsley and rosemary leaves
	¼ cup Fermented Garlic Ginger Sauce (page 34) or 2 tablespoons minced garlic and 2 tablespoons minced ginger	¼ cup Fermented Garlic Ginger Sauce (page 34) or 2 tablespoons minced garlic and 2 tablespoons minced ginger	¼ cup Fermented Garlic Ginger Sauce (page 34) or 2 tablespoons minced garlic and 2 tablespoons minced ginger

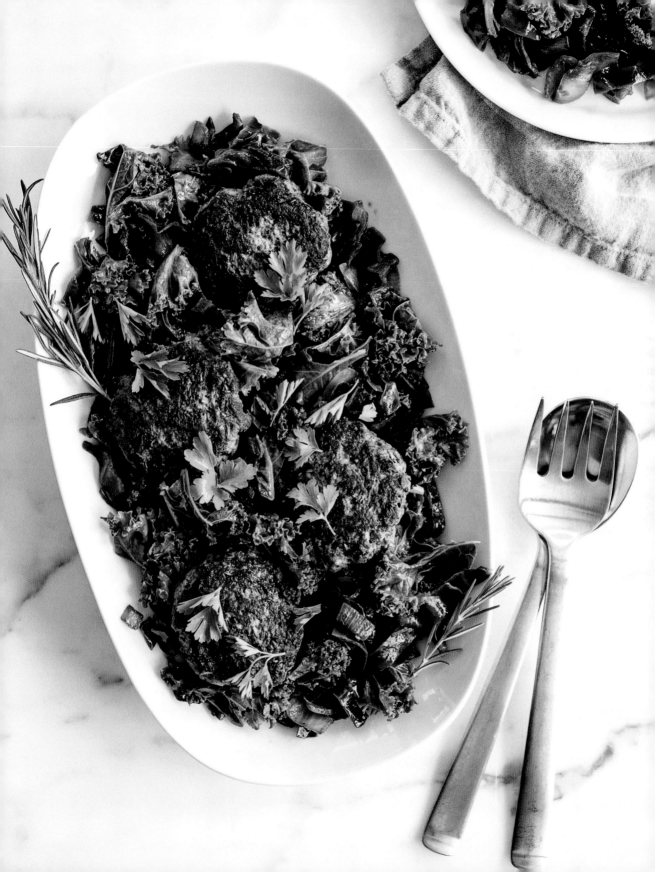

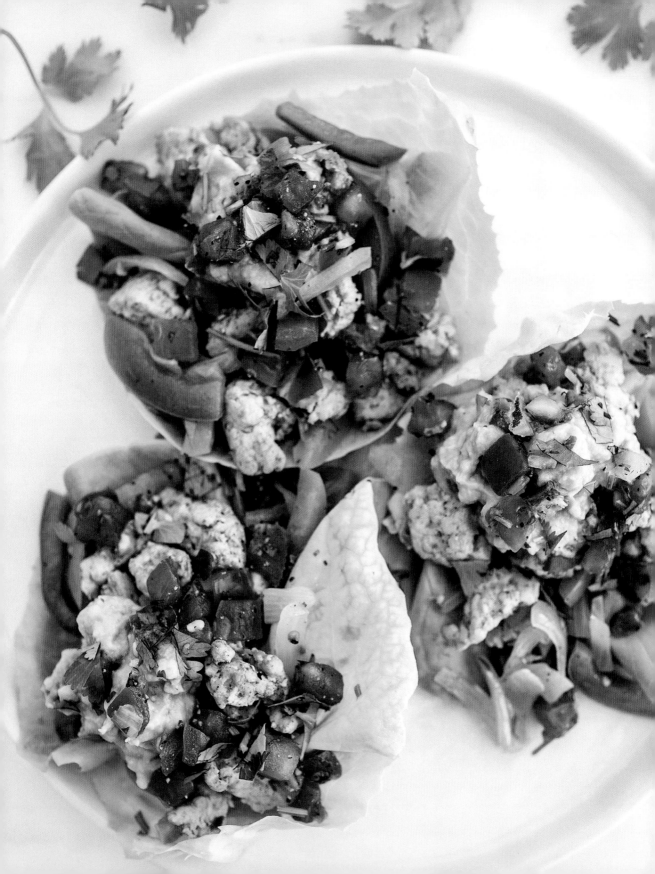

This recipe isn't a typical skillet recipe because instead of preparing your greens with the other ingredients in a stockpot or large skillet, you use the greens as a taco "shell." Butter lettuce and Boston lettuce or other greens, like mature curly kale or collard leaves (which you can eat raw for this recipe) work well.

TURKEY TACOS

MAKES 4 SERVINGS
1 serving = 2½ Wahls veg/fruit cups
1 serving = 3 Wahls Paleo veg/fruit cups
1 serving = 1¾ Wahls Paleo Plus veg/fruit cups

TO MAKE: Heat the ghee in a stockpot or large skillet over medium-high heat. Add the ground turkey, taco seasoning, bell peppers, garlic, and onions. Cook until the turkey is browned and the vegetables are tender, 10 to 12 minutes. Serve the cilantro and hot sauce on the side, or stir them directly into the skillet. Divide the taco filling among eight large leaf wrappers (lettuce, kale, or collards). Add salsa and/or guacamole. Roll up or fold up and enjoy. Alternatively, serve the filling on a bed of greens as a taco salad.

Cooking Tip: You don't need to add water or broth to the fat when you are cooking the meat for this meal.

RECIPE CONTINUES

	WAHLS DIET	WAHLS PALEO	WAHLS PALEO PLUS
MEAT	1 pound ground turkey	1½ pounds ground turkey	1 pound ground turkey
VEGETABLES/ GREENS	3 cups thinly sliced bell peppers	4 cups thinly sliced bell peppers	2 cups thinly sliced bell peppers
	3 cups thinly sliced onion	4 cups thinly sliced onion	2 cups thinly sliced onion
	3 garlic cloves, minced	3 garlic cloves, minced	3 garlic cloves, minced
	8 large lettuce, kale, or collard leaves	8 large lettuce, kale, or collard leaves	8 large lettuce, kale, or collard leaves
FAT	2 tablespoons ghee	2 tablespoons ghee	¼ cup coconut oil
SEASONINGS	1 tablespoon taco seasoning (read the label closely to be sure no gluten or flavorings are listed, or use my recipe on page 45)	1 tablespoon taco seasoning (read the label closely to be sure no gluten or flavorings are listed, or use my recipe on page 45)	1 tablespoon taco seasoning (read the label closely to be sure no gluten or flavorings are listed, or use my recipe on page 45)
	½ cup chopped fresh cilantro	½ cup chopped fresh cilantro	½ cup chopped fresh cilantro
	Hot sauce (optional—use any kind you like that is gluten-free)	Hot sauce (optional—use any kind you like that is gluten-free)	Hot sauce (optional—use any kind you like that is gluten-free)
	Fresh Salsa (page 45) and/or Wahls Guacamole (page 48)	Fresh Salsa (page 45) and/or Wahls Guacamole (page 48)	Fresh Salsa (page 45) and/or Wahls Guacamole (page 48)

WAHLS WARRIORS SPEAK

My husband, Larry, was diagnosed in the fall of 2013 with stage 4 head and neck cancer. It started in his tonsil, spread into the surrounding lymph nodes, and then metastasized to his lungs. We started on the Wahls Protocol even before Larry began treatment, which consisted of eight months of a combination of "the big guns" (chemo and radiation therapy) since his prognosis wasn't very good at that time. Larry was able to stay in ketosis for almost the entire treatment period, which we believe helped strengthen his body throughout the very harsh treatment. Happily, I am able to report that Larry has now been cancer-free for over two years!

After the treatment was complete, we began to add a few more carbs to Larry's diet, but he is still eating a diet free of dairy, wheat, and processed foods, and only very small amounts of natural sweeteners (honey, dates, sorghum, and maple syrup). He does enjoy grains other than wheat, like quinoa and brown rice.

Making the transition to this diet was very difficult, I must say. What we would eat on a given day used to be the first thing I thought of upon awakening and the last thing I thought about as I was nodding off to sleep. But because Larry's prognosis was so poor, I really felt that making this transition to better eating was a matter of life or death for Larry. Now that we've both been eating this way for nearly three years, it has become much easier, and making food for the day seems part of the routine. I shop in a different way than I did before, at different stores with more organic foods. I use "The Clean 15" as a guide for buying fruits and vegetables to try to keep things affordable. We start each day with a big smoothie made in the Vitamix with lots of greens and a few fruits. This gives us a jump start on getting enough vegetables and fruits in each day.

Some other tips that may be helpful to others:

Make small changes. Don't try to give up everything at once.

Use Pinterest and Google to find new recipes. Most have reviews you can check out in advance to see how others might have tweaked a recipe to make it even better.

Many recipes call for heavy cream or milk. It is easy to substitute coconut milk. We don't notice much difference. I also substitute ghee for butter and make my own fresh tomato sauce in the Vitamix instead of buying canned.

Put some extra effort into making your plate of food *look* appealing as well as taste good. It takes time to cook, so I want our food to satisfy our visual sense as well as our appetite. I do this by making sure there are a lot of colorful fruits and vegetables, as well as a pleasing serving dish.

Dessert is important to us. It's different now than what it used to be, but we rarely skip dessert and find we are satisfied with only a little bit of something sweet, such as a small dish of chia pudding, pistachios, or maybe just a couple of dates to satisfy the sweet tooth.

I make large quantities and then freeze portions to pull out for easy meals during the week.

I find we eat more spicy and ethnic recipes than we had previously. The extra spice makes the food more interesting and many spices, such as turmeric, are especially good for cancer prevention.

I *love* our Vitamix! We use it every day.

—Wahls Warriors SARAH AND LARRY

BRATS SKILLET

MAKES 4 SERVINGS

1 serving = 3 Wahls and Wahls Paleo veg/fruit cups

1 serving = 2 Wahls Paleo Plus veg/fruit cups

TO MAKE: Boil the brats for 10 minutes, then slice them. Heat the fat in a large skillet or stockpot over medium-high heat. Add the mushrooms, onion, and sliced brats and sauté until the mushrooms are soft and the onions are translucent, 2 to 5 minutes. Add the garlic and cook, stirring, for 2 minutes. Add the cabbage and cook for 5 minutes more. Remove from the heat and stir in the mustard greens and oregano. Cover and let the skillet sit for 2 minutes.

Serve with sriracha or spicy kimchi, if desired.

	WAHLS DIET	WAHLS PALEO	WAHLS PALEO PLUS
MEAT	4 bratwursts (to equal about 1 pound)	6 bratwursts (to equal about 1½ pounds)	4 bratwursts (to equal about 1 pound)
VEGETABLES/ GREENS	1 cup sliced shiitake mushrooms	1 cup sliced shiitake mushrooms	½ cup sliced shiitake mushrooms
	½ cup coarsely chopped onion	½ cup coarsely chopped onion	½ cup coarsely chopped onion
	8 garlic cloves, minced or put through a garlic press	8 garlic cloves, minced or put through a garlic press	4 garlic cloves, minced or put through a garlic press
	2 cups chopped red cabbage	2 cups chopped red cabbage	½ cup chopped red cabbage
	4 cups chopped mustard greens	4 cups chopped mustard greens	4 cups chopped mustard greens
	½ cup chopped fresh oregano	½ cup chopped fresh oregano	½ cup chopped fresh oregano
FAT	2 tablespoons ghee	2 tablespoons ghee	¼ cup coconut oil
SEASONINGS	Sriracha or spicy kimchi (optional)	Sriracha or spicy kimchi (optional)	Sriracha or spicy kimchi (optional)

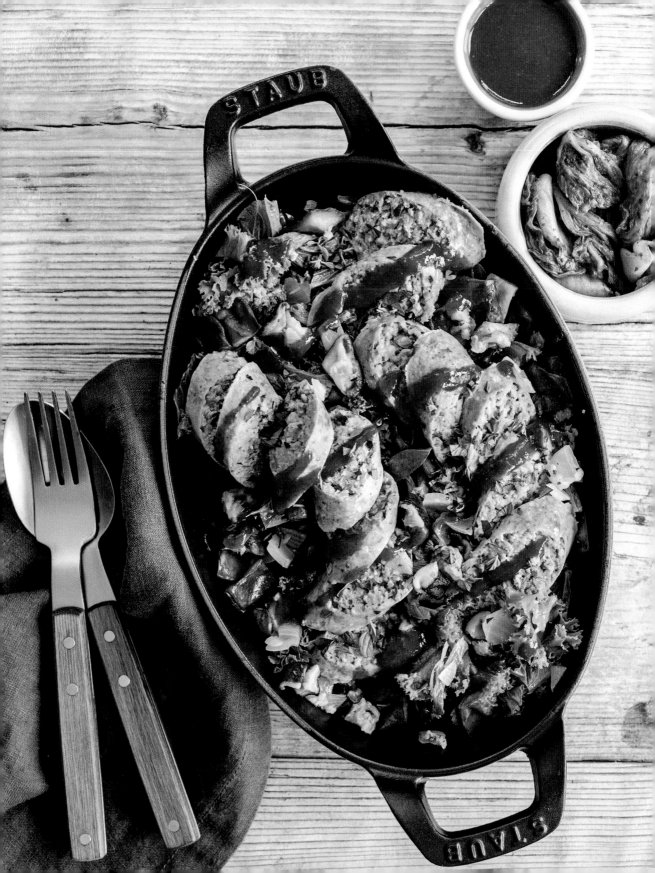

PORK CHOP SKILLET

MAKES 4 SERVINGS

1 serving = 3 Wahls and Wahls Paleo veg/fruit cups

1 serving = 2 Wahls Paleo Plus veg/fruit cups

TO MAKE: Heat 1 tablespoon of the fat, plus two tablespoons water (or broth if you have it) to keep the cooking temperature lower, in a large stockpot or skillet over medium heat. Add the pork chops and cook for about 5 minutes on each side (if you have a meat thermometer, cook them until they register 140°F). Season with half the salt and pepper, and remove them from the heat. Set aside on a plate and tent with aluminum foil. Let stand for 10 to 15 minutes. (The meat will continue to cook and the temperature will rise another 5 degrees as it stands.)

Meanwhile, heat the remaining fat, water, or broth in a pot or skillet and sauté the asparagus and onions until the asparagus is bright green and tender, and the onions are translucent, 2 to 5 minutes. Season with the remaining salt and pepper. Turn off the heat, add the spring greens, and stir for about 1 minute. Divide the asparagus mixture among four plates.

Put the ingredients for the sauce in a Vitamix or other high-speed blender and blend until well combined. Put the pork chops on top of the asparagus mixture. Drizzle the sauce over the pork chops and vegetables. Serve immediately.

	WAHLS DIET	WAHLS PALEO	WAHLS PALEO PLUS
MEAT	4 pork chops (to equal about 1 pound; weight can be higher if you get them with the bones)	4 pork chops (to equal about 1½ pounds; weight can be higher if you get them with the bones)	4 pork chops (to equal about 1 pound; weight can be higher if you get them with the bones)
VEGETABLES/ GREENS	4 cups chopped asparagus, cut into 1-inch pieces	4 cups chopped asparagus, cut into 1-inch pieces	3 cups chopped asparagus, cut into 1-inch pieces
	4 cups coarsely chopped onion	4 cups coarsely chopped onion	1 cup coarsely chopped onion
	4 cups spring greens	4 cups spring greens	4 cups spring greens
FAT	2 tablespoons ghee	2 tablespoons ghee	2 tablespoons coconut oil
SEASONINGS	½ teaspoon sea salt	½ teaspoon sea salt	½ teaspoon sea salt
	Freshly ground black pepper	Freshly ground black pepper	Freshly ground black pepper
	For the sauce:	For the sauce:	For the sauce:
	¼ cup extra-virgin olive oil	¼ cup extra-virgin olive oil	2 tablespoons extra-virgin olive oil
	1 garlic clove, minced	1 garlic clove, minced	2 tablespoons coconut oil
	2 tablespoons chopped fresh chives	2 tablespoons chopped fresh chives	1 garlic clove, minced
			2 tablespoons chopped fresh chives

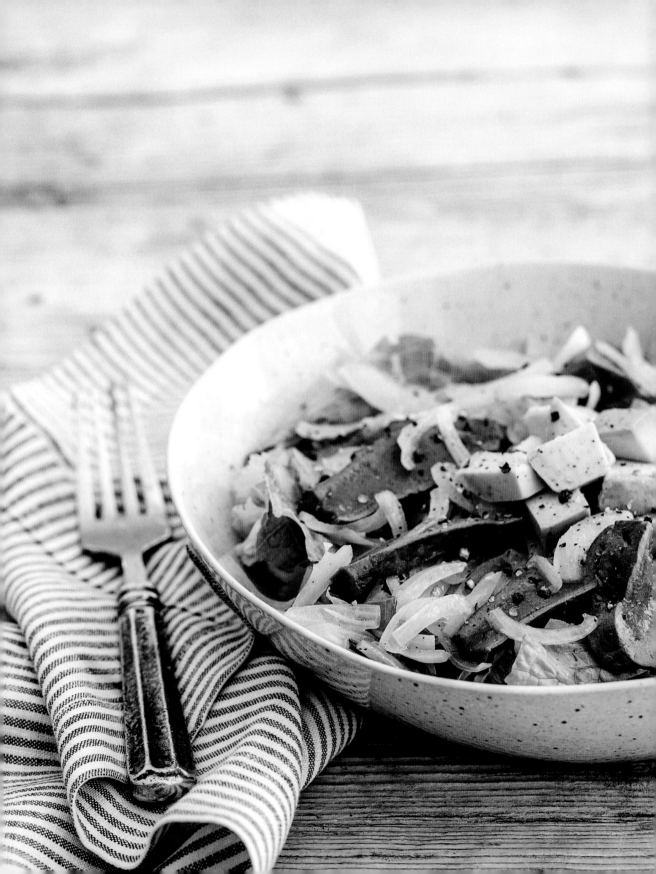

Not everybody loves liver, but I really enjoy it now. I make this recipe with bison liver, but it can be difficult to find, and may not be to everyone's taste. Chicken liver is the mildest of all the available types of liver, so if you are a liver newbie, start with chicken liver and see how you like it in this recipe. The flavors, especially the onion, mellow the taste of the liver and make it more palatable. Lamb liver is also very mild. It is important that the liver be organic, however. Conventionally grown animals will more likely have metabolic syndrome and a less healthy liver. They are also more likely to have toxins stored in the fat and in the liver.

It's preferable nutritionally to cook liver until medium-rare. It should be a little pink in the middle. If you overcook the liver it becomes leathery, dry, and difficult to eat. That's the texture most people associate with liver, but if you cook it well (as opposed to well-done), it is tender and very tasty. In this recipe, the onions really bring a great flavor to the dish. Note that whenever I make liver, I also make twice the amount I need and use the rest to make Wahls Pâté (page 40).

BISON LIVER SKILLET WITH SAUTÉED ONIONS

MAKES 4 SERVINGS
1 serving = 4¼ Wahls and Wahls Paleo veg/fruit cups
1 serving = 2¾ Wahls Paleo Plus veg/fruit cups

TO MAKE: If the liver is not already sliced, slice it into ½- to 1-inch-thick slices. Heat the fat in a large skillet or soup pot over medium-high heat. Add the onions and half the salt and pepper, and cook until tender and translucent, about 5 minutes. Transfer the onions to a bowl and cover, then add the liver to the skillet, adding more fat as needed if the pan is dry. Add the ginger and remaining salt and pepper. Cook for about 5 minutes, until medium-rare, flipping occasionally but watching closely to avoid overcooking. Stir the garlic in with the liver after it is cooked, then return the onions to the pan.

Divide the lettuce among four plates or bowls. Top with the liver and onions, and top the liver with avocado slices.

RECIPE CONTINUES

	WAHLS DIET	WAHLS PALEO	WAHLS PALEO PLUS
MEAT	1 pound bison, lamb, beef, pork, or chicken livers	1½ pounds bison, lamb, beef, pork, or chicken livers	1 pound bison, lamb, beef, pork, or chicken livers
VEGETABLES/ GREENS	4 cups sliced yellow onion (2 large onions)	4 cups sliced yellow onion (2 large onions)	2 cups sliced yellow onion (1 large onion)
	6 garlic cloves, minced or put through a garlic press	6 garlic cloves, minced or put through a garlic press	6 garlic cloves, minced or put through a garlic press
	8 cups romaine lettuce, torn into bite-size pieces	8 cups romaine lettuce, torn into bite-size pieces	4 cups romaine lettuce, torn into bite-size pieces
	2 avocados, pitted, peeled, and sliced	2 avocados, pitted, peeled, and sliced	2 avocados, pitted, peeled, and sliced
FAT	1 tablespoon coconut oil	1 tablespoon coconut oil	¼ cup coconut oil
	1 tablespoon ghee	1 tablespoon ghee	
SEASONINGS	1 teaspoon sea salt	1 teaspoon sea salt	1 teaspoon sea salt
	Freshly ground black pepper	Freshly ground black pepper	Freshly ground black pepper
	1 (2-inch) piece fresh ginger, peeled and grated	1 (2-inch) piece fresh ginger, peeled and grated	1 (2-inch) piece fresh ginger, peeled and grated

BACK BACON WITH GREENS, CRANBERRIES, AND BALSAMIC VINEGAR

MAKES 4 SERVINGS

1 serving = 3 Wahls and Wahls Paleo veg/fruit cups

1 serving = 2 Wahls Paleo Plus veg/fruit cups

TO MAKE: Cook the bacon in a skillet or stockpot for about 10 minutes or until it is as crispy as desired. Remove with a slotted spoon and drain up to half the rendered fat from the skillet. Add the coconut oil to the skillet, stir in the garlic and cranberries, and cook for 1 minute. Remove from the heat and stir in the greens, vinegar, and cooked bacon. Stir until the greens have wilted. Serve immediately.

	WAHLS DIET	WAHLS PALEO	WAHLS PALEO PLUS
MEAT	1 pound back bacon, cut into ½-inch cubes or coarsely chopped	1½ pounds back bacon, cut into ½-inch cubes or coarsely chopped	1 pound back bacon, cut into ½-inch cubes or coarsely chopped
VEGETABLES/ GREENS	8 garlic cloves, minced	8 garlic cloves, minced	4 garlic cloves, minced
	2 cups fresh or thawed frozen cranberries, coarsely chopped	2 cups fresh or thawed frozen cranberries, coarsely chopped	1 cup fresh or thawed frozen cranberries, coarsely chopped
	6 cups dandelion greens or mustard greens	6 cups dandelion greens or mustard greens	5 cups dandelion greens or mustard greens
FAT	2 tablespoons coconut oil or ghee	2 tablespoons coconut oil or ghee	¼ cup coconut oil
SEASONINGS	2 tablespoons balsamic vinegar	2 tablespoons balsamic vinegar	2 tablespoons fresh lime juice

Cooking Tip: Do not use water or broth when browning the bacon, as it could cause the rendered fat to spatter. Also, you want the bacon to get crispy, and liquid will prevent this.

PORK SAUSAGE WITH CABBAGE AND YAMS

MAKES 4 SERVINGS
1 serving = 3 Wahls and Wahls Paleo veg/fruit cups
1 serving = 2½ Wahls Paleo Plus veg/fruit cups

TO MAKE: Brown the pork sausage in a stockpot or large skillet over medium heat until no pink remains, about 6 minutes. Stir in the garlic and cook for 1 minute. Stir in the yams (see note for Wahls Paleo Plus), cabbage, ginger, coconut aminos, fennel seeds, lime juice, and black pepper. Cook until everything is tender but not mushy, about 5 minutes. Serve immediately.

	WAHLS DIET	WAHLS PALEO	WAHLS PALEO PLUS
MEAT	1 pound ground pork sausage or plain ground pork	1½ pounds ground pork sausage or plain ground pork	1 pound ground pork sausage or plain ground pork
VEGETABLES/ GREENS	8 garlic cloves, minced or put through a garlic press	8 garlic cloves, minced or put through a garlic press	6 garlic cloves, minced or put through a garlic press
	4 cups grated red and/or purple yams	4 cups grated red and/or purple yams	4 cups grated red and/or purple yams (or carrots), stirred in just before serving so they remain raw
	4 cups grated green and/or purple cabbage	4 cups grated green and/or purple cabbage	3 cups grated green and/or purple cabbage
FAT	If the pork is very lean, you may add up to 2 tablespoons ghee or coconut oil	If the pork is very lean, you may add up to 2 tablespoons ghee or coconut oil	If the pork is very lean, you may add up to ¼ cup coconut oil
SEASONINGS	1 (2-inch) piece fresh ginger, peeled and grated	1 (2-inch) piece fresh ginger, peeled and grated	1 (2-inch) piece fresh ginger, peeled and grated
	1 tablespoon coconut aminos	1 tablespoon coconut aminos	1 tablespoon coconut aminos
	2 teaspoons fennel seeds	2 teaspoons fennel seeds	2 teaspoons fennel seeds
	Juice of 1 lime	Juice of 1 lime	Freshly ground black pepper
	Freshly ground black pepper	Freshly ground black pepper	

Note for Wahls Paleo Plus: Add the yams at the very end so that they are still raw when you eat them. Or you can serve the skillet meal over a bed of grated raw yams.

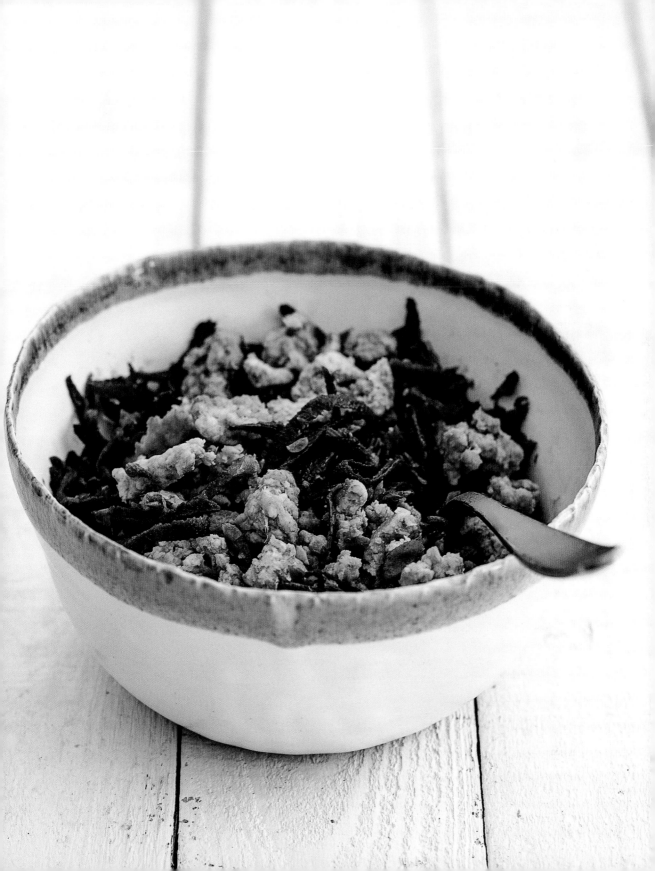

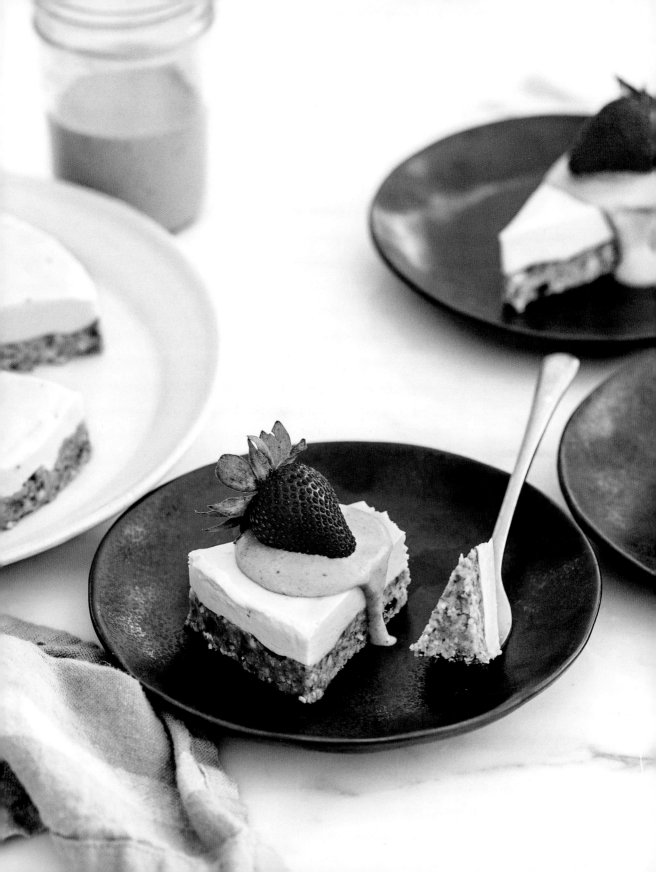

DELECTABLE DESSERTS

SUGAR CAN BE HARD TO RESIST, but we come by the preference naturally. We are programmed to prefer sweet tastes so that we survive. Breast milk is high in fat and milk sugars, so babies come into the world craving sweets, and most of us never lose that early proclivity (one reason why vanilla ice cream is so popular). Yet eating sugar is disruptive to our gut microbiome, encouraging the growth of yeast and bacteria that are less favorable for immune health. This is one of the reasons why I restrict sugars, including natural sugars and simple carbohydrates, at all levels of the Wahls Protocol—and do so even more drastically at the Wahls Paleo Plus level.

Although a more natural diet is one of the goals of the Paleo movement, I see many Paleo food bloggers and authors making delicious, gluten-free, dairy-free, refined-sugar-free desserts that are actually quite sweet. Cakes, cookies, sweet breads, even pies are all delicious and can be "Paleo" (although it is hard for me to imagine a Paleolithic human eating cookies . . .). The problem with these delicious desserts is that they are usually high in calories that come from refined carbohydrates and relatively low in the vitamins, minerals, antioxidants, and micronutrients we need to thrive. Many of these desserts rely on refined white flour (even if it is gluten-free) and fructose-based sweeteners. I'm not that keen on nut-based and other gluten-free flours, or fructose-based sweeteners, as they are not only quite expensive but generally lack the fiber that the good bacteria in our bowels need to flourish. I would much rather people spent their money and time on eating more (and a more diverse selection of) vegetables. Retraining our taste buds is key to achieving the best possible health for you and your family.

After you have escaped the sugar trap, you will find that when you reintroduce even low-sugar fruits like berries, they will taste remarkably sweet and satisfying to you. For my patients who struggle with sugar, I usually suggest a course of two or three months eliminating added sugar (including coconut sugar, date sugar, date syrup, agave syrup, honey, and maple syrup) and even fruit if they want to speed up the process. This elimination helps starve out the sugar-loving bacteria and yeast (*Candida albicans*) and allows your taste to acclimate. I also recommend avoiding all artificial sweeteners, including so-called healthful sweeteners with very few calories such as stevia and birch xylitol, so the brain as well as the taste buds can adjust to food that is not sweetened. Instead, rely on whole foods—whole vegetables, nuts, seeds, and spices—to create a sweeter experience.

After your no-sweetener period, you can go back to the occasional sweet treat, including fruit or any of the desserts in this chapter. You will find your taste for them has decreased and you will likely find that your tastes have changed, and that you prefer much less sweetness in your treats. Traditionally sweet desserts may become too sweet for you—that is progress! Let sweets be for special occasions, not for every day, and your body (especially your gut bacteria) will be the better for it.

You may think you will never be able to give up sugar, but fortunately, it is much easier than some people might lead you to believe. The first few days are the hardest, but after that, many of my patients report that, much to their pleasure and astonishment, their tastes do, in fact, change. They appreciate flavors differently and they have lost their cravings for sugar. For some, this transformation occurs within weeks. For others, it takes several months.

You will find that the desserts in this chapter are less sweet than typical sugary desserts. If you have gone through a two-month elimination of sugar or fruit, you may be surprised to discover that you find the Wahls Paleo Plus variations (which do not have any sweeteners) quite satisfying, and that you enjoy them immensely. I do occasionally make the Wahls Diet and Wahls Paleo versions of the desserts in this chapter, even when they have small amounts of sweeteners. It works for me if I don't do it very often. You can decide the level that works best for you and your family.

But at the risk of sounding repetitious, I do encourage you to work to continually reduce the sugar/sweetener content in your diet, and to work toward eliminating them entirely. This one change will be of great benefit to your health. You will quickly starve out disease-promoting yeasts, nourishing a healthier mix of bacteria living in your bowels. You will find that you enjoy the subtle flavors in your foods much more than you did before. You will also find that herbs, spices, and other seasonings that have a bit of heat to them (like mint, cinnamon, ginger, and hot peppers) will cut the bitterness in foods and make them seem sweeter.

It may seem impossible that you will ever get to this point, but the journey away from sweeteners is just that—a journey. Take it one day at a time, move generally in the right direction, and your body will keep healing and working better. (For even more delicious desserts, see chapter 11, the Holiday chapter, which includes seasonal desserts for various occasions.)

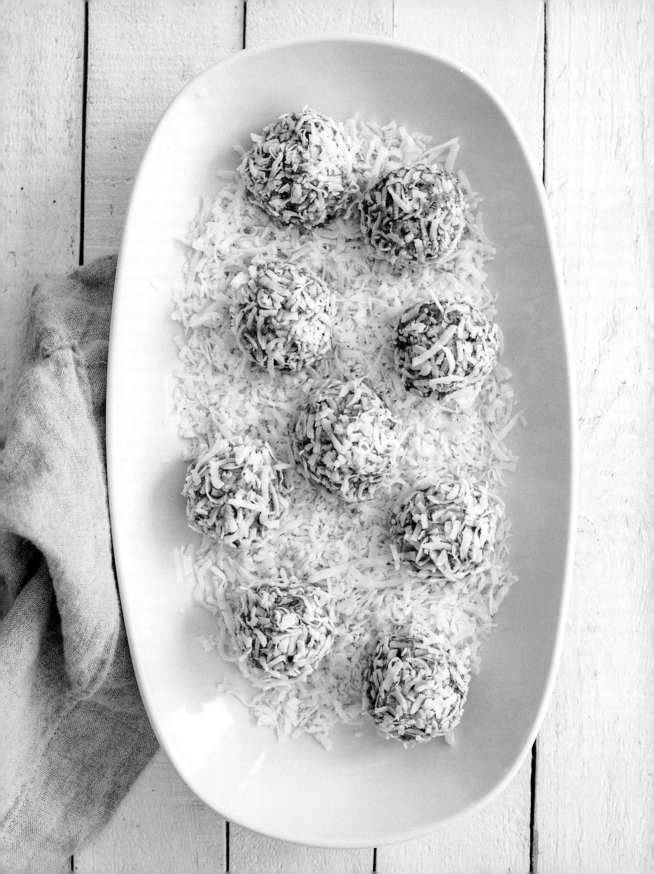

This is a delicious candylike treat, perfect for the holidays or whenever you feel like having something sweet. Make this chocolate version or try the vanilla variation on the next page. You can also vary the spices. Note that the cocoa is bitter, so start with a small amount and increase to taste. As for nut choices, pecans work well in this recipe. Walnuts are also a good choice if they are soaked first, to remove some of the bitter compounds they contain. If you use walnuts, soak them overnight, then drain, rinse, and pat them dry. Use them immediately in this recipe, or, if you aren't going to use them right away, place them in a dehydrator on the lowest setting possible and dehydrate overnight, or dry them in an oven on a baking sheet at the lowest possible setting until they are completely dry. (Stored soaked nuts that are still wet can develop mold.)

CHOCOLATE SNOWBALLS

MAKES 16 PIECES

TO MAKE: Combine all the ingredients except the dried coconut flakes in a food processor and process until thoroughly mixed. Place the mixture in the refrigerator for 10 to 30 minutes to firm it up and make it easier to shape. Form the mixture into small balls (1½ to 2 inches in diameter), then roll them in the coconut flakes. Place them on a baking sheet and freeze for 4 hours and up to overnight to harden. You can also freeze these in mini-muffin tins if you don't want to shape them. It's a faster method and easier to store in the freezer. Serve frozen.

RECIPE CONTINUES

	WAHLS DIET	WAHLS PALEO	WAHLS PALEO PLUS
NUTS	1½ cups pecans or sprouted dehydrated walnuts	1½ cups pecans or sprouted dehydrated walnuts	1½ cups pecans or sprouted dehydrated walnuts
FAT	1 cup ghee or coconut oil	1 cup ghee or coconut oil	1 cup ghee or coconut oil
DRIED FRUIT	½ cup prunes, raisins, or dates	¼ cup prunes, raisins, or dates	None
SEEDS	2 tablespoons chia seeds or freshly ground flaxseeds	2 tablespoons chia seeds or freshly ground flaxseeds	2 tablespoons chia seeds or freshly ground flaxseeds
FLAVORINGS/ SPICES	1 teaspoon to 1 tablespoon unsweetened cocoa powder	1 to 2 teaspoons unsweetened cocoa powder	1 to 2 teaspoons unsweetened cocoa powder
	1 teaspoon ground cinnamon	1 teaspoon ground cinnamon	1 teaspoon ground cinnamon
	¼ teaspoon ground nutmeg (optional)	¼ teaspoon ground nutmeg (optional)	¼ teaspoon ground nutmeg (optional)
	½ teaspoon ground cardamom (optional)	½ teaspoon ground cardamom (optional)	½ teaspoon ground cardamom (optional)
UNSWEETENED DRIED COCONUT FLAKES	1 cup	1 cup	1 cup

Note for Wahls Paleo Plus: Even though you must eliminate the dried fruit, the snowballs will still be tasty and rich, so don't think you can't enjoy this delicious, fudgelike recipe.

Vanilla Variation: Omit the cocoa powder, cinnamon, and nutmeg. Flavor with 1 teaspoon vanilla extract or ⅛ teaspoon vanilla bean seeds and ½ teaspoon ground cardamom.

This is a tangy-sweet and refreshing sorbet. It's one of those recipes that is not appropriate for Wahls Paleo Plus, but if you follow the Wahls Diet or Wahls Paleo, give it a try. This is a sweet one, with not much oil to accommodate the natural sugar, so limit your sweeteners for the rest of the day.

CHERRY SORBET

| MAKES 4 SERVINGS

1 cup frozen cherries

2 tablespoons coconut oil

1 to 2 tablespoons honey, maple syrup, or date syrup

Optional spices: 1 teaspoon ground cinnamon, ½ teaspoon ground cardamom, ½ teaspoon chili powder, ¼ teaspoon ground nutmeg, or ¼ teaspoon cayenne pepper

1 to 1½ cups ice cubes

TO MAKE: Combine all the ingredients except the ice cubes in a Vitamix or other high-speed blender. Add ½ cup water. Blend on high speed until well combined, then continue to blend on high as you add the ice cubes, a few at a time, until the mixture looks thick and creamy and continues to move in the blender jar. You may need to use the tamper to mix the ice cubes into the mixture as it thickens. When the mixture develops four mounds in the corners of the blender jar that are smoothly and continuously falling into the center (as it would for a thick smoothie), the sorbet is done. Pour into decorative serving dishes, top with fresh berries, and serve immediately.

Giving up dairy means one thing to some people: *No ice cream!* But don't despair—ice cream needn't contain dairy. There are many nondairy frozen desserts available in stores, but they tend to be high in sugar. You can make your own more nutrient-dense "ice cream" at home with much less sweetener. Feel free to add your favorite flavors—vanilla beans, cocoa, or fresh fruit, or get even more creative. Try raw cacao nibs, fresh garden herbs, or whatever fruits are fresh at the farmers' market (or in season in your own yard). Recently I added a little cayenne pepper to my ice cream—it was delightfully spicy!

BASIC FROZEN COCONUT "ICE CREAM" TEMPLATE

MAKES 8 SERVINGS

TO MAKE: Combine all the ingredients except the ice cubes in a Vitamix or other high-speed blender. Blend on high speed until well combined, then continue to blend on high as you add the ice cubes, a few at a time, until the mixture looks thick and creamy and continues to move in the blender jar. You may need to use the tamper to mix the ice cubes into the mixture as it thickens. When the mixture develops four mounds in the corners of the blender jar that are smoothly and continuously falling into the center (as it would for a thick smoothie), the ice cream is done. Pour into decorative serving dishes, top with fresh berries, and serve immediately.

	WAHLS DIET	WAHLS PALEO	WAHLS PALEO PLUS
FULL-FAT COCONUT MILK	1 (14-ounce) can	1 (14-ounce) can	1 (14-ounce) can
FAT	¼ cup coconut oil or ghee, softened (not melted)	¼ cup coconut oil or ghee, softened (not melted)	¼ cup coconut oil, softened (not melted)
SWEETENER	2 tablespoons honey or maple syrup	1 tablespoon honey or maple syrup	None
FLAVORINGS/ SPICES (choose any you think would work well together)	1 teaspoon vanilla extract, or ¼ teaspoon vanilla bean seeds	1 teaspoon vanilla extract, or ¼ teaspoon vanilla bean seeds	1 teaspoon vanilla extract, or ¼ teaspoon vanilla bean seeds
	Options:	Options:	Options:
	1 cup fresh or frozen fruit	½ cup fresh or frozen fruit	Up to ½ cup fresh or frozen berries
	1 can pumpkin puree	Up to 1 cup pumpkin puree	Up to 1 tablespoon unsweetened cocoa powder
	Up to 1 tablespoon unsweetened cocoa powder	Up to 1 tablespoon unsweetened cocoa powder	1 teaspoon ground cinnamon
	1 teaspoon to 2 tablespoons ground cinnamon	1 teaspoon ground cinnamon	½ teaspoon ground cardamom
	½ teaspoon ground cardamom	½ teaspoon ground cardamom	Pinch of cayenne or chili powder (if you dare!)
	Pinch of cayenne or chili powder (if you dare!)	Pinch of cayenne or chili powder (if you dare!)	
ICE CUBES	4 cups	4 cups	4 cups

Coconut Ice Cream Variation: You can also make ice cream in your freezer, which will create a denser, richer ice cream that you can serve like an ice cream cake. Simply omit the ice cubes and combine all the other ingredients in a saucepan. Warm the mixture over low heat, stirring until combined. Pour the mixture into a springform pan with a nut crust (page 268; or just pour it into the pan without a crust) and wrap the bottom of the pan in foil to prevent leakage. You could also pour the filling into individual serving dishes (like custard cups or ramekins) and freeze until firm, at least 4 hours or overnight. Serve sprinkled with grated chocolate, drizzled with chocolate or fruit-flavored balsamic vinegar, or topped with fresh berries or a spoonful of Whipped Coconut Cream (see page 264). Remove from the freezer and let the cake soften at room temperature for 20 to 30 minutes if using a cake pan or 5 to 10 minutes if using individual cups.

This is one of the most popular recipes from *The Wahls Protocol*, so I felt that it would be nice to include it in this cookbook with an added variation for white fudge. Wahls Fudge tastes like an indulgent, sweet treat but it's much more nutritionally dense than candy, pastries, or other sweet desserts. In my house, Wahls Fudge makes any day feel like a holiday! Wahls Fudge is calorically dense, so it's excellent for those who are losing too much weight. If you are trying to lose weight, enjoy it sparingly. If you are following Wahls Paleo Plus, omit the raisins and step back on the cocoa to keep the fudge from becoming too bitter.

WAHLS FUDGE

MAKES 20 SERVINGS

TO MAKE: Combine all the ingredients in a food processor. Process until smooth, then press the mixture into an 8 × 8-inch glass baking dish and refrigerate or place in a freezer for 30 minutes to firm up the fudge. Cut into 20 squares and enjoy. I usually store it in the refrigerator so it stays firm (it keeps for about 3 days, but it rarely lasts that long).

	WAHLS DIET AND WAHLS PALEO	WAHLS PALEO PLUS
FAT	1 cup coconut oil	1 cup coconut oil
	1 medium avocado, pitted and peeled	1 medium avocado, pitted and peeled
DRIED FRUIT	1 cup raisins (use golden raisins for the white chocolate fudge version)	None
NUTS	1 cup walnuts, preferably sprouted	1 cup walnuts, preferably sprouted
DRIED UNSWEETENED COCONUT	½ cup	½ cup
FLAVORING	1 teaspoon unsweetened cocoa powder	1 teaspoon to 1 tablespoon unsweetened cocoa powder

Mexican Chocolate Variation: **Add 1 teaspoon ground cinnamon for a Mexican Chocolate flavor.**

White Chocolate Variation: **The avocado is optional for this variation. Omit the cocoa powder. Add 1 teaspoon vanilla extract or ¼ teaspoon vanilla bean seeds.**

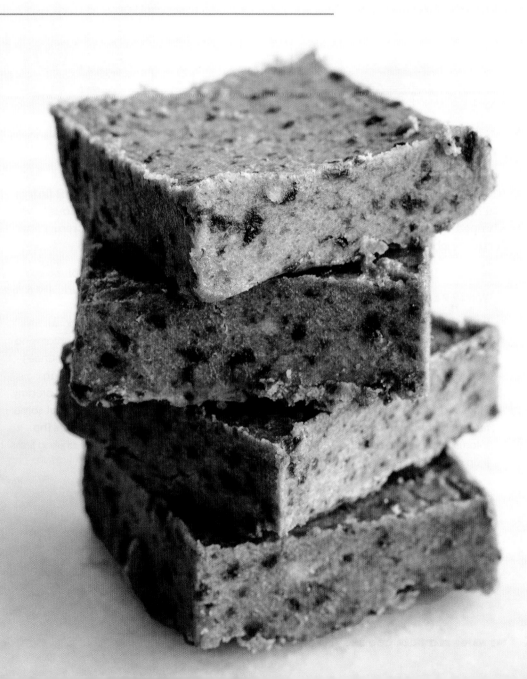

WAHLS CHEEZCAKE

Cheesecake is a classic American dessert, but if you have eliminated grains and dairy from your diet, it may seem a distant memory for you. Fortunately, you can still enjoy cheesecake—or let's call it "cheezcake," since cheese has nothing to do with it! Full-fat coconut milk mixed with gelatin firms up nicely when chilled. With a basic template, you can add your favorite flavors—mix in cocoa powder, garnish with grated chocolate, drizzle with a coconut milk–berry puree, or whatever you like. The wonderful thing about this recipe is it's *excellent* without any sweetener at all. (That's how I prefer it—no sweetener, flavored with spices, and topped with a few berries.) So, for those on Wahls Paleo Plus, you're in for a treat.

Also note that the crust for this recipe is made with nuts and dates, but the Wahls Paleo Plus version doesn't require any dried fruit. It still tastes delicious.

VEGETARIAN GELATIN

Gelatin and collagen are animal-based products, so if you are a vegetarian or vegan, you may not want to use them. Yet you can still have cheezcake! Agar-agar is a tasteless, seaweed-based product that gels just like gelatin, and you can substitute it for gelatin in equal amounts in any recipe. Agar-agar is available in flake and powder form (1 tablespoon flakes = 1 teaspoon powder). It's a good vegetarian baking staple to have in your cupboard.

You can create variations of this cheezcake with whatever flavors and garnishes you like. It is a plain but delicious canvas. (See photo on page 252.)

BASIC CHEEZCAKE TEMPLATE

MAKES 8 TO 12 SERVINGS

TO MAKE: Heat the coconut milk in a saucepan over medium-low heat. Sprinkle in the gelatin and stir until it has dissolved. Remove from the heat and stir in the sweetener (if using) and flavorings. Line an 8½-inch springform or tart pan with the nut crust. Pour in the filling and freeze until firm. Before serving, add any garnishes, toppings, and/or drizzles you wish.

	WAHLS DIET	WAHLS PALEO	WAHLS PALEO PLUS
FULL-FAT COCONUT MILK	1 (14-ounce) can	1 (14-ounce) can	1 (14-ounce) can
GELATIN/ AGAR-AGAR	2 tablespoons powder	2 tablespoons powder	2 tablespoons powder
SWEETENER	¼ cup honey or maple syrup	2 tablespoons honey or maple syrup	None
FLAVORINGS	Up to 1 tablespoon fresh citrus juice, 1 teaspoon flavored extract, or 2 teaspoons unsweetened cocoa powder and/or ground spices like cinnamon, cardamom, etc.	Up to 1 tablespoon fresh citrus juice, 1 teaspoon flavored extract, or 2 teaspoons unsweetened cocoa powder and/or ground spices like cinnamon, cardamom, etc.	Up to 1 tablespoon fresh citrus juice, 1 teaspoon flavored extract, or 2 teaspoons unsweetened cocoa powder and/or ground spices like cinnamon, cardamom, etc.
CRUST	1 recipe Basic Nut Crust (page 268)	1 recipe Basic Nut Crust (page 268)	1 recipe Basic Nut Crust (page 268)
GARNISH/ TOPPING/ DRIZZLE	Fruit, grated dark chocolate, and/or coconut milk–berry drizzle, all optional, as desired	Fruit, grated dark chocolate, and/or coconut milk–berry drizzle, all optional, as desired	Fruit, grated bittersweet or unsweetened chocolate, and/or coconut milk–berry drizzle, all optional, as desired

This recipe uses nuts and dried fruit with fat and spices to make a delicious pie crust without any grain. I use this for all kinds of things—for cheezcake (pages 267, 270, and 271), fresh or cooked fruit, coconut custard, or some combination of these. I don't specify a type of date to use in this recipe because although there are several different types of dates, any of them will work for the Basic Nut Crust. However, Medjool dates, which tend to be the most expensive, are soft and blend easily (they are also the sweetest, so while they work well in this recipe, they are not typically my preference in other recipes). Other types of dates may be much firmer. If the dates you have seem hard and dry, just soak them in warm water for about 20 minutes before blending. Also, if your dates have pits, be sure to remove them before using them in food. The pits are very hard and indigestible.

BASIC NUT CRUST TEMPLATE

MAKES 1 CHEEZCAKE OR TART CRUST

TO MAKE: Combine all the ingredients in a food processor and pulse until moist and well combined. Press evenly into an 8½-inch springform or tart pan.

	WAHLS DIET	WAHLS PALEO	WAHLS PALEO PLUS
NUTS	2½ cups any nuts or seeds	2½ cups any nuts or seeds	2½ cups any nuts or seeds
DRIED FRUIT	½ cup pitted dates or raisins	½ cup pitted dates or raisins	None
FAT	3 tablespoons ghee or coconut oil	3 tablespoons ghee or coconut oil	⅓ cup coconut oil
FLAVORINGS	1 tablespoon ground cinnamon, unsweetened cocoa powder, ground cardamom, or a combination	1 tablespoon ground cinnamon, unsweetened cocoa powder, ground cardamom, or a combination	1 tablespoon ground cinnamon, unsweetened cocoa powder, ground cardamom, or a combination

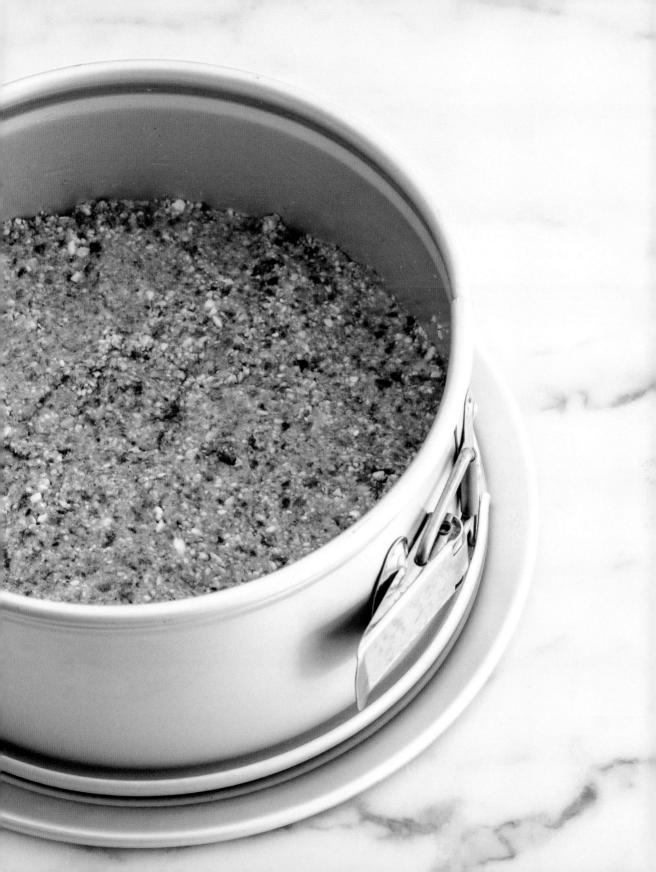

This recipe is flavored subtly with citrus and topped with pineapple and grated coconut.

ISLAND CHEEZCAKE

| MAKES 8 TO 12 SERVINGS

TO MAKE: Heat the coconut milk in a saucepan over medium-low heat. Sprinkle in the gelatin and stir until it has dissolved. Remove from the heat and stir in the sweetener (if using), citrus juice, and vanilla. Line an 8½-inch springform or tart pan with the nut crust. Pour in the filling and freeze until firm. Before serving, top the cake with the pineapple, coconut, and zest.

	WAHLS DIET	WAHLS PALEO	WAHLS PALEO PLUS
FULL-FAT COCONUT MILK	1 (14-ounce) can	1 (14-ounce) can	1 (14-ounce) can
GELATIN/ AGAR-AGAR	2 tablespoons powder	2 tablespoons powder	2 tablespoons powder
SWEETENER	3 tablespoons honey or maple syrup	2 tablespoons honey or maple syrup	None
FLAVORINGS	1 tablespoon fresh lime or lemon juice	1 tablespoon fresh lime or lemon juice	1 tablespoon fresh lime or lemon juice
	½ teaspoon vanilla extract, or ⅛ teaspoon vanilla bean seeds	½ teaspoon vanilla extract, or ⅛ teaspoon vanilla bean seeds	½ teaspoon vanilla extract, or ⅛ teaspoon vanilla bean seeds
CRUST	1 recipe Basic Nut Crust (page 268)	1 recipe Basic Nut Crust (page 268)	1 recipe Basic Nut Crust (page 268)
GARNISH/ TOPPING/ DRIZZLE	½ cup chopped fresh pineapple	½ cup chopped fresh pineapple	½ cup unsweetened shredded or flaked coconut
	½ cup unsweetened shredded or flaked coconut	½ cup unsweetened shredded or flaked coconut	1 teaspoon lime or lemon zest
	1 teaspoon lemon or lime zest	1 teaspoon lime or lemon zest	

Note for Wahls Paleo Plus: Omit the fresh pineapple topping. Your cheezcake will have a delicious subtle tart flavor from the citrus zest and juice.

This is a nice special-occasion cheezcake for chocolate lovers. The spices make it a good recipe for the winter holidays, but you could also serve it with fresh strawberries in the spring or raspberries in the summer.

CHOCOLATE SPICE CHEEZCAKE

MAKES 8 TO 12 SERVINGS

TO MAKE: Heat the coconut milk in a saucepan over medium-low heat. Sprinkle in the gelatin and stir until it has dissolved. Remove from the heat and stir in the sweetener (if using), cocoa powder, cardamom, and nutmeg. Line an 8½-inch springform or tart pan with the nut crust. Pour in the filling and freeze until firm. For a fancy presentation, frost with Whipped Coconut Cream and decorate with grated chocolate and/or berries.

	WAHLS DIET	WAHLS PALEO	WAHLS PALEO PLUS
FULL-FAT COCONUT MILK	1 (14-ounce) can	1 (14-ounce) can	1 (14-ounce) can
GELATIN/ AGAR-AGAR	2 tablespoons powder	2 tablespoons powder	2 tablespoons powder
SWEETENER	¼ cup honey or maple syrup	2 tablespoons honey or maple syrup	None
FLAVORINGS	1 to 2 teaspoons unsweetened cocoa powder	1 to 2 teaspoons unsweetened cocoa powder	1 to 2 teaspoons unsweetened cocoa powder
	1 teaspoon ground cardamom	1 teaspoon ground cardamom	1 teaspoon ground cardamom
	¼ teaspoon ground nutmeg	¼ teaspoon ground nutmeg	¼ teaspoon ground nutmeg
CRUST	1 recipe Basic Nut Crust (page 268)	1 recipe Basic Nut Crust (page 268)	1 recipe Basic Nut Crust (page 268)
GARNISH/ TOPPING/ DRIZZLE	Whipped Coconut Cream, for frosting (optional, page 264)	Whipped Coconut Cream, for frosting (optional, page 264)	Whipped Coconut Cream, for frosting (optional, page 264)
	Unsweetened grated chocolate or cacao nibs (optional)	Unsweetened grated chocolate or cacao nibs (optional)	Unsweetened grated chocolate or cacao nibs (optional)
	Berries (optional)	Berries (optional)	Berries (optional)

WAHLS PUDDING

Pudding is a creamy and satisfying comfort food that is a delicious finish for any meal. The secret to making a healthy pudding is chia seeds. These fiber-rich, nutritious seeds soak up liquid (in this recipe, coconut milk) and form a pudding-like base that you can flavor any way you like. You can also use freshly ground flaxseeds instead of chia seeds; flaxseeds have a similar texture but a slightly stronger flavor. Both have great health benefits. Flax and chia have omega-3 fatty acids, which are great support for your cells, as they make cell membranes and the myelin insulation on the wiring between brain cells. In addition, both flax and chia contain phytoestrogens, which are plant-based compounds that gently stimulate receptors for the estrogen hormones that occur in brain, heart, and bone cells—but not breast cells. The science supports including flax and chia in the diet of women who are menopausal and looking for gentle estrogen support for their brain, heart, and bones without stimulating the estrogen receptors in their breasts (potentially increasing the risk of developing breast cancer). So enjoy flaxseeds and chia seeds often—especially in Wahls Pudding!

Note that the yields for each level of the Wahls Protocol seem quite variable. This is because the declining amount of water at each level increases the amount of fat and therefore affects the serving size.

BASIC WAHLS PUDDING TEMPLATE

TO MAKE: Combine all the ingredients in a blender and blend on low speed until combined. Let the pudding sit for 30 minutes to thicken.

	WAHLS DIET (makes about six 1-cup servings or twelve ½-cup servings)	WAHLS PALEO (makes about four 1-cup servings or eight ½-cup servings)	WAHLS PALEO PLUS (makes four ½-cup servings)
MILK	1 (14-ounce) can full-fat coconut milk 42 ounces unsweetened boxed nut or seed milk, such as almond, hazelnut, or hemp, or water, or a combination (or just fill the empty coconut milk can with nut milk or water or a combination, three times)	1 (14-ounce can) full-fat coconut milk, plus an equal amount of water	1 (14-ounce can) full-fat coconut milk
CHIA SEEDS/ FRESHLY GROUND FLAXSEEDS	⅔ cup	½ cup	⅓ cup
SWEETENERS	1½ tablespoons maple syrup, honey, or glycine, or ½ cup dried fruit (such as raisins or prunes)	1 tablespoon maple syrup, honey, or glycine	None
FLAVORINGS	Any of the following: 1 to 2 tablespoons fresh lemon or lime juice 1 teaspoon to 1 tablespoon spices (such as unsweetened cocoa powder, ground cinnamon, ground nutmeg, or ground cardamom) 1 cup berries (optional) 1 (15-ounce) can pumpkin puree (optional, and note that this will increase the yield by about 1½ cups)	Any of the following: 1 to 2 tablespoons fresh lemon or lime juice 1 teaspoon to 1 tablespoon spices (such as unsweetened cocoa powder, ground cinnamon, ground nutmeg, or ground cardamom) 1 cup berries (optional) 1 (15-ounce) can pumpkin puree (optional, and note that this will increase the yield by about 1½ cups)	Any of the following: 1 to 2 tablespoons fresh lemon or lime juice 1 teaspoon to 1 tablespoon spices (such as ground cinnamon, ground nutmeg, or ground cardamom) ½ cup berries (optional)

RECIPE CONTINUES

Note for Wahls Diet: You may substitute 7 cups (56 ounces) total boxed unsweetened nut or seed milk or boxed coconut milk if you don't want to use the canned coconut milk.

Note for Wahls Paleo: You may substitute a total of 3 1/3 cups boxed nut or seed milk or boxed coconut milk for the canned coconut milk and water.

GLYCINE: THE SWEET AMINO ACID

Glycine is sweetener you might not have heard about. It is an amino acid beneficial for building connective tissue and improving sleep. You can buy it in powder form and use up to 1 teaspoon per day (as you would use sugar, honey, or maple syrup). You'll see I've listed it as a sweetener option in some of the desserts in this chapter. But do not use glycine if you are trying to break your body's cravings for sweetness, because your tongue and your brain will still experience the taste as sweet. However, if you're able to eat sweets occasionally, glycine is a healthier sweetener than sugar.

Note: If you are following Wahls Paleo Plus, I recommend you limit your glycine along with all other sweeteners to stay in ketosis.

This is a special and decadent-seeming dessert but is actually quite nutritious.

CHIA BERRY DARK COCOA PUDDING

TO MAKE: Combine all the ingredients except the berries in a blender and blend on low speed until combined. Pour the pudding into bowls, top with the berries, and serve.

	WAHLS DIET (makes about six 1-cup servings or twelve ½-cup servings)	WAHLS PALEO (makes about four 1-cup servings or eight ½-cup servings)	WAHLS PALEO PLUS (makes four ½-cup servings)
MILK	1 (14-ounce) can full-fat coconut milk 42 ounces unsweetened boxed nut or seed milk, such as almond, hazelnut, or hemp, or water, or a combination (or just fill the empty can with nut milk or water or a combination, three times)	1 (14-ounce can) full-fat coconut milk, plus an equal amount of water	1 (14-ounce) can full-fat coconut milk
CHIA SEEDS/ FRESHLY GROUND FLAXSEEDS	⅔ cup	½ cup	⅓ cup
SWEETENER	1½ tablespoons maple syrup, honey, or glycine	1½ tablespoons maple syrup, honey, or glycine	None
FLAVORINGS	1 teaspoon to 1 tablespoon unsweetened cocoa or cacao powder 1 cup blueberries, raspberries, or cherries, for topping	1 tablespoon unsweetened cocoa or cacao powder 1 cup blueberries, raspberries, or cherries, for topping	1½ teaspoons unsweetened cocoa or cacao powder 1 to 2 teaspoons ground cinnamon, 1 teaspoon mint extract, or 2 to 4 drops mint food-grade essential oil ½ cup blueberries, raspberries, or cherries, for topping

RECIPE CONTINUES

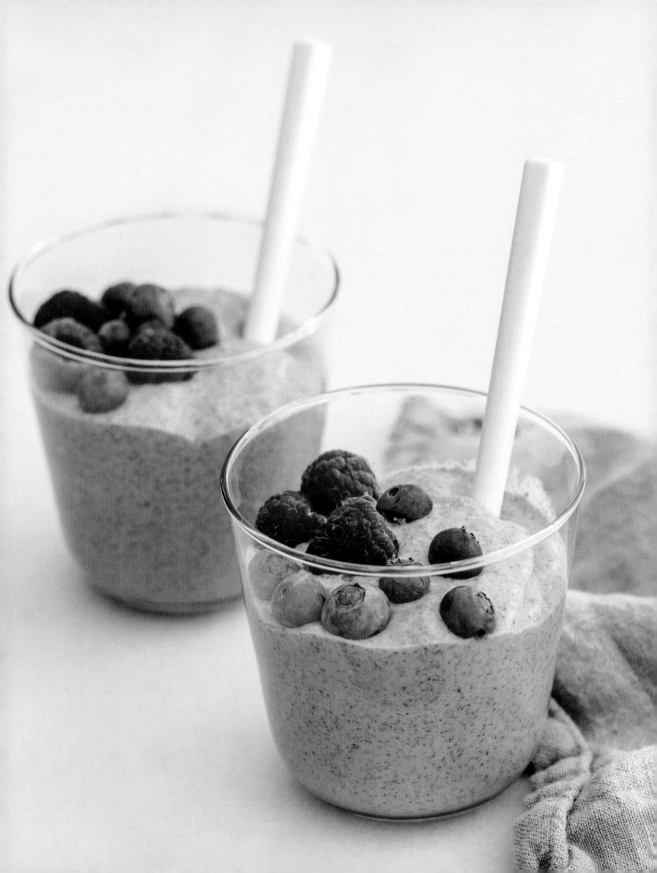

Note for Wahls Diet: **You may substitute 7 cups boxed unsweetened nut or seed milk or boxed coconut milk for the canned coconut milk.**

Note for Wahls Paleo: **You may substitute 3 1/3 cups boxed nut or seed milk or boxed coconut milk for the canned coconut milk and water.**

FERMENTED CHIA PUDDING

Fermented chia pudding is a tasty way to work more fermented foods into your diet. To make it just add 1 to 2 tablespoons fresh lemon or lime juice to the coconut milk when you make your chia pudding. Blend on high speed for 1 to 2 minutes to be sure the coconut milk is thoroughly mixed. Add the chia seeds and blend gently on low speed until well combined. Do not use any other spices, as they could inhibit the growth of beneficial bacteria. Open a probiotic capsule and dump it into the well-blended mixture and stir by hand or blend on low speed for 30 seconds. Pour the mixture into two wide-mouth glass jars and cover with a towel. Let them sit at room temperature for 24 hours, then put the lids on the jars. Refrigerate until cold, then serve with optional fresh berries and a spoonful of Whipped Coconut Cream (see page 264), or other garnishes as listed in the template. Use within 3 days of chilling.

WAHLS WARRIORS SPEAK

I cannot tell you how much I appreciate the community you have built and all the Warriors who keep up the fight on the health front while having fun. I was fifty and teaching mathematics when I learned I had arthritis. After a while, I was sitting in an armchair in pain. Raw food brought me out of the pain and out of the chair. My head worked great, and I was able to return to school. However, because I wasn't eating meat I became anemic, so I went back to the pan-fried liver and steaks that I love. (According to my mother, my ancestor Attila the Hun used to soften his steaks under the saddle, so my love of rather raw steaks is understandable.) However, I slowly returned to a standard American diet. It was not until I found Terry Wahls and the energetic community of Warriors that I stepped back on the path of healing. For a mathematician, every little word can be a clue to a treasure of information, and Terry's writing is concise and clear. Every word is a diamond in the rough.

—Wahls Warrior LIANA

This pudding is excellent for summer, when blackberries are at their peak.

BLACKBERRY LEMON CHIA PUDDING

TO MAKE: Combine all the ingredients except the berries in a blender and blend on low speed until combined. Pour the pudding into bowls, top with the berries, and serve.

	WAHLS DIET (makes about six 1-cup servings or twelve ½-cup servings)	WAHLS PALEO (makes about four 1-cup servings or eight ½-cup servings)	WAHLS PALEO PLUS (makes four ½-cup servings)
MILK	1 (14-ounce) can full-fat coconut milk 42 ounces unsweetened boxed nut or seed milk, such as almond, hazelnut, or hemp, or water, or a combination (or just fill the empty can with nut milk or water or a combination, three times)	1 (14-ounce can) full-fat coconut milk, plus an equal amount of water	1 (14-ounce) can full-fat coconut milk
CHIA SEEDS/ FRESHLY GROUND FLAXSEEDS	⅔ cup	½ cup	⅓ cup
SWEETENER	1½ tablespoons maple syrup, honey, or glycine	1½ tablespoons maple syrup, honey, or glycine	None
FLAVORINGS	2 tablespoons fresh lemon juice 1 cup blackberries, for topping	2 tablespoons fresh lemon juice 1 cup blackberries, for topping	1 tablespoon fresh lemon juice 1 teaspoon ground cinnamon or mint food-grade essential oil ½ cup blackberries, for topping

Note for Wahls Diet: **You may substitute 5 cups boxed unsweetened nut or seed milk or boxed coconut milk for the canned coconut milk.**

Note for Wahls Paleo: **You may substitute 3⅓ cups boxed nut or seed milk or boxed coconut milk for the canned coconut milk and water.**

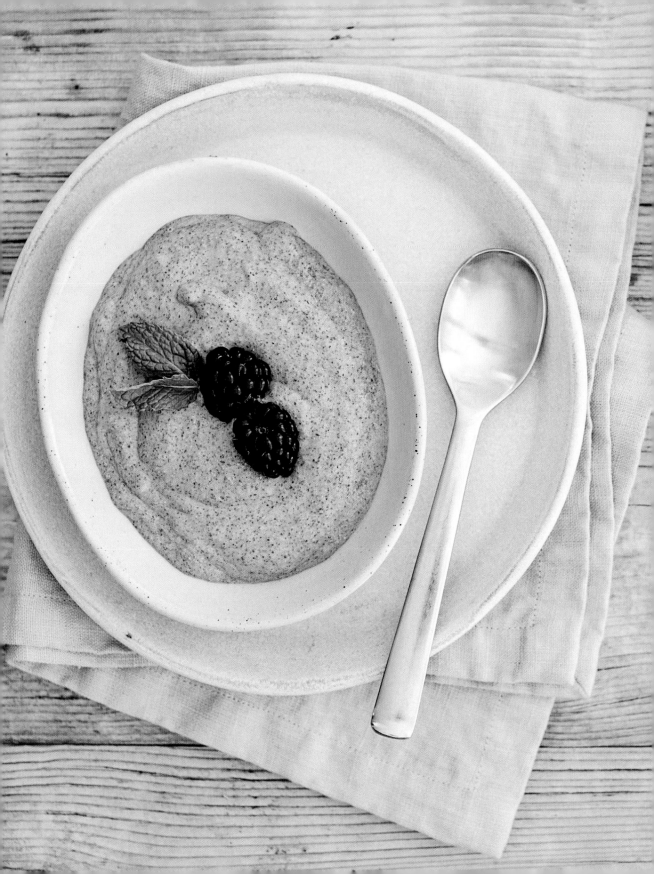

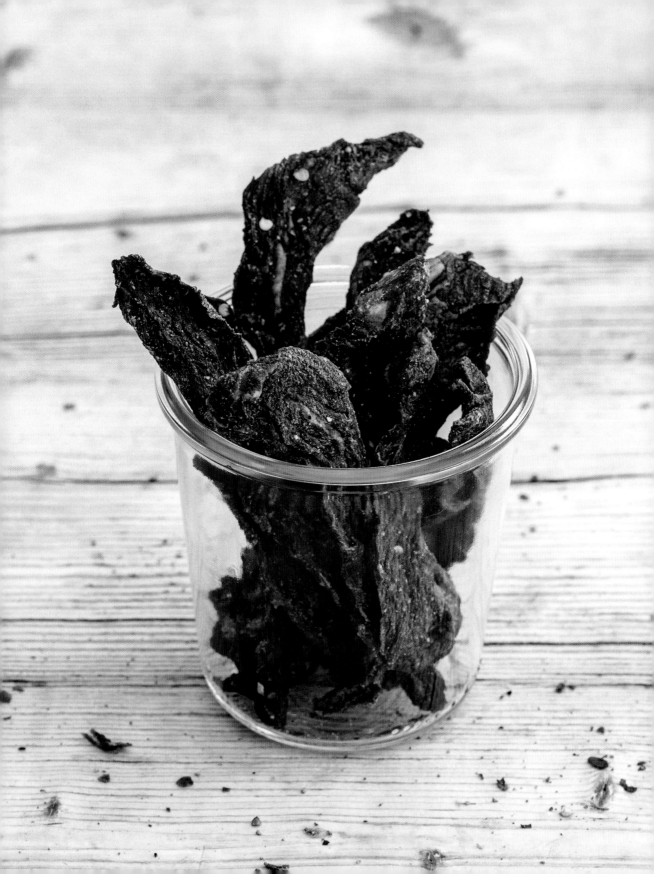

SNACKS
IN A SNAP

SOMETIMES A SNACK IS A NECESSITY. When you can't make it to the next meal, when your body is crying out for sustenance, you need to answer that call—but not with junk food, sugar, industrial oils, or too much salt. Most easy-to-buy snacks are not easy on your health or your attempts to heal, but fortunately, there are quite a few simple snacks you can make at home and have handy to just grab and eat on the go. The snacks I eat most include homemade jerky, homemade vegetable chips, nuts, fruit, raw vegetables, and keto treats. Jerky, dried vegetable chips, and spiced nuts in particular are great for traveling.

Sometimes I'll get a little more ambitious and cook something for a snack (like Brussels sprouts wrapped in bacon), but most of the time, this is simply not necessary. On weekends, I sometimes choose a day to prepare some jerky or keto treats or vegetable chips, and then I am set for a week or more of snacks.

Let this chapter be your inspiration to transform your snacking habits. There is nothing wrong with snacking, as long as your snacks feed your cells and contribute to your vitality.

Jerky is an excellent snack because it is a portable dose of high-quality animal protein. However, store-bought jerky not only contains too much salt, but is usually preserved with chemicals you don't want in your system when you are trying to heal. Instead, make your own jerky at home—it's surprisingly easy, you control the ingredients, and you can be much more creative with your options. Try any good-quality meat, including organ meat and game. Chicken jerky, liver jerky, venison jerky, elk jerky, fish jerky, back bacon jerky—they can all be yours. All you need is a dehydrator (the easiest option) or an oven set on low and some good-quality meat, salt, vinegar, and spices.

Jerky is so easy that I won't give you individual recipes. Just choose options from the template and use what you have, or experiment with flavors that sound tasty.

BASIC JERKY TEMPLATE

MAKES ABOUT 8 SNACK SERVINGS
Note: This jerky recipe is appropriate for all levels of the Wahls Protocol.

TO MAKE: Partially defrost frozen meat, or put unfrozen meat in the freezer just long enough (1 to 2 hours) to get it firm but not frozen solid. This makes it easier to slice. Mix all the marinade ingredients in a small bowl and pour the marinade into a gallon-size plastic zip-top bag or shallow pan with a lid. Thinly slice the meat and add the meat to the marinade. Seal the bag and toss to coat. Refrigerate for 24 hours. Put the meat slices on a dehydrator tray and dehydrate at 140° to 170°F for 6 to 12 hours. Alternatively, preheat the oven to between 140° and 180°F, put the meat slices on a baking sheet, and dry until the meat reaches the texture you like (it will get chewy, then crispy, as it dries), 6 to 12 hours.

FAST-TRACK SNACKS

If you only have a few minutes, grab some celery and fill it with any nut or seed butter you like. Sprinkle with cinnamon or raw cacao nibs, or place blueberries or raspberries along the top, to change up the flavor. This is a filling treat that takes seconds to make, and satisfies both your need to crunch something and your need to have something rich and creamy to hold you over until your next meal.

MEAT

Flank steak

London broil

Chicken breast

Turkey breast

Chicken liver

Beef liver

Venison

Elk

Buffalo/Bison

Any firm-fleshed fish (try salmon, trout, bass, tuna, snapper, or any other good fresh fish)

MARINADE

1 teaspoon sea salt

2 tablespoons coarsely ground black pepper

1 tablespoon vinegar—apple cider vinegar is a good choice

Optional:

Spices of your choice, up to 1 teaspoon of any one type, up to 1 tablespoon total. Some good options include onion powder, garlic granules, curry powder, ground turmeric, ground cumin, and hot pepper flakes.

Teriyaki Variation: Add 1 tablespoon gluten-free tamari, Bragg Liquid Aminos, or coconut aminos. (I realize tamari contains soy, but the amount is negligible.)

Keto Treats are rich, succulent little nuggets of fudgelike joy, but they don't contain any sweetener at all, making them appropriate for any level of the Wahls Protocol. Start with a small amount of spices, maybe ¼ teaspoon per batch, and experiment with increasing to your taste. Freeze in ice cube trays and pop them out whenever you need a treat. They taste almost like candy but will actually nourish your cells and support your health rather than break down your body. My kids love these.

BASIC KETO TREAT TEMPLATE

MAKES 16 TREATS

TO MAKE: Combine the coconut oil, ghee, nut or seed butter, and flavorings in a food processor until well mixed. Fill an ice cube tray with the mixture, put the tray in a zip-top plastic bag to keep the treats fresh, and freeze until firm. Pop out the treats as you need them, or portion the frozen treats into individual bags for a grab-and-go freezer snack. (If you don't have an ice cube tray, you could also drop 2-tablespoon mounds of the mixture on a parchment paper–lined baking sheet and cover with plastic wrap. Freeze, then pack the treats in plastic bags and keep them frozen until serving.)

	WAHLS DIET	WAHLS PALEO	WAHLS PALEO PLUS
FAT	½ cup coconut oil, melted or softened	½ cup coconut oil, melted or softened	1 cup coconut oil, melted or softened
	½ cup ghee, melted or softened	½ cup ghee, melted or softened	
NUT/SEED BUTTER	1 cup	1 cup	1 cup
FLAVORINGS	1 teaspoon to 2 tablespoons of any of the following, to taste:	1 teaspoon to 2 tablespoons of any of the following, to taste:	1 teaspoon to 2 tablespoons of any of the following, to taste:
	Unsweetened cocoa or raw cacao powder	Unsweetened cocoa or raw cacao powder	Unsweetened cocoa or raw cacao powder
	Ground cinnamon	Ground cinnamon	Ground cinnamon
	Ground cardamom	Ground cardamom	Ground cardamom
	Vanilla extract	Vanilla extract	Vanilla extract
	1 or 2 drops food-grade essential oil (peppermint, orange, lemon, or lime)	1 or 2 drops food-grade essential oil (peppermint, orange, lemon, or lime)	1 or 2 drops food-grade essential oil (peppermint, orange, lemon, or lime)

Coconut Variation:
For more texture, add
1 cup unsweetened flaked
or shredded coconut.

Savory Variation:
Add ¼ teaspoon each ground
turmeric, minced fresh ginger,
and ground cumin. Taste and
increase the quantities, if
desired.

VEGETABLE CHIPS

You can make chips out of many different kinds of vegetables. Why limit yourself to potatoes? In fact, potatoes are one of the worst vegetables for making chips because they are high in starch, so they soak up oil easily. Instead, chips made from thick leafy greens like kale and collards or thinly sliced root vegetables or squash are crunchy, salty, and nutritious as well as delicious. Make a big batch and watch them disappear. (Bet you can't eat just one.) Another idea: Dehydrate grated root vegetables in batches (beets, carrots, turnips, etc.), then mix them together for a crunchy snack (add the spices before dehydrating so the spices stay on the chips).

SPICE YOUR CHIPS

Different kinds of vegetable chips taste good with a variety of spices. Here are some great combinations:

- Kale chips or root vegetable chips spiced with turmeric, ground cumin, and ground ginger

- Sweet potato or butternut squash chips with chili powder or smoked paprika

- Summer squash or turnip chips with black pepper, onion powder, garlic powder, and cayenne

- Sweet potato, butternut squash, carrot, or beet chips with ground cinnamon and ground nutmeg

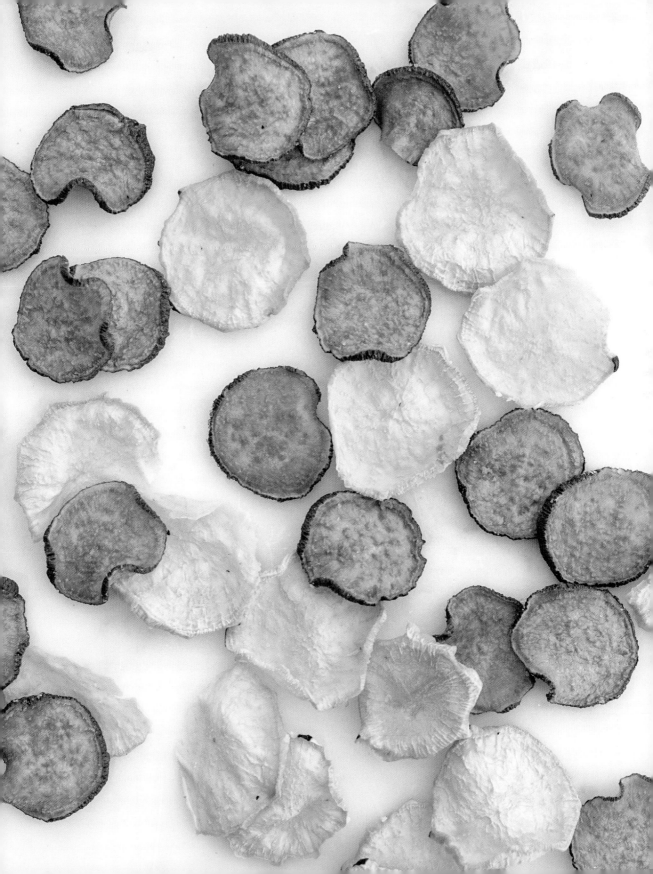

When you are making vegetable chips, it is important to prep the vegetables properly. For root vegetables and squash, a mandoline is a good way to make very thin slices. You could also do this with a sharp knife, but it takes a lot more time and patience (and coordination). Alternatively, you can use a vegetable peeler to create thin slices. If you use other vegetables, like beets, they must also be sliced very thinly. A food processor fitted with a slicing blade, or a mandoline will probably do the job better than you can by hand. Make sure the vegetables are totally dry—any moisture will steam the chips and prevent them from crisping. I like to use my dehydrator for root vegetable and squash chips because they don't burn as easily as they do in the oven. I start the vegetable chips in the evening, and check their crispness in the morning. If they are not crisp enough, I leave them in the dehydrator and go to work. When I get home, they're done. If you don't have a dehydrator, you can dry the chips on a baking sheet in the oven. But I'll say it again: I find it much easier to make chips in the dehydrator because I don't have to worry about burning. If you plan to make chips often, it's probably worth investing in a dehydrator.

BASIC VEGETABLE CHIP TEMPLATE

MAKES 8 SERVINGS
Note for Wahls Paleo Plus: Only use coconut oil in this recipe.

TO MAKE: In a large bowl, toss the vegetables with the fat and flavorings.

If using a dehydrator: Spread the vegetables in a thin layer (don't pile them on top of one another) on a dehydrator tray or baking sheet. Dehydrate at 105°F or below (to keep the enzymes intact) until crispy, 12 to 18 hours, depending on the size of the batch.

If using the oven: Preheat the oven to 250°F. Arrange the vegetables in a single layer on large baking sheets (they will probably fill two jelly-roll-size pans). Dry in the oven for 1 hour. Flip and dry for 1 hour more, or until the edges curl and the chips are crispy. Watch carefully to ensure they do not burn–it can happen in seconds! Remove the chips and allow to cool. If your chips are thicker, you may need to increase the oven temperature to 325°F and watch the chips very closely so that they don't burn.

Store in an airtight container at room temperature to maintain crispness. These will keep for one week, but they are so popular in our home that they are typically gone within days, if not hours.

	WAHLS DIET, WAHLS PALEO, AND WAHLS PALEO PLUS
VEGETABLE	4 cups thinly sliced root vegetables like sweet potatoes, carrots, or turnips, or squash such as butternut, acorn, zucchini, or yellow squash
FAT	Up to 1 tablespoon melted coconut oil or ghee (coconut oil only for Wahls Paleo Plus)
	If using a dehydrator, you could use extra-virgin olive oil and/or flaxseed oil since the temperature is lower
FLAVORINGS	1 tablespoon fresh lemon juice or vinegar, to massage into leafy greens before drying, to tenderize them (optional)
	Up to 1 tablespoon of any other spices, depending on what kind of vegetable you are using
TOPPINGS	Sea salt
	Options:
	Nutritional yeast, for a cheesy flavor
	Ground cinnamon, especially good with carrot, sweet potato, and winter squash chips
	Freshly ground nut meal or flaxseed meal, for a more interesting texture

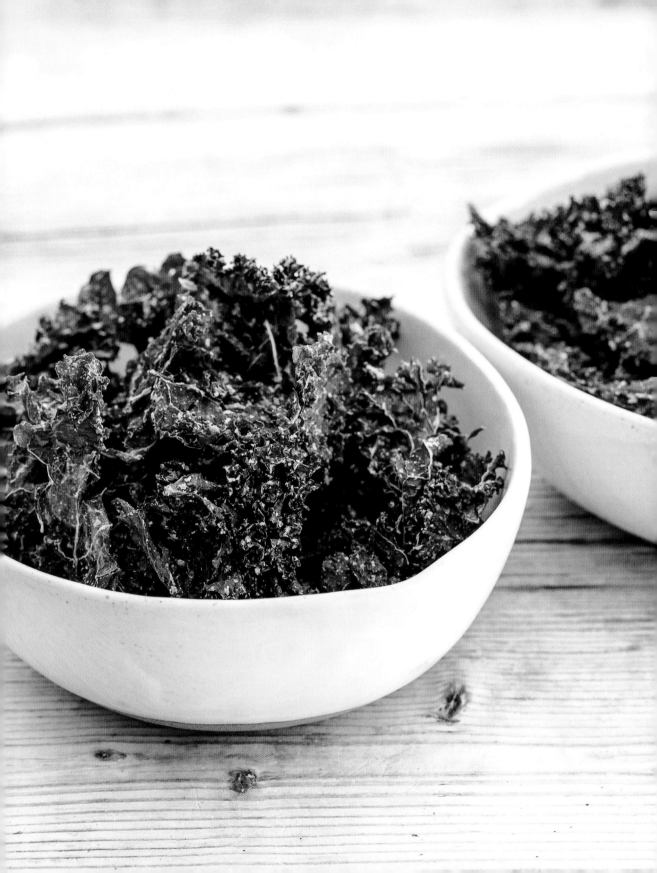

Kale chips are officially a trend—health food stores and regular grocery stores now have them packaged for sale, but most of these contain a lot of salt and flavorings, including sweeteners (even in savory flavors) that aren't good for your health. Luckily, it is easy to make your own.

While I prefer to make veggie chips in the dehydrator, kale and other leafy-green chips are much quicker to prepare in the oven. Just watch them closely because they will go from done to burnt in a flash.

BASIC KALE/COLLARD CHIP TEMPLATE

MAKES 8 SERVINGS
Note for Wahls Paleo Plus: Only use coconut oil in this recipe.

TO MAKE: Remove the thick stems from the kale or collard leaves by slicing down either side of the stem with a sharp knife; cutting the stem out with scissors; or tearing the leaf along the stem to separate them. Keep the leaves whole or tear them into smaller bite-size pieces. (Remember: The pieces will contract during dehydration or roasting.)

In a large bowl, toss the greens with the fat and flavorings. Spread the coated greens in a single layer on large baking sheets (they will probably fill two jelly-roll-size pans). Put them in the oven and turn the heat to 250°F. Dry for about 30 minutes, but keep a close eye on the chips, as the thickness of your greens and temperature of your oven may vary. (For example, kale chips will dry more quickly than thicker collard chips.) As soon as the edges curl and the greens are crispy, they are done. Remove from the oven immediately. If everyone doesn't devour them right away, store them in an airtight container at room temperature to keep them crisp. They can last for a week, but as with the vegetable chips, we like them so much they are typically gone within a few days.

RECIPE CONTINUES

FAST-TRACK SNACKS

Many snacks need virtually no preparation at all. When hunger strikes, get in more of your Wahls-required vegetables and fruits by snacking on fresh raw fruit or raw veggies dipped in nut or seed butter, leftover pâté, salsa, or guacamole.

VEGETABLE 4 cups whole or torn pieces leafy greens like kale or collard greens

FAT Up to 1 tablespoon coconut oil or ghee (coconut oil only for Wahls Paleo Plus)

If using a dehydrator, you could use extra-virgin olive oil and/or flax seed oil since the temperature is lower

FLAVORINGS 1 tablespoon fresh lemon juice or vinegar, to massage into leafy greens before drying, to tenderize them (optional)

Up to 1 tablespoon any other spices, depending on what kind of vegetable you are using

TOPPINGS Sea salt

Options:

Nutritional yeast, for a cheesy flavor

Freshly ground nut meal or flaxseed meal, for a more interesting texture

FAST-TRACK SNACKS

For a quick, hot snack that tastes like a meal, wrap individual Brussels sprouts in strips of bacon, secure with a toothpick, and broil until the bacon is crispy. These also make nice hors d'oeuvres at social events.

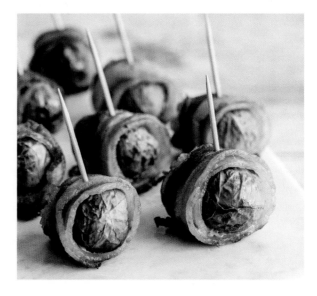

Raw nuts make great snacks at any time, but you can take nuts to the next level if you spice them up.

BASIC SPICED NUTS TEMPLATE

| MAKES 4 SERVINGS

TO MAKE: Put the nuts in a quart jar, add the spices, cover, shake, and enjoy.

WAHLS DIET, WAHLS PALEO, AND WAHLS PALEO PLUS
NUTS — 1 cup (almonds, walnuts, cashews, hazelnuts, pistachios, or a mixture)
SPICES — 1 tablespoon each of your favorite spices.
For a sweet version, try a tablespoon each of unsweetened cocoa powder, ground cinnamon, and a dash of ground nutmeg with almonds
For a savory version, try a tablespoon each of ground cardamom, ground turmeric, ground cinnamon, and unsweetened dried coconut with cashews

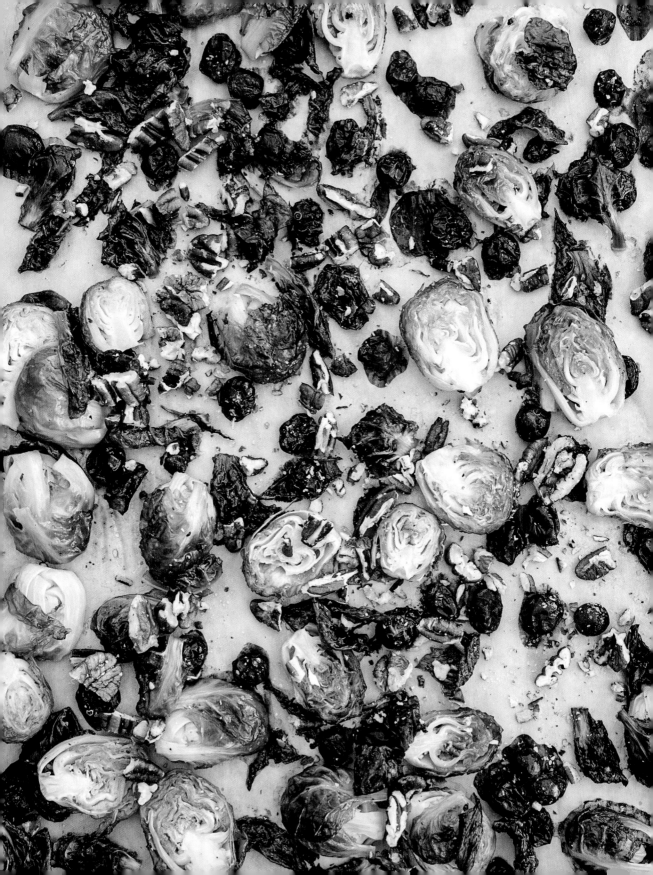

11 WAHLS HOLIDAYS

HOLIDAYS CAN BE PARTICULARLY DIFFICULT when you have a restricted diet, and even though you know your eating plan helps you heal and feel better, it's hard not to cave in "just this once" or temporarily suspend your good habits because it's a holiday. But you don't have to compromise your health to celebrate—not with this chapter. I've constructed three feasts—one for Thanksgiving, one for the winter holiday, and one for spring—along with boxes with ideas for celebrating other holidays, like Halloween, Valentine's Day, birthdays, and summer barbecue season. You can stay true to your cells and avoid a health crash while still having a great time.

Another thing I would also like you to consider is that holidays are not *only* about food. People love to celebrate around food, but the celebrations are really about being with people you love and commemorating events that are meaningful to your culture and life. You can still feel gratitude and give thanks even if you don't have a dinner roll and a mountain of mashed white potatoes. You can still celebrate the winter season or the coming of spring or special spiritual or religious days without eating junk that will make you feel un-celebratory or suffer worsening pain, brain fog, depression, and flare-ups of your chronic disease the following week. Bask in community, spend some quiet time in prayer or meditation, be with your family and/or friends, and, most of all, *enjoy yourself!* Food is just the coconut cream frosting on the grain-free cake.

THANKSGIVING

Give thanks for family, friends, and, yes, food while remaining Wahls compliant with this delicious and filling Thanksgiving Day menu. And don't forget to ask for help with the cooking! Although these recipes are all pretty simple, it's always complicated to make multiple dishes, and it's fun to cook with willing helpers. Even kids can smash up yams, sprinkle cranberries and pecans over a pan of Brussels sprouts, or press the blender button for the Pumpkin Pudding (page 304).

WAHLS THANKSGIVING MENU

Roast Turkey

Stuffing

Mashed Yams

Cooked Greens with Bacon and Mushrooms

Brussels Sprouts, Cranberries, and Pecans

Pumpkin (or Squash or Sweet Potato Pie) Pudding

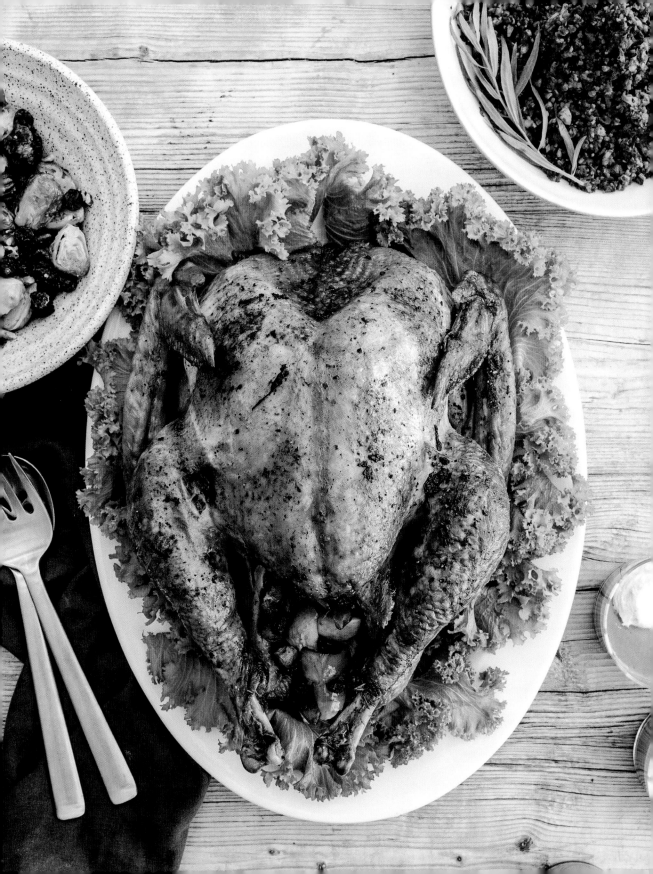

Roasting a turkey is pretty basic. Any roasting instructions will work. However, be sure to choose a turkey that is not injected with any flavorings that contain gluten or sugar. I like to get an organic turkey that hasn't been injected with anything from a local producer. This may be easier in farm country than in some spots, but most cities and towns now have health-food-centric stores that are likely to have organic turkeys.

ROAST TURKEY

TO MAKE: Preheat the oven to 325°F. Remove the giblet packet, if present, from the cavity and pat the turkey dry with paper towels. Rub coconut oil all over the skin. Put the turkey on a rack in a roasting pan and roast for 15 to 20 minutes per pound, until the internal temperature in the breast reaches 160°F (about 3 hours for a 10-pound turkey, but ovens vary quite a bit, so it is safest to use a meat thermometer). Baste the turkey occasionally with the pan drippings, if desired. Remove the turkey from the oven, tent it with foil, and let rest for 10 to 20 minutes. The internal temperature will rise to 165°F or higher as it sits.

BONUS ORGAN MEATS

Organ meats are an important part of Wahls Paleo and Wahls Paleo Plus, and will also benefit you on the Wahls Diet. However, sometimes it is hard to find organ meats. The little packet of giblets stuffed into the cavity of a turkey will provide an extra treat for you. You can cook the giblets in ghee and eat them as an appetizer, or cut up the giblets and use them in soup or for making stock. Or wrap the giblets in bacon and broil until the bacon is cooked as crisp as you like it—usually about 10 minutes. The neck is also good for making turkey stock (see chapter 2).

How do you ruin a perfectly good turkey? By stuffing it full of gluten-filled bread cubes, of course. There are so many interesting ways to stuff a turkey that don't involve bread. You could stuff the turkey with gluten-free bread, of course, or rice, but a serving of bread stuffing contains far more carbs than I recommend for one day.

STUFFING OPTIONS

MAKES 8 SERVINGS
1 serving = ½ Wahls veg/fruit cup, if making the classic stuffing

TO MAKE: For a savory, classically flavored stuffing, stuff the turkey with a mixture of about 4 cups chopped onions, celery, carrots, and sprigs of herbs. Discard the herbs after cooking (or better yet, puree them with the pan juices in a blender for a rich, savory gravy, with or without bits of cooked giblets). This is a good recipe for those following Wahls Paleo Plus.

Personally, I like to make a fruit stuffing of chopped apples, plums, and raisins, just like my grandmother used to make. You could also use pears and a few fresh cranberries. Cut up about 4 cups orchard fruits, add about ½ cup raisins and/or dried cranberries, mix it all together, and stuff the turkey before roasting. Spoon out the fruit stuffing after roasting for a savory-sweet chutney-like treat. This recipe is not appropriate for Wahls Paleo Plus.

Count on one medium yam per person, or one large yam for two people. I recommend keeping the skins on because the skins are where most of the antioxidants are, but if you object to them, you can certainly scoop out the mash and discard the skins.

MASHED YAMS

YIELD VARIES

1 serving = 1½ Wahls veg/fruit cup

Note: This recipe is not appropriate for Wahls Paleo Plus.

TO MAKE: Bake the yam(s) in the oven at 375°F for about one hour, or until soft. Cut into chunks and mash. Add 1 tablespoon coconut oil and/or ghee per yam and season with sea salt and pepper. Serve hot. Adding 1 teaspoon minced garlic and/or chives per yam is also quite tasty.

WAHLS WARRIORS SPEAK

I have secondary progressive MS and I've been wheelchair-bound for five years. I started following the Wahls Diet in November 2014. Soon after, I started standing and was able to reach the top shelves in my kitchen. I went off the diet that Thanksgiving, which was a big mistake; I could no longer stand. I went back on the diet, and by January 30, 2015, I could walk 75 yards with Canadian crutches. It wasn't a stroll in the park, but I was walking. I went to physical therapy and started making great progress. Then they found a tumor in my colon. I had that removed in May 2015. Again, I couldn't walk or stand. It took some time to recover. I stayed on the diet, felt great, and lost 20 pounds of fat. I'm riding an E-stim bike two times a week for 35 minutes each time, and I'm starting to gain weight again in the form of muscles. Walking isn't easy, but I walk at least 100 yards a day, and my bowels and bladder are back to normal. I can sleep all night without going to the bathroom. The food I eat is great; you do pay more for quality food, but it's worth it. I'm lucky that I live in Alaska, where we can catch thirty-five salmon a year, which my daughter gets dip netting. Thank you to Dr. Wahls.

—Wahls Warrior ED

This is another easy and quick recipe.

COOKED GREENS WITH BACON AND MUSHROOMS

MAKES 8 SERVINGS

1 serving = 1 Wahls veg/fruit cup

Note: This recipe is appropriate for all levels of the Wahls Protocol.

1 pound bacon, chopped into bite-size pieces

2 cups sliced mushrooms

1 pound chopped kale or collard greens

TO MAKE: Cook the bacon in a skillet over medium heat until crispy. Add the mushrooms and sauté for about 5 minutes, or until they turn golden brown. Add the kale or collard greens and cook until they are wilted and bright green, about 2 minutes more, mixing everything together as it cooks. Serve hot.

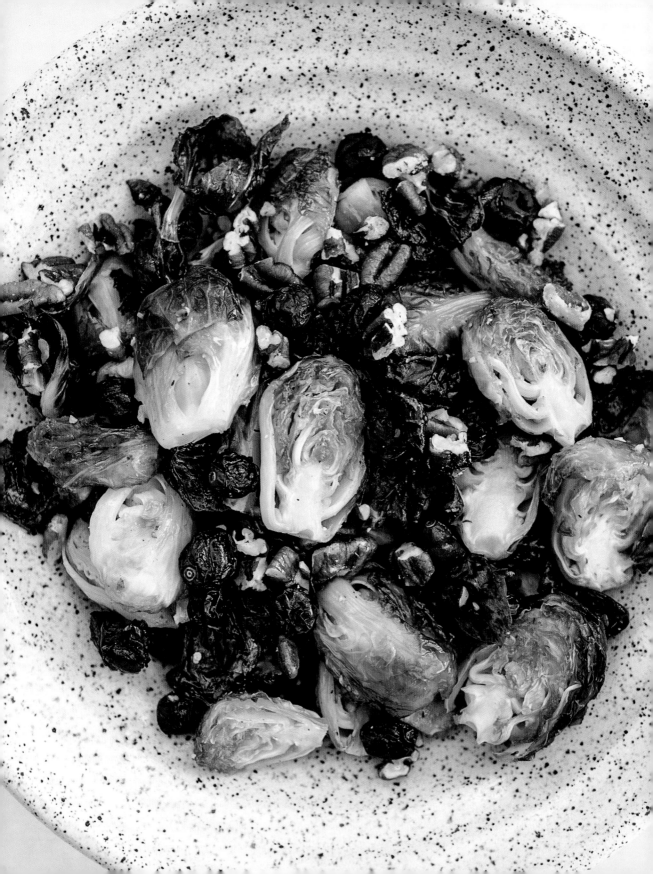

BRUSSELS SPROUTS, CRANBERRIES, AND PECANS

MAKES 6 TO 8 SERVINGS

1 serving = 1 Wahls veg/fruit cup

Note: This recipe is appropriate for all levels of the Wahls Protocol.

1 pound Brussels sprouts

1 tablespoon coconut oil or ghee, melted

Sea salt and freshly ground black pepper

1 cup fresh or thawed frozen cranberries

1 cup chopped pecans

TO MAKE: Preheat the oven to 400°F. Leave the sprouts whole, or halve or quarter them for crispier sprouts. Put them in a large bowl and drizzle with the coconut oil or ghee. Season with salt and pepper. Add the cranberries and toss to combine. Spread out the sprouts and cranberries in a single layer in a large baking pan or two. Bake until the Brussels sprouts are tender and crispy around the edges, about 45 minutes. After baking, transfer the Brussels sprouts and cranberries to a large serving bowl and sprinkle with the pecans.

As much as I love Wahls Paleo Plus, there are some recipes that just can't conform to its low-carb, high-fat requirements. This is one of them. This recipe is very popular with my family, but it is not compliant with Wahls Paleo Plus, and should only be consumed very infrequently on Wahls Paleo. Still, try it for a holiday. I think it's perfect for any fall or winter celebration, and it is truly delicious.

PUMPKIN (OR SQUASH OR SWEET POTATO PIE) PUDDING

MAKES 8 SERVINGS

1 serving = ¼ Wahls veg/fruit cup

Note: This recipe is not appropriate for Wahls Paleo Plus.

1 (14-ounce) can full-fat coconut milk, plus more as needed

1 tablespoon powdered gelatin

2 teaspoons pumpkin pie spice

½ cup raisins or snipped pitted prunes

2 cups pumpkin puree or winter squash or sweet potato puree

Whipped Coconut Cream (see page 264), for serving

8 pecan halves, for serving

TO MAKE: Warm the coconut milk over low heat. Sprinkle the gelatin over the surface and stir until it has dissolved. Place the coconut milk–gelatin mixture in a Vitamix or other high-speed blender, then add the pumpkin pie spice and the raisins. Blend, starting on low speed and gradually increasing to high. Add the pumpkin puree and blend again. If the motor strains, turn off the blender, add 2 to 4 tablespoons more coconut milk, and use the tamper to push everything down into the blender jar. Continue blending until smooth. Pour the mixture into eight individual serving dishes and refrigerate for at least 1 hour. Serve each with a dollop of Whipped Coconut Cream topped with a pecan half.

Note: If you don't have pumpkin pie spice on hand, make your own by combining 1 teaspoon ground cinnamon, ¼ teaspoon ground ginger, ¼ teaspoon ground nutmeg, ⅛ teaspoon ground allspice, and ⅛ teaspoon ground cloves.

WINTER CELEBRATION

Whether you celebrate Christmas, Hanukkah, Kwanzaa, Festivus, or something else, winter is a good time to fire up the oven and have friends and family over to share food and memories, and to celebrate the end of one year and the beginning of the next. Winter celebrations can feature many traditional or non-traditional foods, but this is the kind of menu we enjoy at my house.

WAHLS WINTER CELEBRATION MENU

Beet Kvass

Bacon-Wrapped Dates

Pan-Roasted Duck Breast with Braised Kale

Butternut Squash Soup with Duck Fat and Orange

Cauliflower Cranberry Rice

Snowballs (page 257)

Beet Kvass may sound unusual, but I highly encourage you to make this nutritious traditional eastern European fermented drink for your winter holiday celebration. Not only is it a festive holiday color, but also it will help keep you healthy and help you avoid the winter flu. This recipe is in *The Wahls Protocol,* but I repeat it here because it is so worth including in your diet—not just on a holiday but as often as you can. Be sure to start this recipe two or three days before your holiday feast so it is ready in time.

BEET KVASS

MAKES 4 SERVINGS
1 serving = ¼ Wahls veg/fruit cup
Note: This recipe is appropriate for all levels of the Wahls Protocol.

1 cup coarsely sliced or chopped raw beets (peeling optional)

1 tablespoon grated fresh ginger

1 tablespoon grated orange zest

1 tablespoon sea salt

1 probiotic capsule (such as VSL#3)

2½ cups filtered water, or as needed

TO MAKE: Wash a wide-mouth quart-size canning jar and lid carefully in hot soapy water and rinse well. Place the beet pieces in the jar, sprinkling the ginger, orange zest, and salt in with the beets as you are filling the jar. Open the probiotic capsule and sprinkle the contents over the top. Fill the jar with filtered water. Place a glass filled with water (tap water is fine) or a clean heavy item that fits in the mouth of the jar over the contents to keep the beets submerged underwater. Cover loosely with a clean tea towel and let the mixture sit on the counter for 2 to 3 days. Uncover, seal the jar, and refrigerate. This will keep in the refrigerator for up to three months. When you are ready to serve, pour the brightly colored liquid into a cup or bowl and drink it. You can serve the beets separately, as a side dish, or add them to a smoothie or a salad.

These are easy to make and impressive as an appetizer for guests. When cooked, the salty bacon is the perfect foil for the melt-in-your-mouth sweetness of the warm date and the crunch of the almond.

BACON-WRAPPED DATES

MAKES 12 SERVINGS

Note: This recipe is not appropriate for Wahls Paleo Plus.

8 slices bacon

24 dates

24 whole almonds

TO MAKE: Preheat the broiler. Cut each strip of bacon into three pieces (or two, if the strips are on the short side). Pull the pit out of each date and replace it with an almond. Wrap each date with one piece of bacon and secure with a toothpick. Broil until the bacon is fully cooked, 5 to 10 minutes, depending on the thickness of the bacon and how crisp you like it.

WAHLS WARRIORS SPEAK

After two years of eating Wahls Paleo, I am so grateful for my recovery. I feel blessed that I have the support of my husband and I am feeling so happy that yesterday, after three years, I was finally able to start running again. The impossible is possible, thanks to the Wahls Protocol!

—Wahls Warrior MURIEL

Duck is a richly nutritious meat that is less genetically and chemically manipulated than chicken. It can be expensive, however, so it is the perfect splurge for a holiday meal. You could roast a whole duck in the oven, but I prefer to cook the boneless breasts on the stove, like a pot roast—much less time-consuming and intimidating than roasting a whole duck. This works very well and is a good opportunity to add a lot of vegetables to the pot, increasing the nutrient profile even further. Duck pairs beautifully with cooked greens! It is one of our favorite special meals.

PAN-ROASTED DUCK BREAST WITH BRAISED KALE

MAKES 4 SERVINGS
1 serving = ½ Wahls veg/fruit cup

4 boneless duck breasts

2 tablespoons fresh lemon juice or orange juice

1 bunch lacinato kale, tough ends trimmed

TO MAKE: Score the skin of the duck breasts, being careful not to cut all the way through to the flesh, and put the duck in a cold skillet or stockpot, breast-side down. Cover the pan and set it over medium heat. Cook for 15 to 20 minutes, flipping once halfway through cooking. (The delicious fat will render out of the duck as you cook.) Check the doneness of the duck breasts—I like my duck rare to medium-rare, but if you want your duck more done than that, cook 5 to 10 minutes longer, then remove the meat to a plate and cover.

Add the lemon juice and the kale to the duck fat in the pan and cook for 2 to 3 minutes, until the greens are tender.

Transfer the greens to a serving platter and serve the duck on top. Pour the rendered duck fat and citrus juice into a small pitcher and use it as a sauce. You can also save some of the sauce to serve with Butternut Squash Soup (page 310). (If you have leftover duck fat, save it in the refrigerator, for cooking vegetables or meat at future meals—it adds a unique flavor and texture.)

Butternut squash soup takes on an incredible velvety texture with the addition of liquid gold: duck fat. But many people who have mobility issues balk at the idea of cooking butternut squash because it is so difficult to cut. What you may not realize, however, is that you can roast a butternut squash whole, and then cut it when it is soft. You don't even need to prick the skin before baking! You can also roast more than one at a time if you have a garden or farmers' market bounty and you want a supply of butternut squash puree in your freezer for the winter (and who wouldn't?).

BUTTERNUT SQUASH SOUP WITH DUCK FAT AND ORANGE

MAKES 8 TO 12 SERVINGS
1 serving = ¼ Wahls veg/fruit cup
Note: This recipe is not appropriate for Wahls Paleo Plus.

1 large butternut squash

½ cup duck fat

Juice of 2 oranges

1 teaspoon extra-virgin olive oil

1 teaspoon sea salt

Sprinkle of orange zest

Freshly ground black pepper

TO MAKE: Preheat the oven to 425°F, put the squash in a roasting pan or on a rimmed baking sheet, and roast until it is fork-tender (meaning you can easily pierce it with a fork), 1 hour for a small squash or up to 2 hours for a large one. Alternatively, put the whole squash in a slow cooker and cook on low for approximately 8 hours, or until it is very soft (you can leave it while you go to work and it will be done when you get home). Turn off the slow cooker, let the squash cool, peel it, cut it in half, and scoop out the seeds (all much easier when the squash is cooked). Transfer the squash flesh to a bowl and mash it roughly with a fork.

Measure about 3 cups of mashed butternut squash into a saucepan. Add the duck fat and the orange juice and simmer until warmed through. Pour the soup into bowls. Drizzle with the olive oil and sprinkle with the sea salt, orange zest, and pepper to taste.

Note: If you have a Vitamix or other high-speed blender, you can blend the squash—skin, seeds, and all—with the orange juice and duck fat. A Vitamix is powerful enough to break down the squash seeds. And you will get the fiber from the seed hulls and skins, which will be excellent food for the health-promoting bacteria living in your bowels! It also reduces food waste. If you don't have a high-speed blender like a Vitamix, be sure to peel and seed the squash.

DUCK LIVER AND FAT

If you are lucky enough to get the liver when you buy your duck, or find duck liver in your market, fry it in some coconut oil or ghee and enjoy—duck liver is a special treat! Or wrap it in bacon and broil it. Also, duck fat is highly prized in European kitchens and by chefs, so save any extra duck fat in a jar or ceramic crock and use it for cooking—it's delicious when used to cook skillet recipes!

WAHLS WARRIORS SPEAK

I am so grateful that I am finally recovering from three years of post-viral syndrome. The year 2015 was the year I got back on track, and in 2016 I have three half-marathons already booked in my diary. Go, wellness warriors!

—Wahls Warrior WENDY

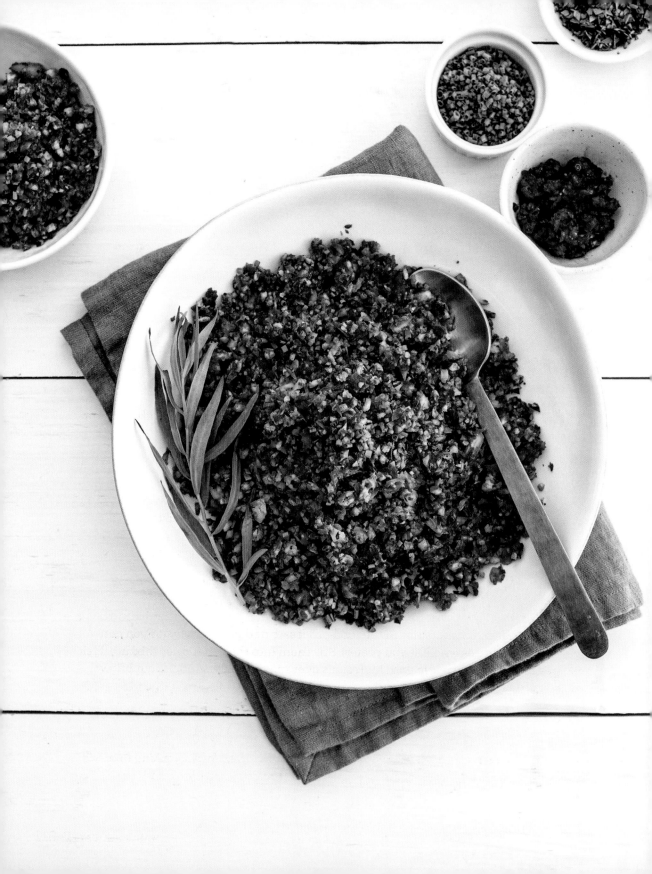

It couldn't be easier to turn cauliflower into "rice." All you need is one head of cauliflower and a food processor. In this recipe, the cranberries and herbs add bright red and green colors—it looks and tastes festive! Don't be afraid to try it—you will be surprised how good it tastes.

CAULIFLOWER CRANBERRY RICE

MAKES 8 TO 12 SERVINGS
1 serving = ¾ Wahls veg/fruit cup
Note: This recipe is appropriate for all levels of the Wahls Protocol.

1 large cauliflower head

¼ cup garlic cloves

¼ cup fresh herbs

2 cups fresh cranberries

1 tablespoon ghee

1 teaspoon sea salt

Freshly ground black pepper

TO MAKE: Quarter the cauliflower head and trim off the tough parts of the stem. Break the cauliflower into pieces and put half in a food processor. Pulse until the cauliflower is chopped into pieces roughly the size of grains of rice. Transfer the riced cauliflower to a large bowl. Repeat with the remaining cauliflower and add that to the bowl, too.

Put the garlic and herbs in the food processor (no need to clean the bowl) and pulse briefly to break them down into small, relatively uniform pieces. Stir them into the cauliflower. Put the cranberries in the food processor and pulse briefly (or you can leave the cranberries whole, if you prefer). Stir them into the cauliflower mixture. Melt the ghee in a large saucepan with high sides over medium heat. Add the cauliflower-cranberry rice and sauté for about 3 minutes, or just until coated with the ghee. Season with the salt and pepper to taste and serve warm.

Variation: You can also make this with grated raw winter squash or yams in place of cauliflower, for an orange and red rice that is bright and festive, too. The cooking time will be slightly longer (5 to 10 minutes) if you use squash or yams to make your rice.

SPRING FEAST

To herald the coming of spring or to celebrate Easter, have a spring feast featuring all the new "baby" vegetables available at this time of year.

WAHLS SPRING FEAST MENU

Bison Roast with Garlic Ginger Rub

Pickled Spring Vegetables with Garden Herbs

Asparagus with Ghee and Lime

Fresh Strawberries Dipped in Coco-Almond Butter Sauce

Greens with Spring Onions and Radishes

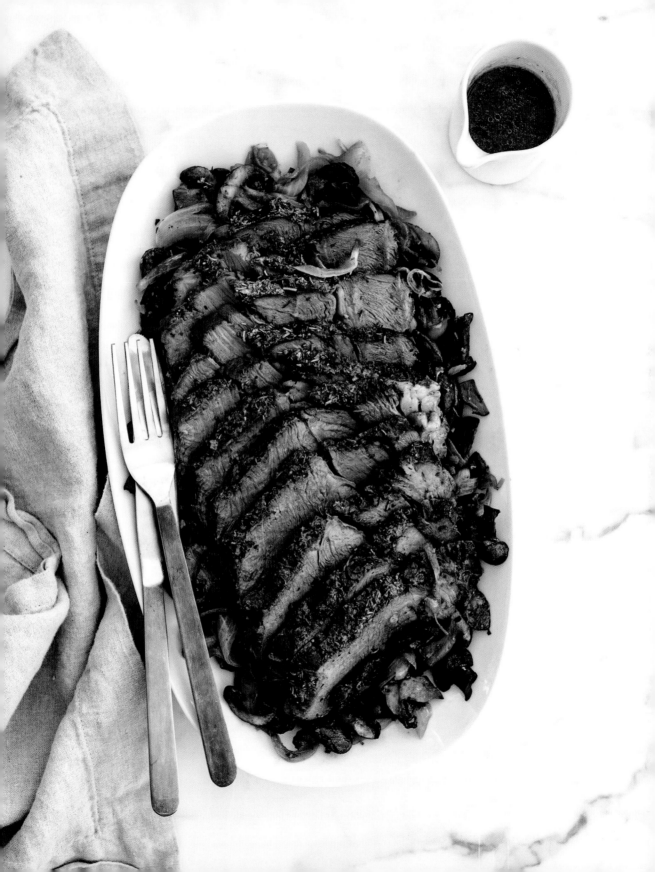

Bison roast can be difficult to find, but it is so worth the search. I get my bison from Tall Grass Bison in Iowa, but you can get grass-fed bison online. Do a search for a farmer near you, or use a farmer who will ship frozen. These two companies will ship within the continental United States: www.grassfedtraditions.com/grass_fed_bison.htm and www.tallgrassbison.com. If you can't find or don't want to make bison roast, you can use grass-fed beef, lamb, or pork.

BISON ROAST WITH GARLIC GINGER RUB

MAKES 8 SERVINGS
1 serving = 1 Wahls veg/fruit cup
Note: This recipe is appropriate for all levels of the Wahls Protocol.

2 to 3 tablespoons herbes de Provence

3 garlic cloves, minced, or 1 tablespoon minced garlic

½ teaspoon grated fresh ginger

½ teaspoon sea salt

Freshly ground black pepper

1 (2-pound) bison roast

2 medium onions, sliced

1 pound mushrooms, sliced

TO MAKE: Preheat the oven to 450°F.

In a small bowl, combine the herbes de Provence, garlic, ginger, salt, and pepper to taste and rub it all over the roast. Put the sliced onions and mushrooms on the bottom of a roasting pan. Set the roast on top. Insert a meat thermometer into the thickest part of the roast.

Put the roast in the oven and cook for 15 minutes, then turn the oven temperature down to 300°F and cook until the internal temperature of the roast reaches 140°F. Remove from the oven, cover tightly with aluminum foil, and let rest for 10 minutes so the juice stays in the meat. (You want a final temperature of 145°F for a rare roast—I use a probe thermometer and set it to alert me when the meat is 140°F, because the temperature will rise 5°F after I take it out of the oven.)

Uncover the roast and slice it. If it is too rare for you, you can put it back in the oven, but watch it closely, as the meat will cook very quickly once it is sliced.

This light, easy ferment is perfect for spring onions and radishes. Colored radishes are fun to use in this recipe—I like to use black radishes, but any will do. Reserve the radish greens for your smoothies or stock.

PICKLED SPRING VEGETABLES WITH GARDEN HERBS

MAKES 4 SERVINGS

1 serving = 1 Wahls veg/fruit cup

Note: This recipe is appropriate for all levels of the Wahls Protocol.

2 to 3 tablespoons sea salt

4 cups filtered water

6 cups sliced mixed spring onions and radishes

1 probiotic capsule (such as VSL#3)

2 tablespoons herbs and whole spices of your choice (such as black peppercorns, chopped dill, caraway seeds, minced garlic, anise, chile peppers, mustard seeds)

1 large cabbage leaf

TO MAKE: Dissolve the sea salt in the water and set aside. Wash a wide-mouth quart-size canning jar and lid carefully in hot soapy water and rinse well with chlorine-free water. Boiling the water for 10 minutes will dissipate the chlorine. Pack the spring onion and radish slices into the jar. Pour the salt water over the vegetables just to cover them. Add the contents of the probiotic capsule and herbs and spices to the jar. Cover the jar with the cabbage leaf and weigh it down with a clean heavy weight that fits in the mouth of the jar, to keep the vegetables submerged. Cover loosely with a towel and let the vegetables sit at 60 to 70°F for 2 to 4 days, then put the lid on the jar and refrigerate. The ferment will keep in the refrigerator for 3 to 6 months. To serve, remove the vegetables with a clean fork to avoid contamination with problematic bacteria. Serve cold.

ASPARAGUS WITH GHEE AND LIME

MAKES 6 TO 8 SERVINGS

1 serving = ½ Wahls veg/fruit cup

1 pound spring asparagus

2 tablespoons ghee

1 tablespoon fresh lime juice

Lime wedges, for serving

TO MAKE: Trim the tough ends off the asparagus. Heat the ghee and lime juice in a skillet over medium heat. Sauté the asparagus 1 to 3 minutes or until tender (thicker asparagus may need a little more time, but a crisp-tender texture is perfect). Transfer to a platter and serve with lime wedges.

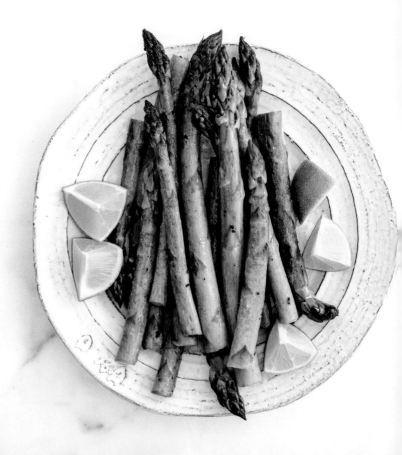

Fresh strawberries usually start appearing in stores in late March and start to taste really good in April and May, and continue through June and sometimes into July. Good strawberries are always a treat for any level of the Wahls Protocol. But for a divine dessert worthy of any special occasion, dip them in Coco–Almond Butter Sauce and chill them (these are also nice for Valentine's Day). The following recipe makes about 1 cup sauce, which is enough to dip about 1 quart strawberries if you cover about half of each berry.

FRESH STRAWBERRIES DIPPED IN COCO–ALMOND BUTTER SAUCE

| MAKES 1 QUART

1 quart strawberries

Coco–Almond Butter Sauce (recipe follows)

TO MAKE: Lightly oil a baking sheet or muffin tin. Wash and dry the strawberries well. Warm the sauce until it has thinned enough for dipping. Dip each strawberry halfway into the sauce, then place them on the baking sheet or in the muffin tin and refrigerate until the sauce is firm. Serve the berries on a chilled plate. The coconut oil and ghee in the sauce are solid below 78°F; in very warm weather, serve the berries over a bed of ice to keep them firm.

COCO–ALMOND BUTTER SAUCE

This sauce turns strawberries into Paleo candy. My family loves it, not just on berries but also drizzled over desserts. It's amazing to eat with a spoon.

| MAKES ABOUT 1 CUP

TO MAKE: Mix all the ingredients by hand in a bowl or in a food processor. Transfer to an airtight container and refrigerate to thicken. To use for dipping, gently warm the sauce to soften and thin it.

RECIPE CONTINUES

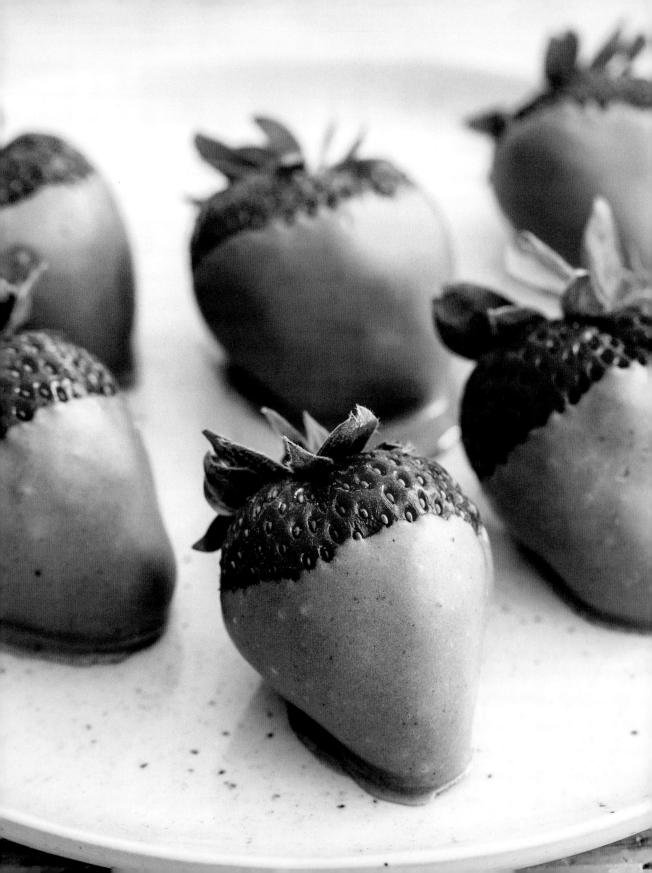

	WAHLS DIET AND WAHLS PALEO	WAHLS PALEO PLUS
NUT BUTTER	½ cup	½ cup
SOFTENED GHEE	¼ cup	¼ cup
SOFTENED COCONUT OIL	¼ cup	¼ cup
SWEETENER	1 tablespoon honey or maple syrup	None
FLAVORINGS	1 tablespoon unsweetened cocoa powder	1 tablespoon unsweetened cocoa powder
	1 teaspoon ground cinnamon	1 teaspoon ground cinnamon

Savory, Spicy Variation: Omit the cocoa powder and add $1/8$ to $1/4$ teaspoon cayenne or ground chile pepper. This variation tastes similar to a Thai peanut sauce and tastes great with bell pepper slices and celery sticks.

BIRTHDAYS THE WAHLS WAY

If it's your birthday, or the birthday of a loved one, you may feel a temporary pang at the loss of the birthday cake tradition. But keep in mind that those white flour, white sugar, fatty-frosting-covered cakes are intensely negative nutritionally for anyone, and for people working actively to improve their health, eating something so devoid of nutrients and so full of inflammatory, disease-flaring ingredients can be really damaging.

Here's the good news: There are delicious desserts in this cookbook that are worthy of a birthday celebration or any other special occasion. Try any of the cheezcakes in the desserts chapter. Or make a nut crust (page 268), fill it with fresh fruit, and frost it with Whipped Coconut Cream (see page 264) or drizzle with Coco–Almond Butter Sauce (page 319). Refrigerate so it firms up to hold candles and you have a festive and special cake.

You can also fill nut crusts with pudding (pages 273–278). When chilled, the pudding will hold birthday candles, too. Or don't worry about the candles and arrange them on the side. There are many festive options. We used to use action figure candles for our birthday celebrations! Happy birthday, indeed!

SUMMER BBQ

A summer barbecue is one of the easiest celebrations to stay Wahls compliant and still have fun. You can enjoy grilled meats of all types; grilled sweet potatoes; grilled vegetables like zucchini, pepper, asparagus, and onions; and even heads of garlic, leafy green salads (skip the croutons and dairy products), raw vegetables, and fresh fruits. If you need a dish to bring, try this easy broccoli salad.

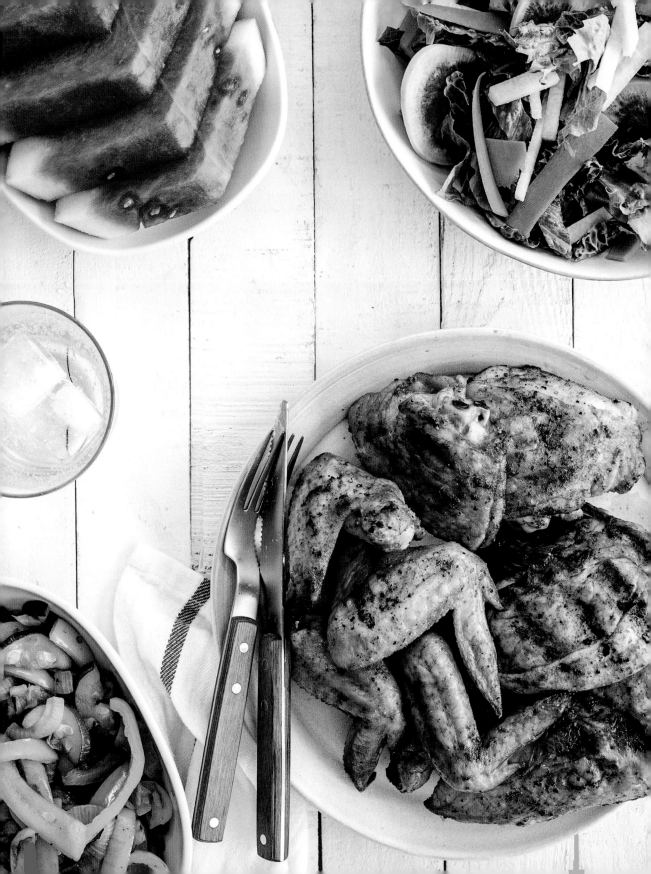

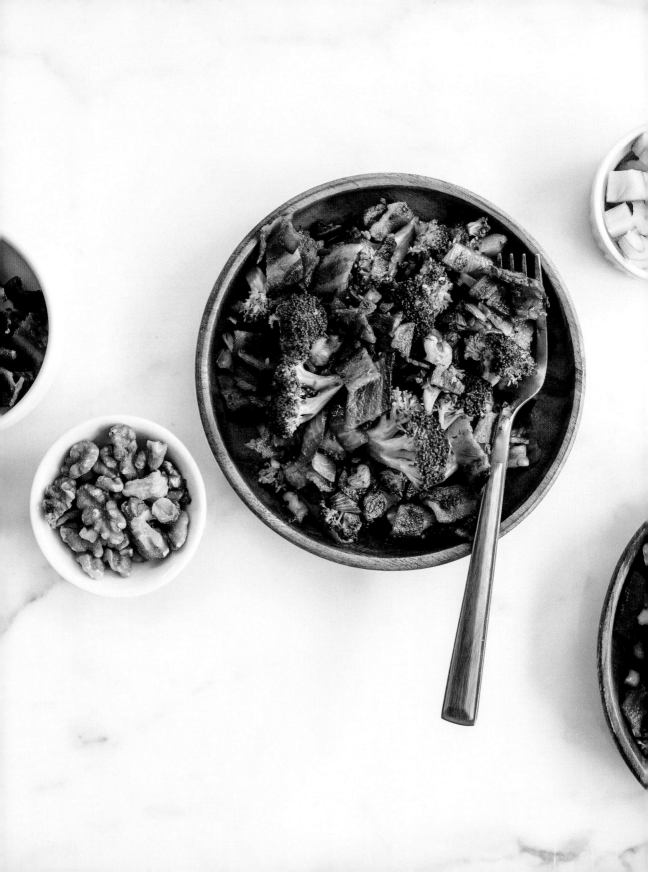

This Wahls-approved recipe is a favorite at picnics—everyone will love it!

BROCCOLI SALAD WITH BACON

MAKES 4 SERVINGS
1 serving = 1¼ Wahls veg/fruit cups

1 pound bacon, chopped into small pieces

½ cup chopped walnuts

1 cup chopped red onion

1 head broccoli, cut into bite-size pieces

½ cup full-fat coconut milk

½ cup golden raisins (omit for Wahls Paleo Plus)

2 tablespoons apple cider vinegar (optional)

TO MAKE: Cook the bacon in a large skillet until crisp. Add the walnuts, onion, and broccoli and cook until the broccoli is crisp-tender, about 10 minutes. Remove from the heat and stir in the coconut milk and raisins (if using). If you want a little more tang, stir in the vinegar. I think it tastes great either way. Toss to coat, cover, and chill until it's time for the party.

WAHLS HALLOWEEN

Halloween can be tough for kids who can't eat gluten or sugar, but it can also be hard for parents who were accustomed to pilfering treats from their kids' stashes. Halloween can seem like it is all about the candy, but you can make it about the spirit of the event. Pumpkin soup, bell peppers carved into jack-o'-lanterns and stuffed with meat and vegetables, and "ghostly" cauliflower rice with shredded coconut and blanched almonds are some meal ideas. But to make your celebration really whimsical and fun, try fruit jigglers.

Fruit jigglers are great for many occasions because you can cut them into different shapes with cookie cutters. You can buy cookie cutters shaped like turkeys, leaves, snowflakes, Christmas trees, dreidels, hearts, bunnies and chicks, stars and flags, and, of course, pumpkins, ghosts, witches, and other scary shapes! Fruit jigglers are so easy to make, you can whip up a batch for every holiday and keep the kids happy and healthy.

FRUIT JIGGLERS

4 cups fruit juice (such as pomegranate, açaí, grape, orange, blueberry, or a mixture of juices to create a blackish color for Halloween)

¼ cup gelatin, ideally from grass-fed animals

TO MAKE: Pour 1 cup of the juice into a saucepan and sprinkle the gelatin over the top. Set aside to soften for 10 minutes. Set the pan over medium heat and warm, stirring, until the gelatin has dissolved. Add the remaining 3 cups juice. Pour the gelatin mixture into a 13 × 9 × 2-inch cake pan and refrigerate overnight. To release the jigglers from the pan, dip the bottom of the pan into warm water for 10 to 15 seconds. Invert the pan onto a cutting board. You can either cut the jigglers into squares or use a cookie cutter to make interesting shapes. Store in an airtight container in the refrigerator for up to 2 days.

Variation: You can also make jigglers using 4 cups of any liquid (such as 2 cups water and 2 cups homemade or purchased kombucha) in place of the juice. If using kombucha, sprinkle the gelatin over water to soften and only stir the kombucha into the gelatin mixture once the temperature is cool enough that it won't kill the kombucha (warm to touch, not hot).

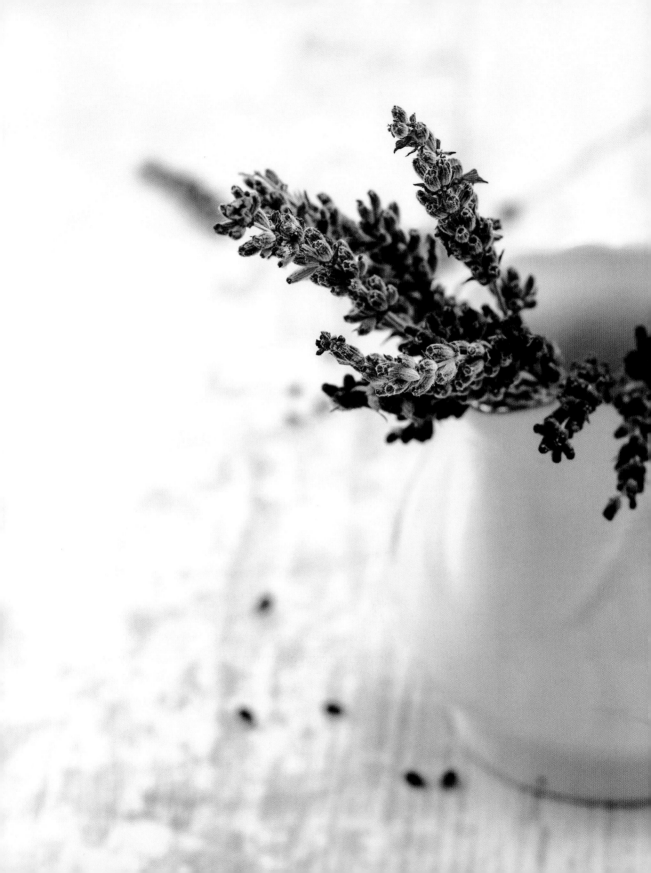

HOUSEHOLD AND PERSONAL CARE RECIPES

AVOIDING TOXINS AND CHEMICALS WHENEVER POSSIBLE is an important part of every level of the Wahls Protocol, but what do you do when you need to wash your hair, moisturize your face, or clean the kitchen? You might be surprised to learn how easy it is to keep your house and your body clean without conventional products that contain chemicals that could have a toxic effect on your cells.

It's true that we live in a toxic world, so it is virtually impossible to live without taking in at least some toxins from air, water, and food. But you can make choices that greatly reduce your toxicity load. If you can clean your home naturally, you will lower the indoor air pollution you experience every day. If you also eliminate toxic chemicals that you use on your body—remember that your skin is porous and takes into your body whatever you put on it—then you will have made a pretty sizable dent in your internal toxicity level, especially over time.

Fortunately, adopting natural products is an easy transition, and much more cost-effective, too. One of the most versatile and inexpensive products you can buy is coconut oil. It's so useful in the kitchen, and it's also an essential product for personal hygiene. When combined with various essential oils, it does as good a job or better than fancy and expensive personal hygiene products from toothpaste to face cream. Add sea salt, extra-virgin olive oil, Epsom salts, and vinegar, and you've got most of your personal and household needs covered.

The DIY tips in this chapter are barely even recipes, they are so simple and basic. Give them a try and enjoy the financial savings as well as the enjoyment of making your own products at home.

PERSONAL CARE PRODUCTS

You can clean your hair, face, and teeth; fight body odor; and keep your skin moisturized and supple with just a few basic ingredients. If you have these on hand, you will be able to cover all your needs. Keep them in your medicine cabinet. You'll have plenty of room when you toss out all those beauty products with ingredients that aren't good for your cells. Here is your personal care shopping list (you probably already have many of these items in your kitchen, which means you can "shop" for them without spending any extra money):

- **Coconut oil:** I buy a big jar just for use in the bathroom.
- **Coconut milk:** Just borrow a can from your kitchen when you need to make shampoo.
- **Extra-virgin olive oil:** I also keep a separate bottle in the bathroom.
- **Ghee and nut oil:** Borrow these from the kitchen, too.
- **Sea salt**
- **Epsom salt**
- **Baking soda**
- **Fresh oregano, lavender, and/or savory leaves:** If you plant a simple herb garden (in your yard or in pots), you will have these available whenever you need them.

- **Liquid castile soap**
- **Your favorite essential oils.** The ones I use most are:
  - Tea tree oil
  - Oregano oil
  - Peppermint oil
  - Clove oil
  - Cinnamon oil
  - Citrus oil (lemon, lime, orange, or grapefruit)
  - Sandalwood oil
  - Chamomile oil
  - Lavender oil

OPTIONAL

- **Bentonite or zeolite clay**
- **Kelp or algae powder**

Shampoo

There are a lot of natural shampoo recipes out there, and some of them work for some people but don't work at all for others. I have no idea why, but a shampoo can make one person's hair look great and another's look unwashed. If you want to make your own shampoo with all-natural ingredients, you may need to experiment a bit with ratios and ingredients, but this is the recipe that I have found works well for me.

½ cup liquid castile soap

½ cup full-fat canned coconut milk

1 teaspoon almond oil

¼ teaspoon of your favorite essential oil, for a nice scent

Mix everything in a jar or bottle and shake well. Pour about 1 tablespoon on top of wet hair and lather, then rinse well. Always shake before using. If you find this shampoo leaves your hair too oily, try rinsing your hair with equal parts apple cider vinegar and water after washing.

Face Wash

To eliminate dirt and oil, rub coconut oil on your face and rinse it off with lukewarm water. Pat your skin dry.

Face Scrub

For a cleansing plus exfoliating effect, mix 1 tablespoon each of extra-virgin olive oil and sea salt in a small cup or bowl. Add a few drops of orange, lavender, or grapefruit essential oil, then scoop it up with your fingers and rub it gently over your face. Rinse with lukewarm water and pat dry.

Face Cream

Plain coconut oil, almond oil, extra-virgin olive oil, and ghee all make excellent night creams to put on before bed.

Natural Facial

Smooth your skin, soothe redness, and look younger with this simple facial. Mix about $1/3$ cup bentonite or zeolite clay, $1/4$ teaspoon kelp or algae, and enough water to make a thick paste. Apply to your face and relax (perhaps in an Epsom salt bath) for 30 minutes. Gently rinse off with luke-warm water. Another option is to add $1/2$ teaspoon turmeric instead of or in addition to the kelp or algae.

CLAY DISPOSAL

When you use clay, don't rinse it down the drain or flush it down the toilet. It can swell or harden and cause serious plumbing issues. Instead, toss it outside on a patch of grass or into your garden. It acts as a natural fertilizer. If you live in a place without your own yard, you can also dispose of it in the garbage (but it will be heavy!).

Clay Foot Soak

Use the same ingredients as you would use for the Natural Facial, but add them to a small tub of warm water and soak your feet for 30 minutes.

Deodorant

Dip your fingers into coconut oil, add a couple drops of essential oil (especially tea tree oil, oregano oil, or Thieves oil), and spread it over your underarms. Rotate various oils so your body's bacteria do not develop a resistance to the effects of any particular oil.

Oil Pulling

Oil pulling is an ancient technique that can dissolve plaque, kill bacteria, and greatly improve your oral hygiene. Swish 1 teaspoon (you can gradually increase to 1 tablespoon) olive, walnut, coconut, or sesame oil in your mouth for 1 minute, then spit it out and brush your teeth. Work up to 5 minutes. Some people like to swish the oil around for up to 20 minutes, but I find I don't usually have time for that.

Toothpaste

All you need to use on your toothbrush is coconut oil. The fat emulsifies the bacterial cell walls, removes stains (most of which are fat soluble), and is very helpful for whitening teeth and reducing periodontal inflammation and gingivitis. Just drag your toothbrush across the oil, coating the top of the brush, then dip the oil-coated toothbrush into a small jar of baking soda to get a little abrasiveness along with the oil. This will help to scrape off plaque. Add a couple drops of essential oil for its antimicrobial properties—I especially like using peppermint, clove, or cinnamon oil for breath freshening.

You will have that same sparkling-clean feeling that you enjoy after getting your teeth cleaned when you use coconut oil, baking soda, and essential oils on your teeth.

If you want to get a little more complicated, you can also mix 1 cup melted coconut oil, ½ cup baking soda, 2 tablespoons cinnamon, 3 or 4 activated charcoal capsules, and 5 mls of your favorite essential oil in a glass jar or container with a lid. I stir this all together and then place in a bath of cold water or ice water and stir the oil mixture intermittently, until it hardens. I keep this in the bathroom, covered, and I use it to brush my teeth and for my oil pulling.

Brushing your teeth with coconut oil and an essential oil will markedly reduce gum irritation and gum infection (gingivitis), and can reduce more serious periodontitis (inflammation involving the roots of the teeth). Note that both gingivitis and periodontitis are associated with higher rates of atherosclerosis, heart disease, and stroke.

Breath Freshening

Chew on fresh oregano, lavender, or savory leaves for an instant breath freshener.

Bath Salts

Soaking in a bath is an excellent way to take in more magnesium, which helps with muscle healing and strength. Mix ½ cup sea salt with ½ cup Epsom salts and pour into a warm bath. Add 4 to 10 drops of your favorite essential oil. I like lavender, sandalwood, or chamomile for a relaxing bath. For more moisture, add 1 tablespoon extra-virgin olive oil to the bathwater.

ICE BATH

To lower inflammation and boost melatonin, try a cold bath. This will feel very uncomfortable at first, but if you gradually make your baths cooler over time, you can ease into it. Cool, cold, or ice baths are excellent for improving sleep. Take your time getting used to this, but I find that the effort is worth it. I sleep much better after a cold or ice bath. Note: Do not use actual ice in your bath if you have Raynaud's disease, which could aggravate the condition.

Detox Bath

Add 1 cup baking soda and 1 cup Epsom salts to a warm bath. For an even more intensive bath that will pull toxins out through the skin, add 1 to 2 tablespoons bentonite clay and/or 1 teaspoon kelp powder. Soak in the bath for as long as you can, then rinse off in the shower.

Note that this is a very small amount of clay in an entire tub of bathwater—you want to be sure that the clay is very dilute if you use it in your bathtub, or it can clog your drain. Also note that if you have a private septic system, taking a dilute clay bathtub soak could void your warranty, so check into this before you try it.

For Restless Legs or Neuropathic Pain

Stir together about 2 tablespoons extra-virgin olive oil or coconut oil, 1 tablespoon sea salt, and 1 tablespoon Epsom salts. Add 20 to 30 drops of frankincense essential oil and massage the mixture over your legs or areas where you are having nerve pain.

HOUSEHOLD CLEANERS

Some of the most toxic chemicals in the average household are found in cleaners. However, you don't need to clean with toxic chemicals. Some basic ingredients from your kitchen and bathroom should take care of most messes. Keep the following ingredients around and you will be ready to clean without fumes:

- Distilled white vinegar
- Isopropyl alcohol
- Plain unscented dish soap

Basic Household Cleaner

Mix equal parts white vinegar and water into a spray bottle. Add 1 teaspoon unscented dish soap and ¼ teaspoon peppermint oil for a fresh scent. Shake gently before using to clean kitchen and bathroom surfaces.

Glass Cleaner

Mix equal parts isopropyl alcohol and water in a spray bottle. Add ½ teaspoon unscented dish soap. Shake gently before using to clean windows and mirrors.

PET CARE

There is a lot of evidence that pets react poorly to grains. Although in the wild, dogs will sometimes eat the contents of their prey's stomachs, those contents are predigested and in small amounts. Their first choice is eating the organ meats. Most dogs need meat and just a hint of greens to thrive, and many do poorly on a grain-based diet, just like humans. Cats in particular do very poorly on grains, and there is a lot of veterinary evidence to suggest that high-grain processed-food diets contribute to the high rates of kidney problems in pet cats. I believe high-grain diets also contribute to the high rates of pet obesity, diabetes, and even anxiety and behavior problems so common to pets today.

Instead, look for grain-free foods for both dogs and cats. Many are available now that more people recognize that grain is not appropriate for dogs and cats. There are also some great books out there that will give you ideas for how to make your own pet food from scratch. If you are eating Wahls Paleo or Wahls Paleo Plus, you can probably share more of your food with your pets as well. Pets should never eat avocado, chocolate, onions, or grapes, but any meat leftovers would be a fine addition to a grain-free kibble or canned food.

For my own pets, I often make venison liver ice cube treats (my neighbors and friends drop off the organs from their hunts—lucky pets!). Simply cut up organ meat into small pieces, drop them in ice cube trays, and freeze. Once frozen, pop the liver ice cubes out and freeze them in a zip-top plastic bag. You will love how this adds more vibrant nutrition to your pet's diet, and your pet will love the treats. (This is an appropriate treat for both dogs and cats.)

FINAL WORDS

THE END OF THIS BOOK is the beginning of the next phase of reclaiming your life. As you work through this book and integrate new habits, foods, and attitudes into your life, you may sometimes stumble. Even as you feel better, you may begin to think that you don't need to eat so well anymore. This happens to many of my patients. I recognize that adopting a new health behavior is challenging for anyone. Sustaining it for the rest of your life is harder still. You will have setbacks. You will make mistakes. You might even get angry at yourself when you "fall off the wagon." Many of my patients tell me how they gave up their healthy habits over the holidays, on vacation, or for some other reason—or sometimes for no other reason than wanting a forbidden food. I understand that. We are all imperfect.

And yet steady progress forward is the key to "youthening," to reclaiming energy and vitality, mobility and strength. It is the key to clearing brain fog and standing up and walking—and even running—again. The trick is not to let so-called failures derail you. Just get back to your healthy habits. Slow and steady wins the race. Crack open this book again and make something you know you love—a simple smoothie or soup, a hearty dinner or luscious dessert, a face cream or an Epsom salt bath. Sit still for a while, breathe, and find your center again. When the food your cells love is also the food your taste buds love, you will have a much easier time eating to support your health rather than to tear it down.

Friends and family who support your food choices are also immensely helpful. Be open and vocal about what you are doing and ask for that support. When the people who love you know it is important to you, they are more likely to stand behind you and avoid sabotaging your good efforts. When they see the changes in you, they will be won over. Having others to talk to and celebrate your successes with is also rejuvenating and inspiring. That is where finding a supportive community can be important to your success. To that end, you may want to follow me on Twitter (@TerryWahls) or Facebook (TerryWahls) to get your daily inspiration, or visit my website, www.terrywahls.com, to see where I will be lecturing next and what programs we have available that may be useful to you to learn more tools to help you reclaim your life. Every August, I have an in-person seminar in Iowa where people come from around the globe to hear me teach about using diet and lifestyle choices to reclaim health and vitality. It is an opportunity to meet other Wahls Warriors who are getting their lives back and to be part of a growing community. Come join us if you can.

Where you go from here is, of course, entirely up to you, but I hope you will let the Wahls Protocol and this cookbook be one important piece in the life you are building. I hope you will let me help you build your health back up, and as you get stronger, more energetic, and more vibrant, I hope you will reach out to help others. Life is a chain, with each of us building the connections when and where we are able. The Wahls Protocol can help you find the strength to live the life you want, and maybe even help you change the food system we all use, even the priorities of our culture. Food is what builds us up or tears us down. I say, let's keep building, and let's do it together.

Keep in touch, and keep eating your vegetables!

Sincerely,

Terry L Wahls

RECIPE LIST

*=Variation   **=Sidebar Recipe

CHAPTER 2

Basic Bone Broth, **page 29**

Chicken Broth*, **page 30**

Fish or Shellfish Broth*, **page 30**

Thicker Broth*, **page 30**

Fermented Red Cabbage, **page 32**

Fermented Garlic-Ginger Sauce**, **page 34**

Nut Milk, **page 37**

Yogurt Milk, **page 38**

Kefir Milk*, **page 38**

Nut or Seed Butter, **page 39**

Wahls Pâté, **page 40**

Rawmesan, **page 42**

Soft Cheez, **page 43**

Fresh Salsa, **page 45**

Wahls Taco Seasoning**, **page 45**

Cilantro Salsa, **page 46**

Watermelon Gazpacho, **page 47**

Tomato-Free Red Sauce, **page 47**

Wahls Guacamole, **page 48**

Slow-Cooker Roasted Root Vegetables, **page 49**

Slow-Cooker Spaghetti Squash, **page 50**

Cauliflower/Broccoli Rice, **page 53**

Herbed Olive Oil, **page 54**

CHAPTER 3

Basic Smoothie Template, **page 65**

Tropical Smoothie, **page 66**

Citrus Smoothie, **page 67**

Strawberry or Raspberry Carrot Smoothie, **page 68**

Apple or Pumpkin Pie Smoothie, **page 71**

Chocolate Smoothie, **page 72**

Carrot Ginger Smoothie, **page 75**

Green Goddess Grape Smoothie, **page 76**

Peach Carrot Smoothie, **page 78**

Orange Smoothie, **page 79**

Blackberry Smoothie, **page 80**

Power Piña Colada**, **page 81**

Beet Mango Smoothie, **page 82**

Watermelon Smoothie, **page 84**

Blackberry Grape Smoothie, **page 85**

CHAPTER 4

Basic Juice Template, **page 94**

Strawberry Orange Juice, **page 95**

Cooling Cucumber Mint Juice,
page 96

Summer Melon Juice, **page 98**

Beet-licious Juice with Ginger and
Orange, **page 101**

Alkalinizing Ginger Lime Juice, **page 103**

Daily Detox Juice with Wild Greens,
page 106

Basic Spritzer Template, **page 109**

Citrus Spritzer, **page 110**

Berry Spritzer, **page 111**

Green Happy Hour Spritzer, **page 113**

Orange Spritzer, **page 114**

Basic Tea/Infusion Template, **page 118**

Detoxifying Turmeric Pepper Cream
Tea, **page 119**

Rosemary Ginger Tea, **page 120**

Wild Greens Tea**, **page 120**

Herbal Rise-and-Shine Tea, **page 121**

Ginger Lemon Infusion, **page 122**

Yerba Mate with Calendula, **page 123**

Chamomile and Coconut Milk Tea,
page 124

Red Clover Tea, **page 125**

CHAPTER 5

Basic Granola Template, **page 130**

Cinnamon Orange Granola, **page 132**

Seedy Flax Granola, **page 133**

Coco-Nutty Granola, **page 134**

Harvest Nut and Spice Granola, **page 137**

Basic Porridge Template, **page 140**

Hemp Heart Porridge, **page 141**

Everything Porridge, **page 142**

Coconut Almond Porridge, **page 143**

Sunny Peach Porridge, **page 144**

Chia-Almond Porridge with
Cranberries, **page 147**

Golden Quinoa Porridge, **page 148**

Flax Raisin or Berry Porridge, **page 151**

CHAPTER 6

Basic Salad Dressing Template, **page 155**

Mixed Greens Salad Dressing, **page 156**

Simple Olive Lemon Vinaigrette, **page 156**

Balsamic Vinaigrette, **page 157**

Wahls Ranch-Style Dressing, **page 157**

Wahls Italian Dressing, **page 158**

Wahls Caesar-Style Dressing, **page 158**

Basic Main Course Salad Template,
page 161

Smoked Oyster Salad, page 162

Fajita Halibut Salad, page 163

Spring Herb Salad with Shrimp, Onions, and Chives, page 165

Grilled Chicken and Purple Potato Salad, page 166

Arugula Chicken Salad with Berries and Lemon, page 168

Garlic Chicken Salad, page 169

Bacon Salad, page 171

Wahls Chicken Caesar Salad, page 172

Poached (or Grilled) Salmon Salad, page 173

Wilted Kale and Duck Salad with Beets, Walnuts, and Soft Cheez, page 174

Basic Side Salad Template, page 177

Light Almond Tomato Salad, page 178

Arugula Salad with Fresh Lemon Vinaigrette, page 179

Beet, Carrot, and Rutabaga Matchstick Salad with Fresh Cilantro, page 181

Watercress Cucumber Salad with Avocado and Orange Slices, page 182

Wild Salad, page 184

Basic Wrap Template, page 189

Drive-Through Wrap, page 191

Deli Sandwich Wrap, page 192

Citrus Salad**, page 193

Berry Melon Salad**, page 193

Mixed Berries**, page 193

CHAPTER 7

Basic Soup Template, page 197

Beef Marrow Broth, page 199

Potassium Broth, page 200

Red Potassium Broth*, page 200

Mushroom Broth, page 201

Old-Fashioned Chicken Soup, page 202

Quick Chicken Broth**, page 202

Kale, Sausage, and Yam Soup with Coconut Milk, page 207

Cauliflower Carrot Garlic Healing Soup, page 208

Bouillabaisse with Leeks, Mushrooms, and Saffron, page 211

Fava Bean and Bacon Soup, page 212

Lamb Meatball Soup, page 215

Tomato Sauce for Freezing, page 218

Basic Tomato Soup Template, page 219

Nightshade-Free "Tomato" Soup**, page 220

Avocado, Dill, and Nut Milk Chilled Cream Soup, page 222

Carrot Gazpacho, page 223

Tomato Gazpacho, page 223

CHAPTER 8

Basic Skillet Template, page 227

Chicken-Potato Skillet, page 229

Steak and Mushroom Skillet, page 230

Turkey Meatball Skillet, page 233

Ground Bison Skillet, **page 235**

Lamb Burger Skillet, **page 236**

Turkey Tacos, **page 239**

Brats Skillet, **page 242**

Pork Chop Skillet, **page 244**

Bison Liver Skillet with Sautéed Onions, **page 247**

Back Bacon with Greens, Cranberries, and Balsamic Vinegar, **page 249**

Pork Sausage with Cabbage and Yams, **page 250**

CHAPTER 9

Chocolate Snowballs, **page 257**

Cherry Sorbet, **page 259**

Basic Frozen Coconut "Ice Cream" Template, **page 260**

Coconut Ice Cream*, **page 261**

Wahls Fudge, **page 262**

Chocolate Avocado Mousse, **page 264**

Whipped Coconut Cream**, **page 264**

Basic Cheezcake Template, **page 267**

Basic Nut Crust Template, **page 268**

Island Cheezcake, **page 270**

Chocolate Spice Cheezcake, **page 271**

Basic Wahls Pudding Template, **page 273**

Chia Berry Dark Cocoa Pudding, **page 275**

Fermented Chia Pudding**, **page 277**

Blackberry Lemon Chia Pudding, **page 278**

CHAPTER 10

Basic Jerky Template, **page 282**

Fast Track Snack: Celery with Nut Butter**, **page 282**

Basic Keto Treat Template, **page 284**

Basic Vegetable Chip Template, **page 288**

Basic Kale/Collard Chip Template, **page 291**

Fast Track Snack: Raw Veggies with Nut Butter, Pâté , Salsa, or Guacamole**, **page 291**

Fast Track Snack: Brussels Sprouts Wrapped in Bacon**, **page 292**

Basic Spiced Nuts Template, **page 293**

CHAPTER 11

Roast Turkey, **page 298**

Stuffing Options, **page 299**

Mashed Yams, **page 300**

Cooked Greens with Bacon and Mushrooms, **page 301**

Brussels Sprouts, Cranberries, and Pecans, **page 303**

Pumpkin (or Squash or Sweet Potato Pie) Pudding, **page 304**

Beet Kvass, **page 307**

Bacon-Wrapped Dates, **page 308**

Pan-Roasted Duck with Braised Kale, **page 309**

Butternut Squash Soup with Duck Fat and Orange, **page 310**

Cauliflower Cranberry Rice, **page 313**

Bison Roast with Garlic Ginger Rub, **page 316**

Pickled Spring Vegetables with Garden Herbs, **page 317**

Asparagus with Ghee and Lime, **page 318**

Fresh Strawberries Dipped in Coco–Almond Butter Sauce, **page 319**

Coco–Almond Butter Sauce, **page 319**

Wahls Birthday Cake**, **page 321**

Broccoli Salad with Bacon, **page 325**

Fruit Jigglers, **page 327**

CHAPTER 12

Shampoo, **page 331**

Face Wash, **page 331**

Face Scrub, **page 332**

Face Cream, **page 332**

Natural Facial, **page 332**

Clay Foot Soak, **page 332**

Deodorant, **page 332**

Oil Pulling, **page 333**

Toothpaste, **page 333**

Breath Freshening, **page 334**

Bath Salts, **page 334**

Detox Bath, **page 334**

For Restless Legs or Neuropathic Pain, **page 335**

Basic Household Cleaner, **page 335**

Glass Cleaner, **pagte 336**

Venison Liver Ice Cube Treats**, **page 336**

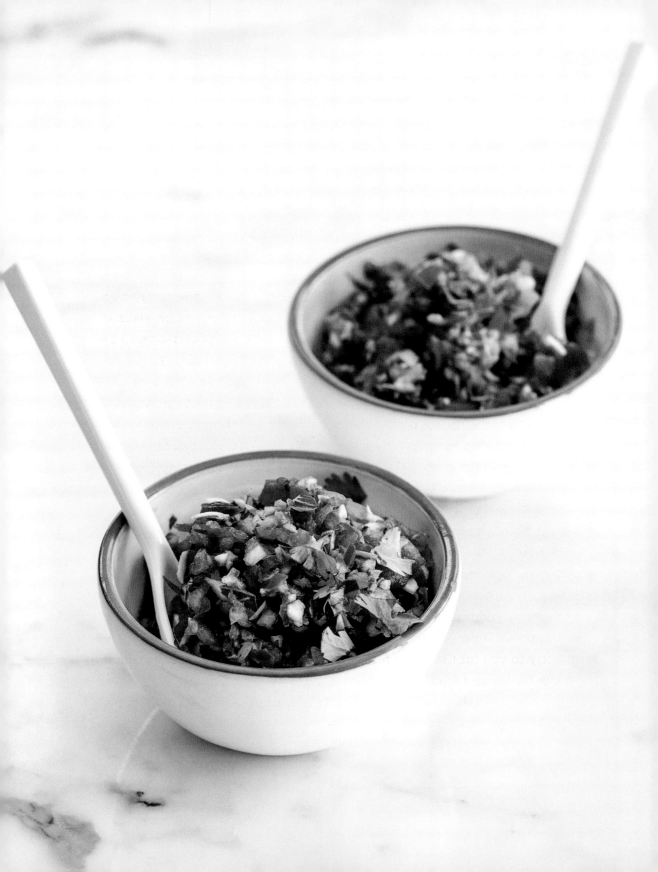

RESOURCES

I have a variety of programs detailed on my website, www.terrywahls .com, for those who are looking for additional support. Look at my website "Shop" page for more information about the various options, as well as information about future seminars and lectures. You can also sign up for the newsletter, so you will be kept abreast of the latest developments!

If you don't already have my book *The Wahls Protocol*, please consider purchasing it, as it is the foundation for this cookbook and contains much more information about the scientific basis of the protocol. You can order a signed copy from Prairie Lights bookstore in Iowa City, Iowa, at www.prairielightsbooks.com/book/9781583335215.

You might also be able to find my first book, *Minding My Mitochondria*, although it is now out of print.

I am excited to announce that you can now purchase Wahls Protocol–compliant food from Pete's Paleo. I partnered with Pete's Paleo to develop meals that are fully compliant with Wahls Paleo and personally approved every recipe. The meals can be shipped directly to you (in the lower forty-eight states only). This is an excellent way to have some food on hand that is the highest-quality nutrition when you can't or just don't want to prepare something yourself. Find out more at https://petespaleo.com/wahls.

Here are the other resources mentioned throughout this book:

https://petespaleo.com/wahls

For sea vegetable products, Maine Seaweed Company tests for heavy metals:
www.seaveg.com/shop

For more information on greens that are low in oxalates:
http://lowoxalateinfo.com/guide-to-low-oxalate-greens

For grass-fed bison: Grass Fed Traditions,
www.grassfedtraditions.com/grass_fed_bison.htm;
Tall Grass Bison,
www.tallgrassbison.com

For grass fed meats: US Wellness Meats,
http://grasslandbeef.com

For wild-caught fish from Alaskan waters:
Vital Choice, http://terrywahls.com/shop/vital-choice

FORAGING AND GARDENING RESOURCES

Square Foot Gardening Foundation: http://squarefootgardening.org

Wild Man Steve Brill: www.wildmanstevebrill.com

Wild Edible: www.wildedible.com

Superfoods for Superhealth: www.superfoods-for-superhealth.com/
wild-edible-greens.html

Wild Food Girl blog: http://wildfoodgirl.com

OCCUPATIONAL THERAPY RESOURCES

Life Solutions Plus: www.lifesolutionsplus.com/kitchen-aids-c-30.html?page

BLENDERIZED DIET ADDITIONAL INFORMATION AND RESOURCES

If you are feeding a child, do work with your medical team to assist you in designing your feedings. Ideally you can ask for a referral to a dietitian with experience with blenderized diets. The child should be older than six months and not immune-compromised. The key is knowing the amount of water and calories needed for your child, given their age and weight. You should also know how many servings of vegetables, berries, nuts, and high-quality protein are recommended each day for the patient. Once you have settled on a food protocol acceptable to all, the food needs to be blended in a high-powered blender such as a Vitamix with sufficient liquid that it can easily pass through a 14 French G tube or J tube. The feeding tube must be 14 French in diameter or larger to prevent clogging. A 60ml syringe or larger syringe is often used to deliver the feeding. Foods that thicken up in the feeding tube include avocados, potatoes, yams, rice, flaxseed, chia seeds, and oatmeal. Keeping the feeding thin enough to pass through the tubing is essential to success. You will also need access to a refrigerator to store the extra formula until it is ready to use. Don't keep pureed food longer than 24 hours. Check if you can get a medical discount for purchasing a Vitamix or high-speed blender because you are making a blenderized diet for a patient.

Here are some resources for more information:

Ancestralize Me blog: www.ancestralizeme.com/using-a-homemade-blenderized-tube-feeding-diet-my-interview-with-krisi-brackett

Children's Hospital of Los Angeles blenderizing information sheet: www.kintera.org/atf/cf/%7B1CB444DF-77C3-4D94-82FA-E366D7D6CE04%7D/GROW%202015%20Blenderized%20Diet.pdf

Article from *Today's Dietitian* about the benefits, risks, and strategies relevant to blenderized food for home tube feeding: www.todaysdietitian.com/newarchives/011315p30.shtml

Slide show about blenderized feeding: www.slideshare.net/lauraschoenfeld/the-use-of-blenderized-tube-feeding-in-pediatric-patients-evidence-and-guidelines-for-dietetic-practice

Pediatric Feeding News: http://pediatricfeedingnews.com/using-a-homemade-blenderized-tube-feeding-diet-interview-with-laura-schoenfeld-mph-rd/

RCNi *Nursing Children & Young People:* http://journals.rcni.com/doi/10.7748/ncyp.27.6.14.s16

Article in *Nutrition Issues in Gastroenterology:* https://med.virginia.edu/ginutrition/wp-content/uploads/sites/199/2014/06/Parrish-Dec-14.pdf

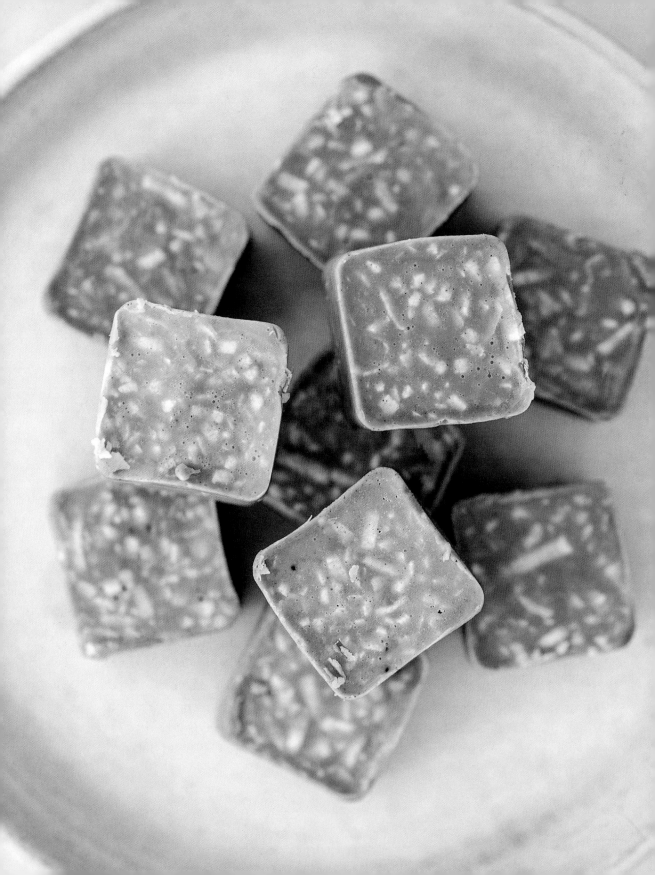

ACKNOWLEDGMENTS

I got my life back. I wrote this book to help you and your family get yours back, too. But this book and my work would not have been possible without the love and help of my wife, Jackie, who is such a gift in my life. Jackie, your support of my mission to take this message to everyone has made it possible for me to lecture around the world and develop the recipes in this book. You also help keep me biking, hiking, foraging, and gardening. It is such a privilege to have you in my life!

Thank you to Cliff Missen, the chief architect of the TEDx event in November 2011. My talk, *Minding Your Mitochondria*, went viral, getting more than 2.5 million views. Because of that talk, I was able to get the first book contract for *The Wahls Protocol* in 2012. The success of that book led to the contract for this one.

But I could not have faced writing another book in the midst of my busy professional life without an extremely talented and efficient coauthor. Eve Adamson makes the task of writing a book in the midst of my busy clinical and research practice so much more manageable. Eve, you are a joy to work with! I can't imagine working with any other writer.

To my editor, Lucia Watson, and your assistant, Nina Caldas, thank you! I very much appreciate your guiding me through the process of getting the photographer lined up as well as editing the manuscript. The food photography by Ashley McLaughlin is spectacular. The design team at Penguin made all those beautiful photos come to life in a most delicious way.

I thank the publicity team at Penguin, Lindsay Gordon and Farin Schlussel, and Jonathan Jacobs at Digital Natives Group for managing social media and assisting with the book launch.

I have had several people help me with my website, the Wahls Protocol Seminar, and our membership program: Naomi Wahls, Zach Wahls, Callie Reger, Annette Reed, and Samantha Ferm. Thank you, your efforts have made it possible for us to offer the public more ways to get support as they embark on using the Wahls Protocol to get their lives back.

In the three years since *The Wahls Protocol* was published, I have continued to work to spread the message that diet and lifestyle choices are powerful determinants of health. I continue to work at the university and the VA seeing patients, conducting our research studies, presenting the findings, and submitting and publishing our research papers. I am grateful to both the VA and the University of Iowa for providing a supportive environment in which to do this work.

I also thank the Wahls Foundation and the University of Iowa Foundation for sustaining this research mission. Allison Ingman, you are so excellent at cultivating and maintaining our relationships with our many generous donors. Dr. Nicholas LaRocca at the National MS Society, thank you for your encouragement and help as I worked on my grant rewrites. Doctors Babita Bisht, Warren Darling, Jen Lee, Linda Rubenstein, Ruth Grossman, and Linda Snetselaar, and Ms. Cathy Chenard, Michaela Fowler, and Amanda Irish, thank you for your tireless support of our research program.

Finally, I must thank you, the reader. Without the faithful support of the public, neither of my books would have ever happened. It was you who created the excitement about my work. And it was your use of social media that created the awareness of the power of diet and lifestyle to restore health. It was you who helped the National MS Society prioritize conducting dietary research. It is all of you who will change the world. You will do it, one delicious meal at time. As you learn how to cook again, you will reclaim your vitality and you will inspire others to begin their journey to health. Together we will create an epidemic of health.

INDEX

Italic page numbers indicate photographs.

Alkalinizing Ginger Lime Juice, 103–4, *105*
almonds
  Basic Spiced Nuts Template, 293
  Bacon-Wrapped Dates, 308
  Berry Melon Salad, 193
  Chia-Almond Porridge with Cranberries, *146, 147*
  Coconut Almond Porridge, 143
  Coco-Nutty Granola, 134–35, *135*
  Light Almond Tomato Salad, 178
  Orange Smoothie, 79
  Strawberry or Raspberry Carrot Smoothie, 68
Apple or Pumpkin Pie Smoothie, 70, *71*
Arugula Chicken Salad with Berries and Lemon, 168
Arugula Salad with Fresh Lemon Vinaigrette, 179
asparagus
  Asparagus with Ghee and Lime, 318, *318*
  Chicken-Potato Skillet, 229
  Garlic Chicken Salad, 169
  Ground Bison Skillet, 235
  Pork Chop Skillet, 244–45
avocados
  Basic Salad Dressing Template, 155

Avocado, Dill, and Nut Milk Chilled Cream Soup, 222
Basic Tomato Soup Template, 219–20
Bison Liver Skillet with Sautéed Onions, 246, 247–48
Chocolate Avocado Mousse, 264–65
Fava Bean and Bacon Soup, 212, *213*
Power Piña Colada, 81
Wahls Chicken Caesar Salad, 172
Wahls Fudge, 262, *263*
Wahls Guacamole, 48, *48*
Watercress Cucumber Salad with Avocado and Orange Slices, 182, *183*

bacon
  Back Bacon with Greens, Cranberries, and Balsamic Vinegar, 249
  Bacon Salad, 170, *171*
  bacon-wrapped Brussels sprouts (fast-track snack), 292, *292*
  Bacon-Wrapped Dates, 308
  Broccoli Salad with Bacon, 324, *325*
  Cooked Greens with Bacon and Mushrooms, 301
  Deli Sandwich Wrap, 192
  Fava Bean and Bacon Soup, 212, *213*

Balsamic Vinaigrette, 157
basics. *See* kitchen tips; staple recipes; Wahls Protocol
Bath Salts, 334
beef. *See* meats
beets
  Bacon Salad, 170, *171*
  Beet, Carrot, and Rutabaga Matchstick Salad with Fresh Cilantro, *180, 181*
  Beet Kvass, 307
  Beet-licious Juice with Ginger and Orange, *100,* 101–2
  Beet Mango Smoothie, 82, *83*
  Nightshade-Free "Tomato" Soup, 220
  potassium broth (variation), 200
  Tomato-Free Red Sauce, 47
  Wilted Kale and Duck Salad with Beets, Walnuts, and Soft Cheez, 174, *175*
berries. *See also* cranberries
  Arugula Chicken Salad with Berries and Lemon, 168
  Berry Melon Salad, 193
  Blackberry Grape Smoothie, 85
  Blackberry Lemon Chia Pudding, 278, *279*
  Blackberry Smoothie, 80
  celery with nut butter (fast-track snack), 282
  Chia Berry Dark Cocoa Pudding, 275–77, *276*

berries (continued)
Flax Raisin or Berry Porridge, 151
Fresh Strawberries Dipped in Coco-Almond Butter Sauce, 319–21, 320
Golden Quinoa Porridge, 148–49, 149
Mixed Berries, 193
Strawberry Orange Juice, 95
Strawberry or Raspberry Carrot Smoothie, 68
beverages. See juices; milks; smoothies; spritzers; teas/infusions
bison. See meats
blackberries. See berries
Bone Broth, Basic, 29–30, 31
Bouillabaisse with Leeks, Mushrooms, and Saffron, 210, 211
Brats Skillet, 242, 243
Brazil nuts
Apple or Pumpkin Pie Smoothie, 70, 71
Basic Smoothie Template, 65
Beet Mango Smoothie, 82, 83
Blackberry Grape Smoothie, 85
Citrus Smoothie, 67
Orange Smoothie, 79
Strawberry or Raspberry Carrot Smoothie, 68
Tropical Smoothie, 66
Watermelon Smoothie, 84
broccoli
Broccoli Salad with Bacon, 324, 325
Cauliflower/Broccoli Rice, 52, 53
Ground Bison Skillet, 235
broths. See soups/broths
Brussels sprouts
Bacon Salad, 170, 171
bacon-wrapped (fast-track snack), 292, 292
Brussels Sprouts, Cranberries, and Pecans, 302, 303
Burger Skillet, Lamb, 236, 237
Butternut Squash Soup with Duck Fat and Orange, 310–11

cabbage
Brats Skillet, 242, 243
Fermented Red Cabbage, 32–34, 35
kimchi (variation), 34
Lamb Burger Skillet, 236, 237
Pork Sausage with Cabbage and Yams, 250, 251
potassium broth (variation), 200
Turkey Meatball Skillet, 232, 233–34
Caesar Salad, Wahls Chicken, 172
Caesar-Style Dressing, Wahls, 158
Calendula, Yerba Mate with, 123
carrots
Beet, Carrot, and Rutabaga Matchstick Salad with Fresh Cilantro, 180, 181
Carrot Gazpacho, 223
Carrot Ginger Smoothie, 74, 75
Cauliflower Carrot Garlic Healing Soup, 208, 209
Peach Carrot Smoothie, 78
Strawberry or Raspberry Carrot Smoothie, 68
Cauliflower and Cranberry Rice, 312, 313
Cauliflower/Broccoli Rice, 52, 53
Cauliflower Carrot Garlic Healing Soup, 208, 209
Chamomile and Coconut Milk Tea, 124
Cheez, Soft, 43
Cheezcake, Chocolate Spice, 271
Cheezcake, Island, 270
Cheezcake Template, Basic, 252, 267
cherries
Cherry Sorbet, 259
Chia Berry Dark Cocoa Pudding, 275–77, 276
Chocolate Smoothie, 72, 73
chia seeds/flaxseeds
Basic Porridge Template, 140
Basic Wahls Pudding Template, 273
Blackberry Lemon Chia Pudding, 278, 279
Chia-Almond Porridge with Cranberries, 146, 147

Chia Berry Dark Cocoa Pudding, 275–77, 276
Chocolate Snowballs, 256, 257–58
Coconut Almond Porridge, 143
Everything Porridge, 142
Fermented Chia Pudding, 277
Flax Raisin or Berry Porridge, 151
Hemp Heart Porridge, 141
Seedy Flax Granola, 133
Sunny Peach Porridge, 144, 145
chicken
Arugula Chicken Salad with Berries and Lemon, 168
bone broth (variation), 30
Chicken-Potato Skillet, 229
Garlic Chicken Salad, 169
Grilled Chicken and Purple Potato Salad, 166–67
Old-Fashioned Chicken Soup, 202–3
Quick Chicken Broth, 202
Wahls Chicken Caesar Salad, 172
chocolate
Chia Berry Dark Cocoa Pudding, 275–77, 276
Chocolate Avocado Mousse, 264–65
Chocolate Smoothie, 72, 73
Chocolate Snowballs, 256, 257–58
Chocolate Spice Cheezcake, 271
Coco-Nutty Granola, 134–35, 135
Cilantro Salsa, 46
Cinnamon Orange Granola, 132
Citrus Salad, 193, 193
Citrus Smoothie, 67
Citrus Spritzer, 110
Clay Foot Soak, 332
Cleaner, Basic Household, 335
Cleaner, Glass, 336
Coco-Almond Butter Sauce, 319–21, 320
coconut flakes/chips/shreds
Basic Granola Template, 130
Berry Melon Salad, 193
Chocolate Snowballs, 256, 257–58
Cinnamon Orange Granola, 132

Coconut Almond Porridge, 143
coconut keto treat (variation), 285
Coco-Nutty Granola, 134–35, 135
Flax Raisin or Berry Porridge, 151
Golden Quinoa Porridge, 148–49, 149
Harvest Nut and Spice Granola, 136, 137
Island Cheezcake, 270
Seedy Flax Granola, 133
Sunny Peach Porridge, 144, 145
Wahls Fudge, 262, 263
coconut milk
    to emulsify cream and dilute, 64
    Fermented Nut or Coconut Milk, 38
    in Wahls Paleo Plus diet, 18–19
    Yogurt Milk, 38
Coco-Nutty Granola, 134–35, 135
collard greens. See kale/collards
Cooling Cucumber Mint Juice, 96, 97
cranberries
    Back Bacon with Greens, Cranberries, and Balsamic Vinegar, 249
    Brussels Sprouts, Cranberries, and Pecans, 302, 303
    Cauliflower and Cranberry Rice, 312, 313
    Chia-Almond Porridge with Cranberries, 146, 147
    Old-Fashioned Chicken Soup, 202–3
    Stuffing Options, 299
Cucumber Mint Juice, Cooling, 96, 97
Cucumber Watercress Salad with Avocado and Orange Slices, 182, 183

dates
    Bacon-Wrapped Dates, 308
    Basic Nut Crust Template, 268, 269
    Chocolate Snowballs, 256, 257–58
Deli Sandwich Wrap, 192
Deodorant, 332–33

desserts
    Basic Cheezcake Template, 252, 267
    Basic Frozen Coconut "Ice Cream" Template, 260–61
    Basic Nut Crust Template, 268, 269
    Basic Wahls Pudding Template, 273
    Berry Melon Salad, 193
    Blackberry Lemon Chia Pudding, 278, 279
    Cherry Sorbet, 259
    Chia Berry Dark Cocoa Pudding, 275–77, 276
    Chocolate Avocado Mousse, 264–65
    Chocolate Snowballs, 256, 257–58
    Chocolate Spice Cheezcake, 271
    Citrus Salad, 193, 193
    Fermented Chia Pudding, 277
    Fresh Strawberries Dipped in Coco-Almond Butter Sauce, 319–21, 320
    Island Cheezcake, 270
    Mixed Berries, 193
    Pumpkin (or Squash or Sweet Potato Pie) Pudding, 304, 305
    sweeteners in, 139, 254–55, 274
    vanilla snowballs (variation), 258
    Wahls Fudge, 262, 263
    Whipped Coconut Cream, 264
Detox Bath, 334–35
Detoxifying Turmeric Pepper Cream Tea, 119
Detox Juice with Wild Greens, Daily, 106–7
dressings. See salad dressings
Drive-Through Wrap, 190, 191
duck
    Butternut Squash Soup with Duck Fat and Orange, 310–11
    liver and fat, 311
    Pan-Roasted Duck Breast with Braised Kale, 309
    Wilted Kale and Duck Salad with Beets, Walnuts, and Soft Cheez, 174, 175

dulse/kelp
    adding to recipes, 214
    Basic Bone Broth, 29–30, 31
    bouillabaisse (variation), 210, 211
    Cauliflower Carrot Garlic Healing Soup, 208, 209
    Fava Bean and Bacon Soup, 212, 213
    Fermented Red Cabbage, 32–34, 35
    Mushroom Broth, 201
    Potassium Broth, 200

Everything Porridge, 142

Face Cream, 332
Face Scrub, 332
Face Wash, 331
Facial, Natural, 332
Fajita Halibut Salad, 163
Fava Bean and Bacon Soup, 212, 213
fermented foods
    Beet Kvass, 307
    Fermented Chia Pudding, 277
    Fermented Garlic-Ginger Sauce, 34
    Fermented Nut or Coconut Milk, 38
    Fermented Red Cabbage, 32–34, 35
    kefir milk (variation), 38
    kimchi (variation), 34
    kombucha, in Fruit Jigglers (variation), 327
    Pickled Spring Vegetables with Garden Herbs, 317
    probiotic capsules for, 18, 35
    salt in, 33
    Soft Cheez, 43
    Yogurt Milk, 38
fish/shellfish
    bone broth (variation), 30
    Bouillabaisse with Leeks, Mushrooms, and Saffron, 210, 211
    Fajita Halibut Salad, 163
    Poached (or Grilled) Salmon Salad, 173
    Smoked Oyster Salad, 152, 162
    Spring Herb Salad with Shrimp, Onions, and Chives, 164, 165

flaxseeds. See chia seeds/
  flaxseeds
Fruit Jigglers, 327, *327*
fruit salads, 193
Fudge, Wahls, 262, *263*

Garlic Chicken Salad, 169
Garlic-Ginger Sauce,
  Fermented, 34
Gazpacho, Carrot, 223
Gazpacho, Watermelon, 47
ginger
  Alkalinizing Ginger Lime
    Juice, 103–4, *105*
  Beet-licious Juice with Ginger
    and Orange, *100*, 101–2
  Bison Roast with Garlic Ginger
    Rub, *315*, 316
  Carrot Ginger Smoothie, 74, *75*
  Ginger Lemon Infusion, 122
  Rosemary Ginger Tea, 120
Glass Cleaner, 336
Golden Quinoa Porridge, 148–49,
  149
granola
  Basic Granola Template, 130
  Cinnamon Orange Granola,
    132
  Coco-Nutty Granola, 134–35,
    135
  guidelines, 127–29
  Harvest Nut and Spice
    Granola, *136*, 137
  Seedy Flax Granola, 133
Grape Blackberry Smoothie, 85
Grape Smoothie, Green Goddess,
  76, *77*
Green Happy Hour Spritzer, 112,
  113
greens. See also kale/collards;
  salads
  Back Bacon with Greens,
    Cranberries, and Balsamic
    Vinegar, 249
  Basic Soup Template, 197–98
  Basic Tomato Soup Template,
    219–20
  Bison Liver Skillet with
    Sautéed Onions, *246*,
    247–48
  Brats Skillet, *242*, 243
  Chicken-Potato Skillet,
    229
  Cooked Greens with Bacon and
    Mushrooms, 301

Daily Detox Juice with Wild
  Greens, 106–7
Fava Bean and Bacon Soup,
  212, *213*
foraging, 106, 186–87,
  186–87
Greens with Spring Onions
  and Radishes, 317
Ground Bison Skillet, 235
  kidney stones and, 154
Lamb Meatball Soup, 215–17,
  216
nutritional benefits, 153
Old-Fashioned Chicken Soup,
  202–3
Pork Chop Skillet, 244–45
Potassium Broth, 200
Power Piña Colada, 81
  in smoothies, 60–62
Steak and Mushroom Skillet,
  230, 231
Turkey Tacos, *238*, 239–40
Wild Greens Tea, 120
Wild Salad, 184
Guacamole, Wahls, 48, *48*

Halibut Salad, Fajita, 163
Happy Hour Spritzer, Green,
  112, *113*
Harvest Nut and Spice Granola,
  136, 137
Hemp Heart Porridge, 141
Herbal Rise-and-Shine Tea,
  121
Herbed Olive Oil, 54, *55*
holiday foods
  Asparagus with Ghee and
    Lime, 318, *318*
  Bacon-Wrapped Dates, 308
  Beet Kvass, 307
  Bison Roast with Garlic Ginger
    Rub, *315*, 316
  Broccoli Salad with Bacon,
    324, 325
  Brussels Sprouts, Cranberries,
    and Pecans, *302*, 303
  Butternut Squash Soup with
    Duck Fat and Orange,
    310–11
  Cauliflower and Cranberry
    Rice, 312, *313*
  Chocolate Snowballs, *256*,
    257–58
  Cooked Greens with Bacon and
    Mushrooms, 301

Fresh Strawberries Dipped
  in Coco-Almond Butter
  Sauce, 319–21, *320*
Fruit Jigglers, 327, *327*
Greens with Spring Onions
  and Radishes, 317
Mashed Yams, 300
menus and ideas, 296, 306, 314,
  321, 322, 323, 326
Pan-Roasted Duck Breast with
  Braised Kale, 309
Pickled Spring Vegetables with
  Garden Herbs, 317
Pumpkin (or Squash or Sweet
  Potato Pie) Pudding, 304,
  305
Roast Turkey, 297, *298*
Stuffing Options, 299
Household Cleaner, Basic, 335
hygiene products. See personal
  care products

"Ice Cream" Template, Basic
  Frozen Coconut, 260–61
Indian beef marrow broth
  (variation), 199
infusions. See teas/infusions
Island Cheezcake, 270
Italian beef marrow broth
  (variation), 199
Italian Dressing, Wahls, 158

Jerky Template, Basic,
  282–83
juices
  Basic Juice Template, 94
  Alkalinizing Ginger Lime
    Juice, 103–4, *105*
  Beet-licious Juice with Ginger
    and Orange, *100*, 101–2
  Cooling Cucumber Mint Juice,
    96, *97*
  Daily Detox Juice with Wild
    Greens, 106–7
  guidelines, 88–93
  Strawberry Orange Juice, 95
  Summer Melon Juice, 98

kale/collards. See also greens
  Bacon Salad, 170, *171*
  Basic Kale/Collard Chip
    Template, 290, 291–92
  Drive-Through Wrap, *190*, 191
  Green Goddess Grape
    Smoothie, 76, *77*

Kale, Sausage, and Yam Soup
with Coconut Milk, 206,
207
Lamb Burger Skillet, 236, 237
Pan-Roasted Duck Breast with
Braised Kale, 309
Turkey Meatball Skillet, 232,
233–34
Turkey Tacos, 238, 239–40
Wilted Kale and Duck Salad
with Beets, Walnuts, and
Soft Cheez, 174, 175
kefir milk (variation), 38
Keto Treat Template, Basic,
284–85, 285
kimchi (variation), 34
kitchen tips
coconut milk, 64
coffee, 117
essential oils and extracts, 61
extra-virgin olive oil, 54
fresh ginger and turmeric,
106
glycine sweetener, 274
lacto-fermentation, 18
matcha, 24
MCT oil, 26
pantry staples, 25–27
probiotic capsules for food
prep, 35
seaweed, 214
soaked nuts and seeds, 131
3-cup measurement, 15
tools and equipment, 24–25
vegetarian gelatin, 266

Lamb Burger Skillet, 236, 237
Lamb Meatball Soup, 215–17, 216
Lemon, Arugula Chicken Salad
with Berries and, 168
Lemon Blackberry Chia
Pudding, 278, 279
Lemon Ginger Infusion, 122
Lemon Olive Vinaigrette, Simple,
156
Lime Juice, Alkalinizing Ginger,
103–4, 105
liver. See meats

mangos
Beet Mango Smoothie, 82, 83
Citrus Smoothie, 67
Tropical Smoothie, 66
Meatball Skillet, Turkey, 232,
233–34

Meatball Soup, Lamb, 215–17, 216
meats. See also bacon; chicken;
duck; turkey
Basic Jerky Template, 282–83
Basic Tomato Soup Template,
219–20
Beef Marrow Broth, 199
Bison Liver Skillet with
Sautéed Onions, 246,
247–48
Bison Roast with Garlic Ginger
Rub, 315, 316
Brats Skillet, 242, 243
Deli Sandwich Wrap, 192
Drive-Through Wrap, 190, 191
Ground Bison Skillet, 235
Kale, Sausage, and Yam Soup
with Coconut Milk, 206,
207
Lamb Burger Skillet, 236, 237
Lamb Meatball Soup, 215–17,
216
organ meats, 213, 298, 311
Pork Chop Skillet, 244–45
Pork Sausage with Cabbage
and Yams, 250, 251
Steak and Mushroom Skillet,
230, 231
venison liver treats for pets,
336
Wahls Pâté, 40, 41
milks
Fermented Nut or Coconut
Milk, 38
kefir milk (variation), 38
Nut Milk, 36, 37
Yogurt Milk, 38
Mousse, Chocolate Avocado,
264–65
mushrooms
Bouillabaisse with Leeks,
Mushrooms, and Saffron,
210, 211
Cooked Greens with Bacon and
Mushrooms, 301
Mushroom Broth, 201
Steak and Mushroom Skillet,
230, 231
My Sauce, 159

Natural Facial, 332
Nightshade-Free "Tomato" Soup,
220
nightshade vegetable
substitutions, 46

nuts/nut butter. See also
almonds; Brazil nuts;
pecans; walnuts
Basic Granola Template, 130
Basic Keto Treat Template,
284–85, 285
Basic Nut Crust Template, 268,
269
Basic Salad Dressing
Template, 155
Basic Spiced Nuts Template,
293
celery with (fast-track snack),
282
Cinnamon Orange Granola,
132
Coco-Almond Butter Sauce,
319–21, 320
for granola and porridge, 128
Harvest Nut and Spice
Granola, 136, 137
Nut Milk, 36, 37
Nut or Seed Butter, 39
soaking nuts, 131

Old-Fashioned Chicken Soup,
202–3
oranges/orange juice
Beet-licious Juice with Ginger
and Orange, 100, 101–2
Beet Mango Smoothie, 82, 83
Butternut Squash Soup with
Duck Fat and Orange,
310–11
Carrot Gazpacho, 223
Carrot Ginger Smoothie, 74, 75
Citrus Salad, 193, 193
Orange Smoothie, 79
Orange Spritzer, 114, 114
Strawberry Orange Juice, 95
Watercress Cucumber Salad
with Avocado and Orange
Slices, 182, 183
Oyster Salad, Smoked, 152, 162

Pâté, Wahls, 40, 41
Peach Carrot Smoothie, 78
Peach Porridge, Sunny, 144, 145
pecans
Brussels Sprouts, Cranberries,
and Pecans, 302, 303
Chocolate Snowballs, 256,
257–58
Coco-Nutty Granola, 134–35,
135

pecans (continued)
Pumpkin (or Squash or Sweet
Potato Pie) Pudding, 304,
305
personal care products
basic ingredients, 330
Bath Salts, 334
breath fresheners, 334
Clay Foot Soak, 332
Deodorant, 332–33
Detox Bath, 334–35
Face Cream, 332
Face Scrub, 332
Face Wash, 331
ice bath, 334
Natural Facial, 332
oil pulling technique, 333
for restless legs or neuropathic
pain, 335
Shampoo, 331
Toothpaste, 333–34
pet care, 336
Pickled Spring Vegetables with
Garden Herbs, 317
pineapple
Berry Melon Salad, 193
Island Cheezcake, 270
Power Piña Colada, 81
pork. See bacon; meats
porridge
Basic Porridge Template, 140
Chia-Almond Porridge with
Cranberries, 146, 147
Coconut Almond Porridge, 143
Everything Porridge, 142
Flax Raisin or Berry Porridge,
151
Golden Quinoa Porridge,
148–49, 149
guidelines, 127–29
Hemp Heart Porridge, 141
Sunny Peach Porridge, 144,
145
Potassium Broth, 200
potatoes
Chicken-Potato Skillet, 229
Grilled Chicken and Purple
Potato Salad, 166–67
resistant starch in, 167
substitutions, 46
puddings
Basic Wahls Pudding
Template, 273
Blackberry Lemon Chia
Pudding, 278, 279

Chia Berry Dark Cocoa
Pudding, 275–77, 276
Fermented Chia Pudding, 277
Pumpkin (or Squash or Sweet
Potato Pie) Pudding, 304,
305
pumpkin puree
Apple or Pumpkin Pie
Smoothie, 70, 71
Basic Frozen Coconut "Ice
Cream" Template, 260–61
Basic Wahls Pudding
Template, 273
Nightshade-Free "Tomato"
Soup, 220
Pumpkin (or Squash or Sweet
Potato Pie) Pudding, 304,
305

Quinoa Porridge, Golden,
148–49, 149

radishes
Chicken-Potato Skillet, 229
Greens with Spring Onions
and Radishes, 317
Grilled Chicken and Purple
Potato Salad, 166–67
Pickled Spring Vegetables with
Garden Herbs, 317
raisins
Basic Nut Crust Template, 268,
269
Basic Wahls Pudding
Template, 273
Broccoli Salad with Bacon,
324, 325
Chocolate Snowballs, 256,
257–58
Flax Raisin or Berry Porridge,
151
Golden Quinoa Porridge,
148–49, 149
Harvest Nut and Spice
Granola, 136, 137
Pumpkin (or Squash or Sweet
Potato Pie) Pudding, 304,
305
Seedy Flax Granola, 133
Stuffing Options, 299
Wahls Fudge, 262, 263
Ranch-Style Dressing, Wahls, 157
raspberries. See berries
Rawmesan, 42, 42
Red Clover Tea, 125

Red Sauce, Tomato-Free, 47
Rice, Cauliflower/Broccoli, 52, 53
Rise-and-Shine Tea, Herbal, 121
Root Vegetables, Slow-Cooker
Roasted, 49
Rosemary Ginger Tea, 120
Rutabaga, Beet, and Carrot
Matchstick Salad with
Fresh Cilantro, 180, 181

salad dressings
Basic Salad Dressing
Template, 155
Balsamic Vinaigrette, 157
Mixed Greens Salad Dressing,
156
My Sauce, 159
Simple Olive Lemon
Vinaigrette, 156
Wahls Caesar-Style Dressing,
158
Wahls Italian Dressing, 158
Wahls Ranch-Style Dressing,
157
salads
Basic Main Course Salad
Template, 161
Basic Side Salad Template, 177
Basic Wrap Template, 189
Arugula Chicken Salad with
Berries and Lemon, 168
Arugula Salad with Fresh
Lemon Vinaigrette, 179
Bacon Salad, 170, 171
Beet, Carrot, and Rutabaga
Matchstick Salad with
Fresh Cilantro, 180, 181
Berry Melon Salad, 193
Broccoli Salad with Bacon,
324, 325
Citrus Salad, 193, 193
Deli Sandwich Wrap, 192
Drive-Through Wrap, 190, 191
Fajita Halibut Salad, 163
Garlic Chicken Salad, 169
Greens with Spring Onions
and Radishes, 317
Grilled Chicken and Purple
Potato Salad, 166–67
Light Almond Tomato Salad,
178
Mixed Berries, 193
Poached (or Grilled) Salmon
Salad, 173
simple main course salads, 160

Smoked Oyster Salad, *152, 162*
Spring Herb Salad with
     Shrimp, Onions, and
     Chives, *164, 165*
Wahls Chicken Caesar Salad,
     172
Watercress Cucumber Salad
     with Avocado and Orange
     Slices, 182, *183*
Wild Salad, 184
Wilted Kale and Duck Salad
     with Beets, Walnuts, and
     Soft Cheez, *174, 175*
Salmon Salad, Poached (or
     Grilled), 173
sauces/salsas/seasonings. *See
     also* salad dressings
  black pepper, 77
  Cilantro Salsa, 46
  Coco-Almond Butter Sauce,
     319–21, *320*
  Fermented Garlic-Ginger
     Sauce, 34
  Fresh Salsa, 44, 45
  pesto, 178
  Rawmesan, 42, *42*
  Tomato-Free Red Sauce, 47
  Tomato Sauce for Freezing, 218
  Wahls Taco Seasoning, 45
sausage. *See* meats
seafood. *See* fish/shellfish
seeds/seed butter. *See also* chia
     seeds/flaxseeds
  Arugula Chicken Salad with
     Berries and Lemon, 168
  Basic Granola Template, 130
  Basic Keto Treat Template,
     284–85, *285*
  Basic Nut Crust Template, 268,
     269
  Carrot Ginger Smoothie, 74, 75
  Cinnamon Orange Granola,
     132
  Harvest Nut and Spice
     Granola, *136, 137*
  Light Almond Tomato Salad,
     178
  Nut or Seed Butter, 39
  soaking seeds, 131
Seedy Flax Granola, 133
Shampoo, 331
shellfish. *See* fish/shellfish
Shrimp, Onions, and Chives,
     Spring Herb Salad with,
     164, 165

skillets
  Basic Skillet Template, 227–28
  Back Bacon with Greens,
     Cranberries, and Balsamic
     Vinegar, 249
  Bison Liver Skillet with
     Sautéed Onions, *246,*
     247–48
  Brats Skillet, *242, 243*
  Chicken-Potato Skillet, 229
  Ground Bison Skillet, 235
  Lamb Burger Skillet, *236, 237*
     oven variation, 226
  Pork Chop Skillet, 244–45
  Pork Sausage with Cabbage
     and Yams, 250, *251*
  Steak and Mushroom Skillet,
     230, 231
  Turkey Meatball Skillet, *232,*
     233–34
  Turkey Tacos, 238, *239–40*
Smoked Oyster Salad, *152, 162*
smoothies
  Basic Smoothie Template, 65
  Apple or Pumpkin Pie
     Smoothie, *70, 71*
  Beet Mango Smoothie, *82, 83*
  Blackberry Grape Smoothie, 85
  Blackberry Smoothie, 80
  in blenderized diet, 205
  Carrot Ginger Smoothie, 74, 75
  Chocolate Smoothie, *72, 73*
  Citrus Smoothie, 67
  Green Goddess Grape
     Smoothie, *76, 77*
  guidelines, 60–64
  Orange Smoothie, 79
  Peach Carrot Smoothie, 78
  Power Piña Colada, 81
  Strawberry or Raspberry
     Carrot Smoothie, 68
  Tropical Smoothie, 66
  Watermelon Smoothie, 84
snacks
  bacon-wrapped Brussels
     sprouts (fast-track snack),
     292, 292
  Basic Jerky Template,
     282–83
  Basic Kale/Collard Chip
     Template, 290, 291–92
  Basic Keto Treat Template,
     284–85, *285*
  Basic Spiced Nuts Template,
     293

Basic Vegetable Chip Template,
     288–89
  celery with nut butter (fast-
     track snack), 282
  coconut keto treat (variation),
     285
  Fruit Jigglers, 327, *327*
  raw veggies with dip (fast-
     track snack), 291
  savory keto treat (variation),
     285
  teriyaki jerky (variation),
     283
  vegetable chips, 286–89, *287*
Snowballs, Chocolate (and
     vanilla variation), *256,*
     257–58
Soft Cheez, 43
Sorbet, Cherry, 259
soups/broths
  Basic Bone Broth, 29–30, *31*
  Basic Soup Template, 197–98
  Basic Tomato Soup Template,
     219–20
  Avocado, Dill, and Nut Milk
     Chilled Cream Soup, 222
  Beef Marrow Broth, 199
  in blenderized diet, 205
  Bouillabaisse with Leeks,
     Mushrooms, and Saffron,
     210, 211
  Butternut Squash Soup with
     Duck Fat and Orange,
     310–11
  Carrot Gazpacho, 223
  Cauliflower Carrot Garlic
     Healing Soup, *208, 209*
  chicken bone broth
     (variation), 30
  Fava Bean and Bacon Soup,
     212, 213
  fish or shellfish bone broth
     (variation), 30
  Kale, Sausage, and Yam Soup
     with Coconut Milk, *206,*
     207
  Lamb Meatball Soup, 215–17,
     216
  Mushroom Broth, 201
  Nightshade-Free "Tomato"
     Soup, 220
  Old-Fashioned Chicken Soup,
     202–3
  organ meats in, 213
  Potassium Broth, 200

soups/broths (continued)
  Quick Chicken Broth, 202
  Tomato Gazpacho, 194, 223
  Watermelon Gazpacho, 47
Spaghetti Squash, Slow-Cooker, 50, 51
spinach. See greens
Spring Herb Salad with Shrimp, Onions, and Chives, 164, 165
spritzers
  alcohol in, 110
  Basic Spritzer Template, 109
  Berry Spritzer, 111
  Citrus Spritzer, 110
  Green Happy Hour Spritzer, 112, 113
  Orange Spritzer, 114, 114
staple recipes
  Basic Bone Broth, 29–30, 31
  Cauliflower/Broccoli Rice, 52, 53
  Cilantro Salsa, 46
  Fermented Garlic-Ginger Sauce, 34
  Fermented Nut or Coconut Milk, 38
  Fermented Red Cabbage, 32–34, 35
  Fresh Salsa, 44, 45
  Herbed Olive Oil, 54, 55
  kefir milk (variation), 38
  kimchi (variation), 34
  Nut Milk, 36, 37
  Nut or Seed Butter, 39
  Rawmesan, 42, 42
  Slow-Cooker Roasted Root Vegetables, 49
  Slow-Cooker Spaghetti Squash, 50, 51
  Soft Cheez, 43
  Tomato-Free Red Sauce, 47
  Wahls Guacamole, 48, 48
  Wahls Pâté, 40, 41
  Wahls Taco Seasoning, 45
  Watermelon Gazpacho, 47
  Yogurt Milk, 38
strawberries. See berries
Stuffing Options, 299
Summer Melon Juice, 98
Sunny Peach Porridge, 144, 145
sweet potatoes/yams
  Chicken-Potato Skillet, 229
  Kale, Sausage, and Yam Soup with Coconut Milk, 206, 207
  Mashed Yams, 300
  Pork Sausage with Cabbage and Yams, 250, 251
  Pumpkin (or Squash or Sweet Potato Pie) Pudding, 304, 305
  Turkey Meatball Skillet, 232, 233–34

Tacos, Turkey, 238, 239–40
Taco Seasoning, Wahls, 45
teas/infusions
  Basic Tea/Infusion Template, 118
  black tea versus green tea, 116
  Chamomile and Coconut Milk Tea, 124
  coconut milk in, 116–17
  Detoxifying Turmeric Pepper Cream Tea, 119
  Ginger Lemon Infusion, 122
  Herbal Rise-and-Shine Tea, 121
  matcha, 118
  Red Clover Tea, 125
  Rosemary Ginger Tea, 120
  Wild Greens Tea, 120
  Yerba Mate with Calendula, 123
templates
  Cheezcake, 252, 267
  Frozen Coconut "Ice Cream," 260–61
  Granola, 130
  Jerky, 282–83
  Juice, 94
  Kale/Collard Chip, 290, 291–92
  Keto Treat, 284, 285
  Main Course Salad, 161
  Nut Crust, 268, 269
  Porridge, 140
  Salad Dressing, 155
  Side Salad, 177
  Skillet, 227–28
  Smoothie, 65
  Soup, 197–98
  Spiced Nuts, 293
  Spritzer, 109
  Tea/Infusion, 118
  Tomato Soup, 219–20
  Vegetable Chip, 288–89
  Wahls Pudding, 273
  Wrap, 189

tomatoes
  Basic Tomato Soup Template, 219–20
  Bouillabaisse with Leeks, Mushrooms, and Saffron, 210, 211
  Fresh Salsa, 44, 45
  Light Almond Tomato Salad, 178
  substitutions, 46
  Tomato Gazpacho, 194, 223
  Tomato Sauce for Freezing, 218
Tomato-Free Red Sauce, 47
"Tomato" Soup, Nightshade-Free, 220
Toothpaste, 333–34
Tropical Smoothie, 66
turkey
  giblets, 298
  Roast Turkey, 297, 298
  Turkey Meatball Skillet, 232, 233–34
  Turkey Tacos, 238, 239–40
Turmeric Pepper Cream Tea, Detoxifying, 119

vegetable chips, 286–89, 287
vegetables. See also specific types
  cup equivalents, 27, 57, 226
  gardening, 196
  nightshade substitutions, 46
  peels, 90
  3-cup measurement, 15

Wahls Protocol
  blenderized food, 204–5
  healthful eating, 13
  ketogenic diet, 12
  levels, 11–14
  orthorexia, 21
  sugar cravings, 89, 139, 254–55
  Wahls Diet, 15–16
  Wahls Paleo, 16–18
  Wahls Paleo Plus, 18–20
walnuts
  Basic Spiced Nuts Template, 293
  Broccoli Salad with Bacon, 324, 325
  Chocolate Snowballs, 256, 257–58
  Everything Porridge, 142
  Golden Quinoa Porridge, 148–49, 149

Rawmesan, 42, 42
Wahls Fudge, 262, 263
Wilted Kale and Duck Salad
    with Beets, Walnuts, and
    Soft Cheez, 174, 175
Watercress Cucumber Salad
    with Avocado and Orange
    Slices, 182, 183

watermelon
    Berry Melon Salad, 193
    Summer Melon Juice, 98
    Watermelon Gazpacho, 47
    Watermelon Smoothie, 84
Whipped Coconut Cream, 264
Wild Greens Tea, 120
Wild Salad, 184

Wilted Kale and Duck Salad with
    Beets, Walnuts, and Soft
    Cheez, 174, 175

yams. See sweet potatoes/yams
Yerba Mate with Calendula,
    123
Yogurt Milk, 38

ALSO BY TERRY WAHLS, M.D.

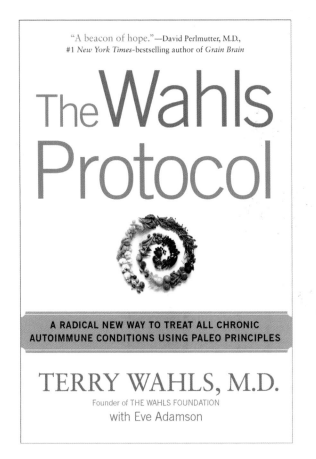

"A beacon of hope." —David Perlmutter, M.D.,
#1 *New York Times*-bestselling author of *Grain Brain*

The Wahls Protocol

**A RADICAL NEW WAY TO TREAT ALL CHRONIC
AUTOIMMUNE CONDITIONS USING PALEO PRINCIPLES**

TERRY WAHLS, M.D.
Founder of THE WAHLS FOUNDATION
with Eve Adamson

A life-changing, integrative approach to healing
chronic autoimmune conditions based on pioneering research
into functional medicine and paleo principles.

terrywahls.com

AVERY